Program Development and Grant Writing in Occupational Therapy

MAKING THE CONNECTION

Joy Doll, OTD, OTR/L

Assistant Professor, Clinical Education
Department of Occupational Therapy
School of Pharmacy and Health Professions
Creighton University
Omaha, Nebraska

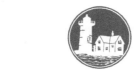

JONES AND BARTLETT PUBLISHERS
Sudbury, Massachusetts
BOSTON   TORONTO   LONDON   SINGAPORE

World Headquarters
Jones and Bartlett Publishers
40 Tall Pine Drive
Sudbury, MA 01776
978-443-5000
info@jbpub.com
www.jbpub.com

Jones and Bartlett Publishers Canada
6339 Ormindale Way
Mississauga, Ontario L5V 1J2
Canada

Jones and Bartlett Publishers International
Barb House, Barb Mews
London W6 7PA
United Kingdom

Jones and Bartlett's books and products are available through most bookstores and online booksellers. To contact Jones and Bartlett Publishers directly, call 800-832-0034, fax 978-443-8000, or visit our website, www.jbpub.com.

Substantial discounts on bulk quantities of Jones and Bartlett's publications are available to corporations, professional associations, and other qualified organizations. For details and specific discount information, contact the special sales department at Jones and Bartlett via the above contact information or send an email to specialsales@jbpub.com.

The author, editor, and publisher have made every effort to provide accurate information. However, they are not responsible for errors, omissions, or for any outcomes related to the use of the contents of this book and take no responsibility for the use of the products and procedures described. Treatments and side effects described in this book may not be applicable to all people; likewise, some people may require a dose or experience a side effect that is not described herein. Drugs and medical devices are discussed that may have limited availability controlled by the Food and Drug Administration (FDA) for use only in a research study or clinical trial. Research, clinical practice, and government regulations often change the accepted standard in this field. When consideration is being given to use of any drug in the clinical setting, the health care provider or reader is responsible for determining FDA status of the drug, reading the package insert, and reviewing prescribing information for the most up-to-date recommendations on dose, precautions, and contraindications, and determining the appropriate usage for the product. This is especially important in the case of drugs that are new or seldom used.

Production Credits
Publisher: David Cella
Acquisitions Editor: Kristine Jones
Associate Editor: Maro Gartside
Editorial Assistant: Teresa Reilly
Production Director: Amy Rose
Production Assistant: Julia Waugaman
Marketing Manager: Grace Richards
Manufacturing and Inventory Control Supervisor: Amy Bacus
Composition: Forbes Mill Press
Cover Design: Scott Moden
Cover, Part Opener, Chapter Opener, and Text Box Image: © Atlantic/Dreamstime.com
Printing and Binding: Malloy Incorporated
Cover Printing: John Pow Company

Library of Congress Cataloging-in-Publication Data
Doll, Joy D.
  Program development and grant writing in occupational therapy : making the connection / by Joy D. Doll.
    p. ; cm.
  Includes bibliographical references and index.
  ISBN-13: 978-0-7637-6065-6 (pbk.)
  ISBN-10: 0-7637-6065-X (pbk.)
  1. Occupational therapy. 2. Proposal writing in medicine. I. Title.
  [DNLM: 1. Occupational Therapy--economics. 2. Occupational Therapy--methods. 3. Community Health Services. 4. Program Development--economics. 5. Program Development--methods. 6. Research Support as Topic--economics. 7. Research Support as Topic--methods. 8. Writing. WB 555 D665p 2010]
  RM735.42.D65 2010
  615.8'515068--dc22
                          2009011054
6048
Printed in the United States of America
13 12 11 10 09   10 9 8 7 6 5 4 3 2 1

Contents

Foreword

This is the first time I have been asked to write a foreword for a book, and I am delighted for three main reasons. First, the book is written by one of my former occupational therapy students at the University of South Alabama. I knew her then as Joy Voltz, and I have followed her career in occupational therapy with great interest, pride, and admiration.

Secondly, I am even more pleased because she has chosen to write about community practice in occupational therapy, a topic near and dear to my heart. When I was an occupational therapy student at Virginia Commonwealth University, Dr. Gary Kielhofner nurtured my interest in community practice. Now I am thrilled to pass the torch to Joy. If in some small way I enhanced her attraction and commitment to community practice, I am honored.

Finally, the book itself is wonderful, academic, and well researched, as well as practical and useful. The book covers the nuts and bolts of community assessment, program development, grantwriting, and program evaluation. The content reflects the author's extensive experience in community-based practice and the available evidence in the literature. It provides practitioners and students alike with the knowledge and skills to develop, fund, and evaluate community-based occupation-based programs. This is important as the shift from hospital-based care to community-based care continues to grow. The federal government's health agenda, *Healthy People 2020*, is designed to enhance the health and wellbeing of Americans, and this text provides a blueprint for occupational therapy involvement in community and public health efforts.

The book is both scholarly and pragmatic, a difficult synthesis to achieve. I commend Joy Doll for her work on this text. It no doubt will further enhance the role and skills of current and future occupational therapy practitioners in community-based settings.

Marjorie E. Scaffa, PhD, OTR/L, FAOTA

Acknowledgments

I would like to thank my parents for their ongoing support and belief in me no matter what. I also have to thank Mike for always believing in me no matter what happens and enduring my desire to be with people to better the world.

I would like to dedicate this book to the Omaha Tribe of Nebraska, which has taught me the true meaning of community work and what it means to become part of a community. I also dedicate this book to John Penn, who taught me so much about grant writing and let me be a part of his team.

Introduction

In recent years, the profession of occupational therapy has developed an interest in community practice, and although this area of practice is not well defined, it deserves to be supported and recognized. For occupational therapy practitioners working in community settings rather than in clinical care, the demands are different and unique skills are required for successful practice. The purpose of this book is to be a tool for community practitioners or for any practitioners or students interested in community work, whether full time or as a side project.

Tools for community practice include program development and grant writing. But beyond these, there are challenges in matching a program with a community for true success. This book not only addresses the skills needed for program development and grant writing but also explores successful and sustainable programming in community settings. Success and sustainability are not only tied to grant funding but truly require creative strategies, building on community capacity and buy-in from the people actually benefiting from the services. The components of program development and grant writing are not only for nontraditional practice, and it is my hope that clinicians in all settings will find this book relevant to practice, despite the context.

It is of importance to note that this book outlines strategies for success in community practice, but that each community and program is unique. What leads to success in one community may not do so in another. Occupational therapy practitioners working in the community must utilize their clinical reasoning skills to determine which strategies to apply to their community setting. Strategies for utilizing clinical reasoning in a community practice setting are emphasized throughout the text with case studies and process worksheets. These process worksheets are meant to help readers think through the processes for program development and grant writing in order to lay a foundation for development of occupational therapy practice in these areas.

Another important note to consider is that community practice is an ongoing lesson. Occupational therapy practitioners working in community settings have to be bold and creative in designing strategies. They must constantly reflect critically on the unique community needs to be able to modify the program as necessary. Critical self-reflection and program evaluation are key components. Similar to the model they use in traditional clinical settings, occupational therapy practitioners must be in constant evaluation mode and able to modify the program accordingly. Reflection and evaluation processes are emphasized throughout this book to facilitate the development of these tools for successful community-based practice.

This book focuses on capacity building as an approach to success in community practice. In community practice, needs—especially health-related ones—are often grossly evident and cannot be fully addressed. In the case of working with an underserved or health disparate community, needs can be overwhelming and leave one feeling helpless to address them. However, any community that faces challenges also has strengths that can be utilized to tackle community needs. Some examples include strong cultural ties, a powerful collective faith, and dependable leadership. These factors are the keys to a successful program, and this book focuses on approaches for building and using capacity to develop successful programs.

Healthcare professionals are generally viewed as experts in their practice area. However, in community practice, success relies on a partnership approach instead of an expert approach. This means that for occupational therapy practitioners success often results from being a part of the community and not viewed as outsider consultants. This book takes the approach of community partnership and promotes community immersion as a tactic for success. It is the author's belief and experience that this approach ensures that programs meet authentic needs and facilitate community change.

For occupational therapy practitioners working in community settings, program development and grant writing are a happy couple. Grant writing cannot occur without the process of comprehensive program development, and programs in community settings usually require external funding. In community settings, most grants are geared toward program implementation and program development is typically not supported by external funders. Although there are many resources available on grant writing techniques and strategies, for occupational therapy practitioners in community settings grant proposals are usually irrelevant without a strong program. Therefore, the purpose of this book is to provide a resource for the integration of grant writing and program development. For many community practitioners, these two aspects of community practice provide significant challenges and this book provides tools and strategies for success.

Reviewer Recognition

Joseph Cipriani, EdD, OTR/L
Professor, Department of Occupational Therapy
Misericordia University
Dallas, Pennsylvania

Sandra Barker Dunbar, DPA, OTR/L, FAOTA
Professor, Occupational Therapy Department
Health Professions Division, College of Allied Health and Nursing
Nova Southeastern University
Fort Lauderdale–Davie, Florida

Sue Coppola, MS, OTR/L, BCG, FAOTA
Associate Professor, Division of Occupational Science
University of North Carolina
Chapel Hill, North Carolina

Cristy Daniel, MS, OTR/L
College of Saint Mary
Omaha, Nebraska

Denise Donica, DHS, OTR/L
Assistant Professor, Occupational Therapy Department
East Carolina University
Greenville, North Carolina

Anne M. Haskins, PhD, OTR/L
Occupational Therapy Department
University of North Dakota
Grand Forks, North Dakota

Liane Hewitt, DrPH, OTR/L
Associate Professor Chair, Department of Occupational Therapy
Loma Linda University
Loma Linda, California

Heather Javaherian, OTD, OTR/L
Loma Linda University
Loma Linda, California

Pamela Kasyan-Itzkowitz, MS, OTR/L, CHT
Occupational Therapy Department
Nova Southeastern University
Fort Lauderdale–Davie, Florida

Jane Painter, EdD, OTR/L
Associate Professor, Director, Clinical Education
College of Allied Health Sciences, Occupational Therapy Department
East Carolina University
Greenville, North Carolina

Amy Paul-Ward, PhD, MSOT
Assistant Professor, Department of Occupational Therapy
College of Nursing and Health Sciences
Florida International University
Miami, Florida

Greshundria M. Raines, OTD, MPA, OTR/L
Assistant Professor and Academic Fieldwork Coordinator
Department of Occupational Therapy
Alabama State University
Montgomery, Alabama

Janeene Sibla, OTD, MS, OTR/L
University of Mary
Bismarck, North Dakota

Stacy Smallfield, DrOT, OTR/L
University of South Dakota
Vermillion, South Dakota

Theresa Smith, PhD, OTR, CLVT
Texas Woman's University
Houston, Texas

Beth P. Velde, OTR/L, PhD
Professor, Occupational Therapy Department
Assistant Dean, College of Allied Health Sciences
East Carolina University
Greenville, North Carolina

Callie Watson, OTD, OT/L
College of Saint Mary
Omaha, Nebraska

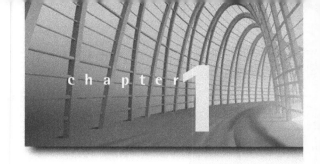

Community Practice in Occupational Therapy: What Is It?

LEARNING OBJECTIVES

By the end of this chapter, the reader will be able to complete the following:

1. Describe the role of the occupational therapy practitioner in community practice.
2. Compare and contrast theoretical approaches to community practice in occupational therapy.
3. Reflect on the skills required to engage in community practice as an occupational therapy practitioner.

Key Terms

- Community
- Community-based participatory research (CBPR)
- Community-based practice
- Community-built practice
- Community capacity building
- Community-centered
- Community partnership
- Community practice
- Health
- Primary health promotion
- Secondary health promotion
- Tertiary health promotion

Overview

This chapter provides a basic introduction to community practice as a foundation for program development and grant writing for occupational therapy practitioners. The premise of this book is that successful grant proposals are based on sound program development. Throughout this book, many of the concepts introduced in this chapter are discussed in greater detail including application and examples. In this chapter, models of community occupational therapy practice are defined and described along with skills and challenges related to community practice. Important concepts of community practice are described as are methods and strategies for building evidence in community practice.

Introduction

Occupations do not occur in a vacuum and, as outlined in the Occupational Therapy Practice Framework (OTPF), occupations are affected by the context in which people live (American Occupational Therapy Association [AOTA], 2008). **Community** is an important context that influences peoples' ability to engage in occupations. Communities can facilitate or inhibit occupational engagement of those with and without disabilities. In this book, the skills of grant writing are thoroughly discussed as applied to community occupational therapy practice. Occupational therapy **community practice** can be initiated and supported by external funding, including grants (Brownson, 1998). Prior to delving into the topic of grant writing, the question must be asked: What is community practice for occupational therapy practitioners?

What Is Community?

Communities provide a unique setting for occupational therapy practice. "Everyday life of a community, its mix of people, their needs, concerns, joys and struggles, offers an unparalleled opportunity to define [the occupational therapy] discipline, research its potential" (Fidler, 2001, p. 8). Communities are individuals tied together by occupational engagement and a collective sense of meaning. Communities are not simply defined by geographic location but refer to a "person's natural environment, that is, where the person works, plays, and performs other daily activities" (Brownson, 1998). Communities are the settings where people reside, build relationships, and engage in health practices (Brownson, 1998; Scaffa, 2001; Grady, 1995). Communities exist as a context in which people define their lives. For some people, identifying membership in a community may be challenging, yet everyone belongs to multiple communities.

> **LET'S STOP AND THINK**
>
> How do you define community? What communities do you belong to? Take some time to write down answers to these questions and reflect on your definition and the communities of importance to you.

The importance and relevance of community practice in occupational therapy have been discussed throughout the profession's history (McColl, 1998). In occupational therapy, an essential conception of community is one that considers groups of people engaged in a collective occupation. In other words, just as individuals have unique occupations, so do communities. The basis of a community is relationships, and communities of people come together "to do something that cannot be easily done in isolation" (Scaffa, 2001, p. 8). Based on this premise, communities have unique cultures, relationships, views of health, and occupations.

Health in the Context of Community

The World Health Organization defines **health** as "a state of complete physical, mental and social well-being and not merely the absence of disease or infirmity" (World Health Organization [WHO], 1998). Health has been comprehensively defined in the profession of occupational therapy as

> the absence of illness, but not necessarily disability; a balance of physical, mental, and social well-being attained through socially valued and individually meaningful occupation; enhancement of capacity and opportunity to strive for individual potential; community cohesion and opportunity; social integration, support, and justice, all within and as part of a sustainable ecology. (Wilcock, 2006, p. 110)

Both definitions acknowledge that health is not only about disease state. These definitions incorporate a holistic view of well-being and the importance of quality of life as a significant component of health. In community practice, occupational therapy practitioners must retain a broad view of health in order to implement successful health-related programs because the extrinsic factors of health cannot be denied. For example, when conducting an occupational therapy evaluation in the home, the practitioner can explore the impact that the environment has on the client's occupational engagement and easily visualize the barriers to transfers or mobility that the client may face in the home.

In the community context of occupational therapy practice, the definition of health moves away from the medical definition. Health is viewed as the ability to engage in occupation (Baum & Law, 1998; Wilcock, 2006). Occupations "demonstrate a community's and an individual's culturally sanctioned intellectual, moral, social and physical attributes. It is only by what they do that people can demonstrate what they are or what they hope to be" (Wilcock, 2006, p. 9). The inability to engage in occupation, whether caused by physical, mental, social, or environmental challenges, leads to many problems with maintenance of health and well-being.

Wilcock (2006) says it best: "Health is remarkably simple and remarkably complex" (p. 3). Perhaps this perception of health can act as an appropriate mantra for occupational therapy practitioners working in the community. Health can be affected by simple factors, such as risk factors, in which people make conscious choices to engage in healthy and unhealthy behaviors that prevent or lead to disease. On the other hand, the health status of an individual and a community may be affected by forces beyond individual or group behaviors. External forces, such as transportation, socioeconomic status, and health disparities, greatly affect the health of a community.

Dr. Paul Farmer (2003), physician and medical anthropologist, discusses the impacts of social and political decisions on public health, acknowledging that these larger systems affect the health of communities and entire countries. Many of the factors that affect the health of groups and communities are out of the autonomous control of the people affected. For example, many underserved communities find their health status affected by oppressive forces outside of their control (Farmer, 2003). Health disparities, unequal treatment of patients, and access to health insurance (including both the uninsured and underinsured) are sociopolitical factors that affect peoples' ability to access and respond to healthcare regimens and how community members define and engage in healthy behaviors.

For example, community members may not walk in the community for exercise because there are no sidewalks and residents fear for their safety when they have to walk in the streets. Although this may sound like an oversimplified problem, many times infrastructure and city planning issues, such as a lack of sidewalks, make community members feel like they are unable to practice healthy behaviors, like walking. In this example, the health determinant actually has nothing to do with the community members' physical ability to engage in health maintenance activities but demonstrates a simple barrier to health and well-being in a community setting. By considering factors such as these, occupational therapy practitioners can explore alternative methods for engaging community members in health maintenance because they understand the complexity of the human experience.

As experts in occupation, occupational therapy practitioners easily identify factors that prevent a person from healing. Skills in activity analysis provide occupational therapy practitioners with a basis for understanding engagement and how activities and occupations are impeded by physical factors. In a community practice setting, occupational therapy practitioners use these same clinical skills to explore the determinants of health beyond the physical by taking a systems approach to understanding health and disease (Wilcock, 2006; McColl, 1998; Scriven & Atwal, 2004). The role of the occupational therapy practitioner in community practice is to explore occupational engagement in a broad sense. Practitioners must apply to the community setting the same clinical skills they use to analyze an activity and how an individual can accomplish it despite a disability (McColl, 1998).

Occupational therapy practitioners must understand the context and conditions beyond physiologic problems that affect health status. Community characteristics, including but not limited to socioeconomic status, culture, political infrastructure, public transportation, availability of healthcare services, and geographic location, affect community health status. Occupational therapy practitioners practicing in the community setting need not fully understand all the factors that create community context but must acknowledge their existence and impact on the health status and well-being of the community and its members. Based on this complexity and interdependence of external factors on health status, occupational therapy practitioners are called to view health in a broader sense (Wilcock, 2006).

The Need for Community Practice

Occupational therapy practitioners recognize that "staying within the medical model deprives society of the full benefits of an occupational approach" (Miller & Nelson, 2004, p. 138). Community practice opens the door for the profession of occupational therapy to grow and apply occupation in its natural settings. Yet communities are complex and dynamic, and addressing health issues in communities is complicated by factors such as reimbursement, community-defined needs, and health disparities. Current healthcare systems lack the ability to adequately address community health issues, health disparities, health promotion, and health behaviors, which lays the ground work for occupational therapy practitioners to actively explore and define roles in community practice (Scaffa, 2001; Fazio, 2008). Because of these challenges in the healthcare system, occupational therapy practitioners can adopt

> a client-centered, community approach that requires practitioners to have the skills to work effectively in individual, dyadic, group, and community interactions to implement restorative as well as preventive and health maintenance programs that enhance the function and well-being of clients. (Baum & Law, 1998, p. 9)

With the drastic changes in healthcare services, the rising costs of health care, and the time constraints on providing health care caused by funding limitations, an increasing demand for community health programs has developed across the disciplines (Merryman, 2002; Fazio, 2008). To meet these demands, communities are turning to healthcare providers for assistance to meet the needs of community members (Baum & Law, 1998; Suarez-Balcazar, 2005). Furthermore, insurance costs have risen drastically, forcing individuals and employers that provide health insurance to explore the role of health maintenance and wellness as a method for reducing costs (Cover the Uninsured, 2008). All of these factors justify the need for occupational therapy practice in community settings.

The profession of occupational therapy is becoming more proactive in addressing health needs that arise, expanding outside a rehabilitation approach. Examples of this include fall prevention programs and driving programs (Dorne & Kurfuerst, 2008). Programs such as these demonstrate a shift in the profession from rehabilitating those who are ill or disabled to facilitating healthy living, aging in place, and quality of life for all. Most of these programs occur in a community setting.

Understanding Community Practice in Occupational Therapy

Defining community practice in occupational therapy is challenging because of its encompassing nature and its differences from traditional practice. In the community setting, occupational therapy practitioners "have no recipe for success in this realm of practice, no standard treatment plans to follow, no scheduled times to perform activities of daily living treatments" (Loukas, 2000). Occupational therapy practice in community settings is broad, and programs are unique to each community and practitioner working in the community. Occupational therapy interventions move "beyond the individual treatment of a client to working with systems that affect the ability of an individual or group to achieve work, leisure, and social goals" (Brownson, 1998, p. 61). According to the Occupational Therapy Practice Framework (OTPF), occupational therapy practitioners must consider clients not only as individuals but also as both organizations and populations within a community (AOTA, 2008). Because communities are collective in nature, occupational therapy practitioners in community practice must explore innovative ways of practicing, not just new venues for practice (Brownson, 1998).

Community practice in occupational therapy explores "the role of occupation in the shaping of a society and a daily life" (Fidler, 2001, p. 7). McColl (1998) proposes that occupational therapy practitioners in community settings "need basic knowledge about the nature and distribution of disability and occupation and about the determinants of successful community living with a disability" (p. 11). But beyond understanding the experience of individuals with a disability living in the community, community practice involves understanding the collective whole. As discussed previously, communities are unique and exhibit collective occupations. Even when addressing individual clients, the impact of the community and relationships within it are instrumental to occupational engagement (Fazio, 2008). Wilcock (2006) suggests that "occupation provides a mechanism for social interaction and societal development and growth, forming the foundation of community" (p. 9). As individuals experience challenges to occupational engagement, so do communities. Occupational therapy practitioners must understand these concepts to apply them in a community setting.

Community practice provides a clear picture of the dynamics that affect a person's ability to practice healthy occupations. The difference between community practice and traditional medical practice is simple: "Community practice exists in the client's 'real life' and 'real world'" (Siebert, 2003, p. 2). In fact, all the aspects that affect health and occupational engagement must be considered in the community setting because this makes therapy more applicable and client-centered (Brownson, 1998). For example, when an occupational therapist completes a home safety assessment, the practitioner can easily view barriers and accessibility issues. Obviously, this approach has an advantage over simply interviewing the client in an inpatient setting about his or her perceived barriers and accessibility issues in the home. Client perceptions are valid and important, yet a discussion about home safety that is conducted in the inpatient setting is removed from the dynamic environment and community context in which the person engages daily. Practicing in community settings provides practitioners with a realistic view of the client's life and promotes better treatment outcomes because suggestions and therapy occur in context.

Fazio (2008) suggests that to engage in community practice successfully, the occupational therapy practitioner must adopt a systems approach (Gray, Kennedy, & Zemke, 1996a; Gray, Kennedy, & Zemke, 1996b). Occupational therapy practitioners are interested in occupation related to "the dynamics of this process within the larger system of environment/community" (Fazio, 2008, p. 25). Communities are complex, with multiple dynamics all interacting and interconnected. Occupational therapy practitioners must find a role that can facilitate positive health changes in this system (Fazio, 2008).

By being in a community, practitioners can perceive community members' barriers and challenges to healthy living. Many factors that affect health are not visible in clinical settings because the environment is controlled by the healthcare system. In the community, many factors affect an individual's ability to live healthily. For example, American Indians living on a reservation typically receive federal food commodities, which dictate food availability. Telling a client to eat healthy is simple, but obviously reservation-based American Indians may find it difficult to comply with this suggestion because of the limited food choices available. Clients are challenged by issues such as nutritional access, and practitioners must take into account these issues when working with communities. When providing services in community settings, practitioners must know the community in order to implement healthcare recommendations and treatments that meet the needs of the community members and that acknowledge challenges to basic health maintenance (Fazio, 2008). Factors such as food access affect the overall health of a community and imply the need for healthcare practitioners to understand the community context to facilitate healthy living.

Communities can be collectively healthy or unhealthy as a result of many factors. For example, in cities with reliable and accessible transportation systems, individuals with physical disabilities can get to work on time. Because of the accessible and reliable transportation system, these community members can make a societal contribution and are able to sustain a living income, which improves quality of life for all members of the community. In communities where transportation is not reliable or accessible, individuals with physical disabilities may not be able to maintain a job and cannot make a living wage. Because of lack of transportation services, individuals with physical disabilities are alienated and may experience a decreased quality of life. This example highlights the impact understanding the role community plays in occupational engagement.

The occupational therapy profession has identified practice settings in which occupational therapy practitioners can provide occupational therapy–related services (Scaffa, 2001); however, the concepts and framework of community practice in occupational therapy have not been formally outlined or accepted in the profession. Because of this lack of a collective professional definition of community practice, occupational therapy practitioners must begin to define community practice. Occupational therapy practitioners have the opportunity to explore the impact of occupational therapy practice in communities and define the specific role the profession will play in community health.

The Roles of Occupational Therapy Practitioners in the Community

It is important for readers to have a basic understanding of the roles of occupational therapy practitioners in community settings. As mentioned, no specific standards for community practice exist; however, because of the nature of community practice, specific roles and responsibilities have emerged and are discussed in the literature. These roles are often not practice-based but describe the general characteristics a practitioner needs to be successful in community settings. These include advocacy, assessment skills, capacity building skills, and the ability to apply the principles of occupation in a community context. Obviously, these roles and responsibilities are broad and each community practitioner will find different activities associated with each of these generalized roles. The following subsections describe these characteristics further.

Advocacy

In community practice, occupational therapy practitioners are required to advocate for clients for multiple reasons. Advocacy is part of the principles and values of the profession (AOTA, 1993). Although advocacy is important in all occupational therapy practice settings, it takes on a unique role in community settings (Jensen & Royeen, 2002) where practitioners address health issues not typically covered by insurance providers and may work with an underserved population that cannot afford services. The practitioner must discover and explore feasible approaches to address health issues in the community, which requires advocacy on many levels, from educating community members on the role of occupational therapy practitioners to advocating for the needs of underserved communities (Herzberg & Finlayson, 2001). For example, identifying a health problem and developing a program to address this problem is a form of advocacy (King et al., 2002; Scaletti, 1999). Writing a grant to fund services is also a form of advocacy.

Practitioners must also advocate for promotion of inclusion of all in the community (Grady, 1995) because community involvement is an important component of quality of life and self-esteem for individuals. Practitioners might sometimes need to advocate in regard to grant funding, especially when funding streams are eliminated or threatened as a result of political debate, economics, trends, or changes in administration (Jensen & Royeen, 2002). In community practice, an occupational therapy practitioner may be called to contact or communicate with political officials to voice support for initiatives.

> **LET'S STOP AND THINK**
>
> Think of a community you belong to that is important to you. Brainstorm ways in which you would engage in advocacy for that community. Think of specific ways you could advocate both as a member of that community and as an occupational therapy practitioner.

TABLE 1-1   OCCUPATIONAL THERAPY ROLES IN ADVOCACY
• Education • Addressing unmet health needs • Serving the underserved through health-related programs • Promoting inclusion • Political advocacy

Assessment Skills

Occupational therapy practitioners in community practice require unique assessment skills. In community program development, most interventions are for a group and not for an individual; therefore occupational therapy practitioners in community practice must learn how to assess groups of people regarding occupational engagement and performance (Brownson, 1998; Fazio, 2008). Some practitioners may find this a challenge because it deviates from the traditional therapist–client relationship and delivery model. Furthermore, community assessment requires skills in multiple data collection methods and data analysis. It requires an understanding of epidemiology and how community data can be used in program development and grant writing (Fazio, 2008; Wilcock, 2006).

In addition to gathering initial assessment data, occupational therapy practitioners in the community must collect ongoing evaluation data. Knowledge and understanding of program evaluation methods are crucial to the success of any program (Suarez-Balcazar & Harper, 2003). Evaluation methods are vital to improve community programs and ensure that programs address their intended purposes. Assessment also helps to build evidence and science-driven approaches that are necessary to justify funding and development of community practice in the field of occupational therapy.

Gaining skills in assessment can be challenging to novice practitioners. Methods and strategies for developing these skills are discussed later in the text. Assessment not only provides feedback on a program's outcomes but can lead to external funding support and potential policy development (Suarez-Balcazar, 2005).

BEST PRACTICE HINT

Outcome data from assessment can be used in advocacy by demonstrating a need and justifying how a program can affect a community's health in a positive and effective way.

Building Community Capacity

Community capacity building can be defined as exploring and understanding a community's potential or ability to address health problems (Chino & DeBruyn, 2006; Goodman et al., 1998). Although all communities have needs, in underserved communities where severe health disparities exist and issues such as access to care permeate, it can be challenging to explore community capacity. Although occupational therapy practitioners have been trained to identify problems or needs, in every community, they must look beyond need to identify capacity and assets for addressing health issues (Fazio, 2008).

To engage community capacity building, occupational therapy practitioners must be **community-centered** and apply client-centered practice to the community. In client-centered practice, practitioners seek to understand the goals of the community members in a similar way as to how they seek to understand the individual client in traditional therapist–client interactions (McColl, 1998). Community interventions that are based on and developed using community-identified needs build upon community strengths and have been successful (Kretzmann & McKnight, 1993; Elliott, O'Neal, & Velde, 2001). Occupational therapy practitioners must understand the occupational profile of the community to develop meaningful interventions that are based on occupational preferences (Brownson, 1998).

> ### LET'S STOP AND THINK
>
> Think of a community you belong to that is important to you. What does the community have to offer that is unique or beneficial? Write down what you identify and reflect on how these capacities could be used in the context of community occupational therapy practice.

Applying Occupation in the Community Context

Occupational therapy practitioners in the community must understand occupation in a community context (Fazio, 2008). Occupational therapy practitioners are experts on occupation and have argued that occupation is a "fundamental prerequisite of wellbeing and linked it to an individual's state of happiness, self-esteem and physical and mental health" (Scriven & Atwal, 2004, p. 427; Wilcock, 2006). However, in community practice, practitioners must understand occupations both on the individual and community levels. Because illness and health are affected by disease as well as external context and health infrastructure, occupational therapy practitioners must transform traditional beliefs about occupation to apply occupation on multiple levels. Occupation can be applied in the community context through program development and grant writing, the focus of this text.

Skills Required for Community Practice

Occupational therapy practitioners in the arenas of community health, public health, community-based practice, and community-built practice require a unique set of skills to achieve success. Fidler (2001) states that "responding to the varied needs, interests and welfare of a community will differ in orientation, attitudinal and knowledge base from the one that currently guides our education and practice" (p. 8). Despite this fact, some skills required for community practice transfer easily from the clinical setting to a community practice setting, whereas others require development and experience.

TABLE 1-2 COMMUNITY OCCUPATIONAL THERAPY PRACTITIONER SKILLS

• Consultancy	• Networking
• Education	• Management skills
• Autonomy	• Program evaluation skills
• Client-centered practice	• Cultural awareness
• Clinical reasoning	• Team skills
• Health promotion	

According to a survey of community occupational therapists conducted by Mitchell and Unsworth (2004), community occupational therapists need to possess the following skills and characteristics: consultancy, education, autonomy, client-centered practice, clinical reasoning, and health promotion. A study by Lemorie and Paul (2001) indicates that community occupational therapy practitioners need to know how to do the following: network, navigate community resources, manage volunteers, evaluate programs, health promotion/disease prevention, and address multicultural practice issues. Fazio (2008) discusses skills required of occupational therapy practitioners including communication skills, ability to develop collaborative relationships, management skills, and leadership skills. Furthermore, occupational therapy practitioners in community settings need to be able to interact with an interprofessional team that includes both professionals and valued community members (Baum & Law, 1998; Paul & Peterson, 2001; Miller & Nelson, 2004).

Occupational therapy practitioners in community settings can find a role in consultancy (Mitchell & Unsworth, 2004; Lysack, Stadnyk, Krefting, Paterson, & McLeod, 1995). For example, an occupational therapy practitioner can serve on the board of directors for a health-related nonprofit or be an active member of a community coalition. In these roles, the occupational therapy practitioner provides advice as an expert in occupation or some other component of the profession. Even though the occupational therapy practitioner does not provide direct service or engage in direct program development, he or she acts as an advisor to these processes, which leads to professional development and knowledge about community practice.

Education is a key component of community practice. Occupational therapy practitioners usually take on an educator role. According to Brownson (2001), community "programs are

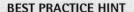

BEST PRACTICE HINT

Many practitioners feel intimidated by community practice. A best practice hint is to seek out a mentor or support group of practitioners that work in the community. By participating in a network, practitioners can develop skills important to community practice.

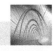

BEST PRACTICE HINT

To explore community practice occupational therapy practitioners can join a board of directors or advisory board of a community organization. Serving in this capacity helps the practitioner learn about the processes of community organizations.

distinguished from clinical services in that programs are primarily educational" (p. 96). Providing education is a significant component of community practice when practitioners explore health promotion and lifestyle modification. Occupational therapy practitioners in community settings need to have strong educative skills (Scaffa, 2001). Perhaps their most significant challenge is to tackle education in a manner that fits the needs of the community, gearing education to the culture and health literacy levels of the community members.

> **LET'S STOP AND THINK**
>
> Consider the multiple theoretical approaches that occupational therapy practitioners in community settings must employ (public health, epidemiology, systems theory, sociology, organizational psychology, and sociology). Identify which aspects from each theoretical approach occupational therapy practitioners might use in community practice.

The tenets of community practice draw from a variety of social sciences including public health, epidemiology, systems theory, sociology, organizational psychology, and sociology (Munoz, Provident, & Hansen, 2004). Occupational therapy practitioners can use elements from each source as tools for community practice. Practitioners in community practice must commit to lifelong learning and make ongoing efforts to experiment and strategize for success.

Models of Practice in the Community

In occupational therapy, there are two main approaches to practice: community-based practice and community-built practice. Occupational therapy practitioners must decide which approach works best for the needs of their practice and the community. In this section, each approach is explored and described as a valuable framework.

Community-Based Practice

Community-based practice is the location in which occupational therapy services are provided. In this model, specific locations within the community context are identified and the skills of and roles that occupational therapy practitioners can play in the setting are described. Examples include adult daycare programs, driving rehabilitation programs, and health promotion programs (Scaffa, 2001; McColl, 1998). According to Wittman and Velde (2001), community-based practice "refers to skilled services delivered by health practitioners using an interactive model with clients" (p. 3).

For community-based practice, occupational therapy practitioners must move away from the medical model and focus on a health promotion and disease prevention approach to healthcare delivery (Scaffa, 2001). Scaffa, Desmond, and Brownson (2001) encourage occupational therapy practitioners to adopt a role in health promotion program development by providing an occupation-based perspective or developing occupation-based programming to complement current health promotion programs.

Program development is a significant component of community practice. It can be compared to the occupational therapy process and includes the following steps:

TABLE 1-3 THEORETICAL FRAMEWORKS UTILIZED IN COMMUNITY-BASED PRACTICE	
Occupational Therapy Theories	**Theories Outside Occupational Therapy**
Model of Human Occupation	Social Learning Theory
Ecology of Human Performance	Health Belief Model
Occupational Adaptation	Precede-Proceed Model
Person-Environment-Occupational Performance Model	Transtheoretical Model of Health Behavior Change

Source: Scaffa, M. (Ed.). (2001). *Occupational therapy in community-based practice settings.* Philadelphia: F. A. Davis.

preplanning, needs assessment, plan development, implementation, evaluation, and institutionalization (Brownson, 2001). Program development will be discussed in further detail in Chapter 2. Community-based practice has been widely accepted in occupational therapy. The community-based practice approach transfers practice skills from the clinical setting to a population-based program development model.

Community-Built Practice

Community-built occupational therapy programs are "open systems in constant interaction with their physical, natural, temporal, social and political environment" (Elliott et al., 2001, p. 106). The basis of the **community-built practice** model is collaboration with a strength-based approach and "ends when the client-defined community has effectively built the capacity for empowerment" (Wittman & Velde, 2001, p. 3). Community-built practice is founded on the following principles:

1. *Each community member and community has strengths.* In the community-built practice model, each community member and community is evaluated for strengths. Practice focuses on health promotion and wellness and recognizes the ability of each individual and community to build capacity for success. It is assumed that the community will embrace the practice and, at some self-defined point, no longer need the occupational therapy services.

2. *Community members are equal partners in program development, implementation, and evaluation.* According to the community-built practice model, community programs can be successful only if they receive the buy-in of community members and involve them in the program planning and implementation. Community members are the experts in the community's culture, dynamics, politics, and health issues and are the strongest resource of any community program. The community-built practice model recognizes this fact and uses it as a strategy for success (Wittman & Velde, 2001).

3. *Community members "own" the program.* The community program should not depend on experts or "outsiders" to be successful but should become embodied by the community. This process takes time and is not well defined in the community-built model because communities vary; but the ultimate goal of community-built practice is for the community to assume responsibility for the program.

4. *The occupational therapy practitioner must be culturally aware for the program to succeed* (Barnard et al., 2004; Wittman & Velde, 2001). In most cases, the occupational therapy practitioner comes from a cultural background different from the community members. Cultural awareness and cultural desire (Campinha-Bacote, 2001) are skills required of the practitioner for the program activities to have an impact.

Community-built practice is an emerging model in occupational therapy practice that is based on community- and capacity-building models in population-based and health promotion practice (Wittman & Velde, 2001).

Community-Based Practice versus Community-Built Practice

Both community-based practice and community-built practice are models used as frameworks for community practice. Although both models focus on community practice, they differ in their approaches and philosophies.

A community-based occupational therapy program takes place in the community context. It focuses on applying the concepts of occupational therapy practice to community settings to develop programs that address occupational needs. Braveman (2001) shares an example of a community-based program for addressing the work rehabilitation needs of individuals with HIV/AIDS. The program, based on the Model of Human Occupation and provided as part of the services offered by a community organization, provides four phases of intervention: Phase 1 focuses on self-assessment and exploration of roles and habits, phase 2 focuses on developing skills required for work, phase 3 includes employment placement with support, and phase 4 provides long-term follow-up and support in the new work role. To develop the program, Braveman (2001) followed a program development model proposed by Grossman and Bortone (1986) and implemented the program within a community context.

Community-built practice utilizes a collaboration model and focuses on the needs and capacities of the community and its members. The community-built model refers to this aspect in its title: *Community* is *built* with the occupational therapy practitioner as facilitator. Barnard and colleagues (2004) in "Wellness in Tillery" describe an example of a community-built model. Tillery is a small, rural town in North Carolina with a large African American population. Students in the East Carolina University Occupational Therapy program were assigned to develop programming following a community-built model. Students were asked to immerse themselves in the community to learn about the people and to face their own biases about the community. Through building relationships, the students were able to collaborate with the older African Americans in the community to develop the Open-Minded Seniors Wellness Program, a program focused on physical activity, spirituality, nutrition education, and cognition activities. Through surveys and feedback, the program was able to increase senior wellness and improve overall quality of life among the community members involved. The program's success is attributed to the concepts of the community-built model, which include collaborative planning and implementation, equal partnerships in program implementation, and a sense of community ownership of the program.

Both models of community practice offer approaches and methods for the occupational therapy practitioner. The community-based model focuses on a variety of health promotion and program development approaches whereas the community-built model provides a structured way of viewing the community and program development. Occupational therapy practitioners must determine which approach best suits their clinical reasoning and the community they plan to partner with. Examples of community-based and community-built practice programs exist in the literature to aid the practitioner in picking a model best suited for practice.

BEST PRACTICE HINT

Explore the literature for models of community-based practice and community-built practice to identify which model best suits you.

Public Health and Occupational Therapy

According to Hildenbrand and Froehlich (2002), the aim of public health is to "mobilize resources to ensure health-supporting conditions for all persons." Wilcock (2006) argues that occupational therapists have a role in public health. On the other hand, Scriven and Atwal (2004) question "whether the profession has the competencies and capacity to join others in the public health workforce with upstream remits and responsibilities" (p. 428; Scaffa, Van Slyke, & Brownson, 2008). Despite the debate, the role of occupational therapy practitioners in community practice follows a traditional public health model.

BEST PRACTICE HINT

Many states have public health organizations similar to state occupational therapy associations. Explore membership in the public health organization of your state to learn more and to network with public health professionals.

Health promotion is a key component of public health. According to the World Health Organization (2008), health promotion is "the process of enabling people to increase control over their health and its determinants, and thereby improve their health." In general, the occupational therapy literature acknowledges that practitioners' roles in community practice are to "work with clients to promote health and overcome a range of physical, social and emotional barriers and problems to maximise the client's quality of life" (Mitchell & Unsworth, 2004, pp. 14–15). For many occupational therapy practitioners, practice may delve into health promotion, which tightly aligns with the tenets of public health (Baum & Law, 1998).

Practitioners who are unfamiliar with the concepts of public health may find it difficult to transition to a public health framework. Hildenbrand and Froehlich (2002) argue that occupational therapy practitioners have a fundamental role to play in public health, including the promotion of health maintenance for individuals with or without disabilities, development of occupation-based community programs, and participation on teams of public health professionals involved in health promotion programming. They encourage occupational therapy practitioners to embrace a role in public health, stating that "public health arenas of health maintenance, disease prevention, and health promotion offer a new vision of opportunity for personal challenge, professional development, and discipline expansion."

According to *The Promotion of Health Statement and the Prevention of Disease and Disability* published by the American Occupational Therapy Association, occupational therapy practitioners can play a role in health promotion through the promotion of healthy living, use of occupation as a vehicle for healing and health maintenance, and the provision of interventions focused on both individuals and populations (Scaffa et al., 2008). The document goes on to state that "because of the inextricable and reciprocal links between people and their environments, larger groups, organizations, communities, populations, and government policymakers must also be considered for intervention" (p. 420).

In community practice, there are three main areas of health promotion as outlined by Scriven and Atwal (2004): primary health promotion, secondary health promotion, and tertiary health promotion. Following traditional definitions of prevention, **primary health promotion** is defined as "activities that target the well population and aim to prevent ill health and disability through, for example, health education and/or legislation." **Secondary health promotion** "is directed at individuals or groups in order to change health-damaging habits and/or to prevent ill health moving to a chronic or irreversible stage and, where possible, to restore people to their former state of health." **Tertiary health promotion** occurs "with individuals who have chronic conditions and/or are disabled and is concerned with making the most of their potential for healthy living" (Scriven & Atwal, 2004, p. 425). Each level of prevention/promotion focuses on a different subset of the population. Primary prevention explores health for all individuals whereas secondary prevention focuses on working with people who have identified risk factors and tertiary prevention focuses on those who already have an existing condition affecting their lives.

Occupational therapy practice is fueled by the belief that wellness and health derive from engagement in occupation (Fazio, 2008). This very fundamental principle defines the role of occupational therapy practitioners in public health and prevention in community settings.

TABLE 1-4 EXAMPLES OF PREVENTION		
Primary Prevention	**Secondary Prevention**	**Tertiary Prevention**
• Wearing helmet while cycling	• Health screenings including cholesterol and blood pressure	• Medications for existing disease
• Obtaining immunizations		
• Wearing a seatbelt while driving		
• Rehabilitation		

Source: Fitzgerald, M. A. (2008). Primary, secondary, and tertiary prevention: Important in certification and practice. Retrieved July 10, 2008, from http://www.fhea.com/certificationcols/level_prevention.shtml

Building Evidence in Community Practice

Community programming in occupational therapy, though at this point not thoroughly researched, has demonstrated a positive impact (Dunn, 2000; Loisel et al., 2003; Scaffa, 2001; Fazio, 2008). Because evidence-based practice is emphasized as a key component for achieving the science-driven goals of the profession, exploring evidence in community practice is crucial. Furthermore, occupational therapy practitioners must continue to add to and develop this evidence.

According to Horowitz and Chang (2004), "preventative community-based occupational therapy lifestyle redesign programs have been found to provide significant benefits in promoting quality of life, physical functioning, and mental health" (p. 48). These community programs have demonstrated an impact not only on physical well-being but the whole person, which is the ultimate goal of authentic occupational therapy.

Much of the evidence regarding community practice actually refers to education of occupational therapy students and exploration of successful strategies for teaching the skills necessary to practice in the community (Lemorie & Paul, 2001; Munoz, Provident, & Hanson, 2004; Miller & Nelson, 2004; Eggers, Munoz, Sciulli, & Crist, 2006; Perrin & Wittman, 2001). In most examples, students have been required to engage in a service learning project with a community partner or to participate in level I fieldwork experiences in a community setting. Students have the opportunity to learn basic community practice skills such as conducting assessments, program development, grant writing, case management, identifying occupations common to the community or population, and basic community-based participatory research (Perrin & Wittman, 2001; Munoz et al., 2004).

Aging in place is an area of practice that uses a health promotion model. Programs such as the Well Elderly Study exemplify the importance of occupational engagement in health promotion programs (Mandel, Jackson, Zemke, Nelson, & Clark, 1999). Community programs targeted at older adults including driving programs and fall prevention programs have evidenced success (Dorne & Kurfuerst, 2008; Siebert, 2003). Evidence is a crucial component of community practice. Occupational therapy practitioners should integrate and disseminate evidence-based approaches when they write grants and develop programs.

Community-Based Participatory Research

In the field of public health, **community-based participatory research (CBPR)** is used to demonstrate the effectiveness of programs that affect communities. The beauty of CBPR is that the framework itself acknowledges the unique needs and values of each community. According to Israel, Eng, Schulz, and Parker (2005), community members and researchers need "jointly to decide on the core values and guiding principles that reflect their collective vision and basis for decision making." Practitioners in the community setting must understand that collaboration is the key to success (Brownson, 1998; Fazio, 2008).

Although CBPR has guiding principles, it allows for the community to drive the research. In most cases, the research team acts as a facilitator, guiding the community toward addressing its own health issues. CBPR empowers communities because it assumes that community members are the experts on their own experience. In a sense, CBPR closely aligns with the occupational therapy principle of client-centered care and provides a forum for using evidence-based practice in the community. CBPR is covered in more detail later in the text.

Challenges to Community Practice

Occupational therapy practitioners face many challenges in working directly with and in communities. First, occupational therapy community practice is not well defined. Currently, resources name the skills required for working in community settings, but a collective definition of community practice for occupational therapy practitioners has not been created. Occupational therapy practitioners in community practice are to "acquire new skills, fill new roles, and use a client-centered approach to treatment" (Lemorie & Paul, 2001, p. 34).

Another significant obstacle to overcome in community practice and program development is funding (Brownson, 1998). In many cases, programs cannot be funded by third parties because the programs and services provided are not considered reimbursable by third-party payers, and the community members being served may not be able to pay for services. Unfortunately, very few planning grants exist and most funders expect infrastructure to be in place so that program implementation can occur upon receipt of funding. For newly developed programs, a lack of external funding can be a challenge and practitioners must realize that work might need to be done without financial support.

Program sustainability is another significant challenge. Grant funding does not last forever. Occupational therapy practitioners must plan for program sustainability from the beginning and explore avenues for garnering financial resources to provide ongoing support for the programming or practice. Throughout this text, sustainability is emphasized and explored in relation to program development and grant writing.

Other challenges may include the pressure to succeed in facilitating behavioral change. In community settings, occupational therapy practitioners find themselves acting as change agents for community health because they are experts in occupations and in transforming lives through health education and engagement. However, changing behavior is a complex process and programs do not always promote the intended or proposed change. The pressure to succeed in changing behavior can be a frustration and challenge that affects community practice, especially when related to grant funding that does not allow enough time or resources for change to occur. Many funders now recognize the challenge of behavioral change (Edberg, 2007). When developing a program or writing a grant proposal, practitioners must provide sufficient time and outcomes and acknowledge the challenges of health behavior change.

Another significant task of community program development is what Mitchell and Unsworth (2004) refer to as "time spent on non-OT work." In program development, occupational therapy practitioners may act in roles outside of their profession and may spend time on what is considered "non-OT work." For some practitioners, this may present difficulties, but for others, it may be a reward of this type of practice.

Finally, achieving success with a program is complicated. An occupational therapy practitioner may develop a great program, but attendance or participation is low. In this case, there may be a disconnect between the program and the community. As part of the evaluation plan, the occupational therapy practitioner must always build in methods for assessing and modifying the program to continue to meet community needs. Strategies for recruitment and promoting program buy-in are discussed later in this text.

Community practitioners must plan and think in ways different from practitioners in traditional practice settings. Despite the complications, occupational therapy practitioners can succeed in community practice and develop successful programs that make a difference. Two strategies for success include community immersion and developing viable partnerships in the community.

The Concept of Community Immersion

To succeed in community practice, practitioners must truly understand the needs and strengths of a community. One way that occupational therapy practitioners can come to understand community needs is through community immersion. They must spend time in the community developing relationships and exploring the impact of occupation in the community (Cooper, Voltz, Cochran, & Goulet, 2007; Cross & Doll, 2008).

One way for practitioners to immerse themselves in the community is through working in a traditional clinical role in the community. Interacting with clients helps the practitioner understand trends of health and health behaviors. Many times, ideas for community practice develop out of patterns observed in clinical practice (Voltz-Doll, 2008).

Another way is to provide pro bono services, perhaps during evenings or on weekends. Through pro bono service practitioners can gain a perspective on the community. Services provided free of charge generally have positive outcomes, but the risk is that community members will assume that services will always be provided for free. Despite this, the advantages of pro bono work include building rapport with community members and the opportunity to build programmatic ideas to address community needs (Voltz-Doll, 2008).

BEST PRACTICE HINT

If you are providing pro bono services with the intention of developing a community program, be upfront with participants so that community members know the purpose and goals of the provided services.

Community immersion is crucial to success in community practice because the practitioner can come to know and understand the community. Knowledge of the community ensures that the practitioner identifies needs and strategies to address health issues that align with community values and culture. Immersion also allows the practitioner insight into system-based issues such as policies or infrastructure that can either promote or inhibit healthy living and occupational engagement.

The Concept of Partnership

In community practice, no one can work alone to solve the complex social problems and all the dynamics that affect health and well-being. A partnership model ensures that the needs of all parties involved are met. Partnerships are in no way perfect and take time to develop. In any partnership there will be misunderstandings, struggles, and frustrations. By following the principles outlined in **Table 1-5**, practitioners can provide a foundation for maintaining a successful **community partnership**. Partnerships are central to community practice in occupational therapy.

In a partnership, all parties come to the table with something to offer and all parties benefit. A partnership approach to community practice ensures success and examines "ways that scientific knowledge and community experiential knowledge can come together to address complex social problems" (Suarez-Balcazar et al., 2005, p. 48; Jensen & Royeen, 2001).

In a partnership model, the community and the healthcare practitioner work together to identify needs and develop the program in collaboration. According to

TABLE 1-5   MAINTAINING A PARTNERSHIP IN COMMUNITY PRACTICE

Principle	Description
Develop relationship based on trust and mutual respect	• Build relationships • Practice collaborative visioning • Develop common agenda
Identify community stakeholders	• Seek out community leaders • Develop relationships with community leaders • Take time to understand the leadership style of the community
Establish reciprocal learning style	• Value knowledge and experience of community members as much as own knowledge
Educate community members	• Educate community members on occupational therapy and the role it can play in the partnership
Develop communication structure	• Use communication styles of the community • Be available to communicate • Encourage partner to always be open and honest
Be present in the community	• Make an investment in the community by attending cultural or community events meaningful to the people
Maximize resources	• Acknowledge the resources of both entities in the partnership
Practice collaborative program development	• Develop programs in collaboration or enable program development to be driven by community members
Use a multimethod approach	• Use multiple approaches to assess and evaluate success
Build cultural competence	• Celebrate diversity • Acknowledge cultural differences • Be aware of how culture affects health beliefs and practices
Share accountability	• Share accomplishments equally
Implement collaborative dissemination	• Include community partner in dissemination

Source: Adapted from Suarez-Balcazar, Y., Hammel, J., Helfrich, C., Thomas, J., Wilson, T., & Head-Ball, D. (2005). A model of university–community partnerships for occupational therapy scholarship and practice. *Occupational Therapy in Health Care, 19*(1/2), 47–70.

Suarez-Balcazar and colleagues (2005), maintaining a partnership requires seven principles: "(a) developing a relationship based on trust and mutual respect, (b) establishing a reciprocal learning style, (c) developing open lines of communication, (d) maximizing resources, (e) using a multi-methods approach, (f) respecting diversity and building cultural competence, and (g) sharing accountability" (p. 51). These principles are neither sequential nor hierarchical, but are all necessary in the partnership process. Other strategies for establishing and maintaining partnerships include identifying community stakeholders, educating the partner on the role of occupational therapy in the community, being present in the community, collaborating on program development, and collaborating on dissemination.

LET'S STOP AND THINK

What challenges to forming a community partnership do you think exist? How would you address these challenges as an occupational therapy practitioner?

Application to the Occupational Therapy Practice Framework

Community practice should be grounded in the concepts and values presented in the Occupational Therapy Practice Framework (OTPF). The OTPF provides guidelines for practitioners engaged in community practice. Community practice ties in to the OTPF by "supporting health and participation in life through engagement in occupation" in the community context (AOTA, 2008, p. 626).

Community is listed as an area of practice in the Framework. The OTPF discusses the importance of community life in the overall health and wellness of human beings, stating that "occupational therapy practitioners are concerned not only with occupations but also the complexity of factors that empower and make possible clients' engagement and participation in positive health-promoting occupations" (AOTA, 2008, p. 629).

Not only is community viewed as a context for practice in the OTPF, but also as an approach in regards to interventions for populations. According to the OTPF, the goal of population-based community interventions is to "enhance the health of all people within the population by addressing services and supports within the community that can be implemented to improve the population's performance" (AOTA, 2008, p. 655). Community programs that work with underserved communities match with the concept of occupational justice working to address health disparities.

Practitioners who follow the OTPF must have many of the skills that are discussed later in this text, including advocacy, consultancy, and education. The Framework promotes the health, participation, and engagement in occupation by members of a community.

Conclusion

Prior to engaging in program development and writing grant proposals to support such programs, occupational therapy practitioners must have a firm grasp of the concept of community practice. This chapter provides a foundation in community practice including basic introductions to the concepts of practice and models of practice. Community practice requires unique skills. The need for and benefit of building evidence in community practice are also important to ensuring that programs remain relevant and impactful.

Glossary

Community Individuals tied together by occupational engagement and a collective sense of meaning

Community-based participatory research (CBPR) A research model in which the community designs the research program and participates in the implementation of research focused on its own health issues

Community-based practice The location in which occupational therapy services are provided

Community-built practice Uses a capacity-based approach to explore the community needs and build programs to address these community-specified needs

Community capacity building Exploring and understanding a community's potential or ability to address health problems

Community-centered Applying a client-centered approach to a community

Community partnership When the community and the healthcare practitioner collaborate on identifying needs and the program is developed in collaboration

Community practice When occupational therapy practitioners use their skills to explore the determinants of health beyond the physical and take on a systems approach to understanding health and disease

Health "A state of complete physical, mental and social well-being and not merely the absence of disease or infirmity" (WHO, 1998)

Primary health promotion Activities for the well population to prevent disease or disability

Secondary health promotion Activities to encourage positive health behaviors to improve health status

Tertiary health promotion Activities to maximize the quality of life of individuals experiencing disease or disability

References

American Occupational Therapy Association. (1993). Core values and attitudes of occupational therapy practice. *American Journal of Occupational Therapy, 47*(12), 1085–1086.

American Occupational Therapy Association. (2008). Occupational therapy practice framework: Domain and process, 2nd edition. *American Journal of Occupational Therapy, 62*(6), 626–683.

Barnard, S., Dunn, S., Reddic, E., Rhodes, K., Russell, J., Tuitt, T. S., et al. (2004). Wellness in Tillery: A community-built program. *Family and Community Health, 27*(2), 151–157.

Baum, C., & Law, M. (1998). Community health: A responsibility, an opportunity, and a fit for occupational therapy. *American Journal of Occupational Therapy, 52*, 7–10.

Braveman, B. (2001). Development of a community-based return to work program for people living with AIDS. *Occupational Therapy in Health Care, 13*(3–4), 113–131.

Brownson, C. A. (1998). Funding community practice: Stage 1. *American Journal of Occupational Therapy, 52*, 60–64.

Brownson, C. A. (2001). Program development: Planning, implementation, and evaluation strategies. In M. Scaffa (Ed.), *Occupational therapy in community-based practice settings.* Philadelphia: F. A. Davis.

Campinha-Bacote, J. (2001). A model of practice to address cultural competence in rehabilitation nursing. *Rehabilitation Nursing, 26*(1), 8–11.

Chino, M., & DeBruyn, L. (2006). Building true capacity: Indigenous models for indigenous communities. *American Journal of Public Health, 96*(4), 596–599.

Cooper, M., Voltz, J. D., Cochran, T. M., & Goulet, C. (2007, April). Focus on rural community engagement: The student perspective of learning in the community. Paper presented at Catching Waves: Using Engagement to Address Critical Issues: The Tenth Annual Continuums of Service Conference. San Jose, CA.

Cover the Uninsured. (2008). Quick facts on the uninsured. Retrieved September 30, 2008, from http://covertheuninsured.org/content/quick-facts-uninsured

Cross, P., & Doll, J. D. (2008). Developing health professional students into rural health care leaders of the future through best practices. In G. M. Jensen & C. D. Royeen (Eds.), *Leadership in rural health interprofessional education and practice.* Sudbury, MA: Jones and Bartlett.

Dorne, R., & Kurfuerst, S. (2008). Productive aging and occupational therapy: A look ahead. *Special Interest Section Quarterly: Gerontology, 31*(1), 1–4.

Dunn, W. (2000). *Best practice occupational therapy in community service with children and families.* Thorofare, NJ: Slack.

Edberg, M. (2007). *Essentials of health behavior: Social and behavior health in public health.* Sudbury, MA: Jones and Bartlett.

Eggers, M., Munoz, J. P., Sciulli, J., & Crist, P. A. (2006). The community reintegration project: Occupational therapy at work in a county jail. *Occupational Therapy in Health Care, 20*(1), 17–37.

Elliott, S., O'Neal, S., & Velde, B. P. (2001). Using chaos theory to understand a community-built occupational therapy practice. *Occupational Therapy in Health Care, 13*(3/4), 101–112.

Farmer, P. (2003). *Pathologies of power: Health, human rights, and the new war on the poor.* Berkeley: University of California Press.

Fazio, L. S. (2008). *Developing occupation-centered programs for the community* (2nd ed.). Upper Saddle River, NJ: Prentice Hall.

Fidler, G. S. (2001) Community practice: It's more than geography. *Occupational Therapy in Health Care, 13*(3/4), 7–9.

Fitzgerald, M. A. (2008). Primary, secondary, and tertiary prevention: Important in certification and practice. Retrieved July 10, 2008, from http://www.fhea.com/certificationcols/level_prevention.shtml

Goodman, R. M., Speers, M. A., McLeroy, K., Fawcett, S., Kegler, M., Parker, E., et al. (1998). Identifying and defining the dimensions of community capacity to provide a basis for measurement. *Health Education and Behavior, 25*, 258–278.

Grady, A. P. (1995). 1994 Eleanor Clarke Slagle Lecture: Building inclusive community: A challenge for occupational therapy. *American Journal of Occupational Therapy, 40*, 300–310.

Gray, J. M., Kennedy, B. L., & Zemke, R. (1996a). Dynamic systems theory: An overview. In R. Zemke & F. Clark (Eds.), *Occupational science: The evolving discipline* (pp. 297–308). Philadelphia: F. A. Davis.

Gray, J. M., Kennedy, B. L., & Zemke, R. (1996b). Application of dynamic systems theory to occupation. In R. Zemke & F. Clark (Eds.), *Occupational science: The evolving discipline* (pp. 309–324). Philadelphia: F. A. Davis.

Grossman, J. & Bortone, J. (1986). Program development. In S.C. Robertson (Ed.), *Strategies, concepts, and opportunities for program development and evaluation.* (pp. 91–99). Bethesda, MD: The American Occupational Therapy Association.

Herzberg, G., & Finlayson, M. (2001). Development of occupational therapy in a homeless shelter. *Occupational Therapy in Health Care, 13*(3/4), 133–147.

Hildenbrand, W., & Froehlich, A. K. (2002). Promoting health: Historical roots, renewed vision. *OT Practice, 7*, 10–15.

Horowitz, B., & Chang, P. F. (2004). Promoting engagement in life and well-being through occupational therapy lifestyle redesign: A pilot study within adult day programs. *Topics in Geriatric Rehabilitation, 20*(1), 46–58.

Israel, B. A., Eng, E., Schulz, A. J., & Parker, E. A. (2005). Introduction to method in community-based participatory research for health. In B. A. Israel, E. Eng, A. J. Schulz, & E. A. Parker (Eds.), *Methods in community-based participatory research for health.* San Francisco: Jossey-Bass.

Jensen, G. M., & Royeen, C. B. (2001). Analysis of academic-community partnerships using the integration matrix. *Journal of Allied Health, 30*, 168–175.

Jensen, G. M., & Royeen, C. B. (2002). Improved rural access to care: Dimensions of best practice. *Journal of Interprofessional Care, 16*, 117–128.

King, M. A., Tucker, P., Baldwin, K., Lowry, J., LaPorta, J. & Martens, L. (2002) A life needs model of pediatric service delivery: Services to support community participation and quality of life for children and youth with disabilities, *Physical and Occupational Therapy in Pediatrics, 22*, 53–77.

Kretzmann, J. P., & McKnight, J. L. (1993). *Building communities from the inside out: A path toward finding and mobilizing a community's assets.* Skokie, IL: ACTA Publications.

Lemorie, L., & Paul, S. (2001). Professional expertise of community-based occupational therapists. *Occupational Therapy in Health Care, 13*(3/4), 33–50.

Loisel, P., Durand, M. J., Diallo, B., Vachon, B., Charpentier, N., & Labelle, J. (2003). From evidence to community practice in work rehabilitation: The Quebec experience. *Clinical Journal of Pain, 19*, 105–113.

Loukas, K. M. (2000). Emerging models of innovative community-based occupational therapy practice: The vision continues. *OT Practice.* Retrieved September 30, 2008, from http://www.aota.org/Pubs/OTP/1997-2007/Features/2000/f-071700.aspx

Lysack, C., Stadnyk, R., Krefting, L., Paterson, M., & McLeod, K. (1995). Professional expertise of occupational therapists in community practice: Results of an Ontario survey. *Canadian Journal of Occupational Therapy, 62*, 138–147.

Mandel, D., Jackson, J., Zemke, R., Nelson, L., & Clark, F. (1999). *The well-elderly study: Implementing lifestyle redesign.* Bethesda, MD: American Occupational Therapy Association.

McColl, M. A. (1998). What do we need to know to practice occupational therapy in community? *American Journal of Occupational Therapy, 52*, 60–64.

McKnight, J. (1995). *Careless society: Community and its counterfeits.* New York: Basic Books.

Merryman, M. B. (2002). Networking as an entrée to paid community practice. *OT Practice.* Retrieved September 30, 2008, from http://www.aota.org/Pubs/OTP/1997-2007/Features/2002/f-051302.aspx

Miller, B. K., & Nelson, D. (2004). Constructing a program development proposal for community-based practice: A valuable learning experience for occupational therapy students. *Occupational Therapy in Health Care, 18*, 137-150.

Mitchell, R., & Unsworth, C. A. (2004). Role perceptions and clinical reasoning of community health occupational therapists undertaking home visits. *Australian Occupational Therapy Journal, 51,* 13–24.

Mu, K., Chao, C. C., Jensen, G. M., & Royeen, C. (2004). Effects of interprofessional, rural training on students' perceptions on interprofessional health care services. *Journal of Allied Health, 33*(2), 125–131.

Munoz, J. P., Provident, I., & Hansen, A. M. (2004). Educating for community-based practice: A collaborative strategy. *Occupational Therapy in Health Care, 18*(1/2), 151–170.

Paul, S., & Peterson, C. Q. (2001). Interprofessional collaboration: Issues for practice and research. *Occupational Therapy in Health Care, 15*(3/4), 1–12.

Perrin, K., & Wittman, P. P. (2001). Educating for community-based occupational therapy practice: A demonstration project. *Occupational Therapy in Health Care, 13,* 11–21.

Scaffa, M. (Ed.). (2001). *Occupational therapy in community-based practice settings.* Philadelphia: F. A. Davis.

Scaffa, M., Desmond, S. & Brownson, C. (2001). Public health, community health and occupational therapy. In M. Scaffa (Ed.), *Occupational therapy in community-based practice settings.* Philadelphia: F. A. Davis.

Scaffa, M., Van Slyke, N., & Brownson, C. (2008). Occupational therapy in the promotion of health and the prevention of disease and disability statement. *American Journal of Occupational Therapy, 62*(6), 694-703.

Scaletti, R. (1999). A community development role for occupational therapists working with children, adolescents and their families: A mental health perspective. *Australian Occupational Therapy Journal, 46,* 43–51.

Scriven, A., & Atwal, A. (2004). Occupational therapists as primary health promoters: Opportunities and barriers. *British Journal of Occupational Therapy, 67*(10), 424–429.

Siebert, C. (2003, June). Communicating home and community expertise: The occupational therapy practice framework. *Home & Community Health Special Interest Section Quarterly,* 1–4.

Stanley, P., & Peterson, C. Q. (2002). Interprofessional collaboration: Issues for practice and research. *Occupational Therapy in Health Care, 15*(3–4), 1–12.

Suarez-Balcazar, Y. (2005). Empowerment and participatory evaluation of a community health intervention: Implications for occupational therapy. *Occupational Therapy Journal of Research, 25*(4), 1–10.

Suarez-Balcazar, Y., Hammel, J., Helfrich, C., Thomas, J., Wilson, T., & Head-Ball, D. (2005). A model of university–community partnerships for occupational therapy scholarship and practice. *Occupational Therapy in Health Care, 19*(1/2), 47–70.

Suarez-Balcazar, Y., & Harper, G. (2003).Community-based approaches to empowerment and participatory evaluation. *Journal of Prevention and Intervention in the Community, 26,* 1–4.

Voltz-Doll, J. D. (2008). Professional development: Growing as an occupational therapist. *Advance for Occupational Therapy Practitioners, 24*(5), 41–42.

Wilcock, A. (2006). *An occupational perspective on health* (2nd ed.). Thorofare, NJ: Slack.

Wittman, P. P., & Velde, B. P. (2001). Occupational therapy in the community: What, why, and how. *Occupational Therapy in Health Care, 13*(3/4), 1–5.

World Health Organization. (1998). Definition of health. Retrieved July 16, 2008, from http://www.euro.who.int/observatory/Glossary/TopPage?phrase=H

World Health Organization. (2008). Promoting health. Retrieved October 20, 2008, from http://www.who.int/healthpromotion/en/

PROCESS WORKSHEET 1-1 **WHERE DO I FIT IN COMMUNITY OCCUPATIONAL THERAPY PRACTICE?**

To consider your role in community-based practice, you can engage in a self-assessment process to facilitate your learning process. Rate yourself based on the following strengths and challenges of community practice.

Strongly Agree	Agree	Undecided	Disagree	Strongly Disagree
5	4	3	2	1

1. I value the concepts of practice in community practice.

5	4	3	2	1

2. I believe that occupational therapists have a valuable role to play in community practice.

5	4	3	2	1

3. I feel confident acting as a consultant in community practice settings.

5	4	3	2	1

4. I enjoy being able to practice using a creative, independent approach.

5	4	3	2	1

5. I have confidence in the principles of health promotion related to occupational therapy practice in the community.

5	4	3	2	1

6. I have implemented health promotion programming successfully in a community.

5	4	3	2	1

7. I enjoy building relationships with others.

5	4	3	2	1

8. I like being part of a collaborative team addressing health concerns.

5	4	3	2	1

9. I enjoy working with people from diverse backgrounds.

5	4	3	2	1

10. I enjoy planning activities for a community.

5	4	3	2	1

Continues

PROCESS WORKSHEET 1-1 **WHERE DO I FIT IN COMMUNITY OCCUPATIONAL THERAPY PRACTICE? (CONTINUED)**

Strongly Agree	Agree	Undecided	Disagree	Strongly Disagree
5	4	3	2	1

11. I prefer to play a consultant role related to occupational therapy over direct clinical practice.

5	4	3	2	1

12. I enjoy learning and applying social science theories to occupational therapy practice.

5	4	3	2	1

13. I do not mind an unpredictable practice environment or outcomes.

5	4	3	2	1

14. I am flexible when outcomes are not what are expected.

5	4	3	2	1

15. I do not mind spending time doing non-OT work.

5	4	3	2	1

Now add up your score to judge your confidence with community practice.

Total Score: _____

Please note: This activity is meant to be used as a tool to help you process your confidence in community practice and does not determine your ability to practice in community settings.

75–50: Confident Community OT

Based on your score, you are confident in the beliefs, skills, and challenges of an occupational therapy practitioner in community practice.

49–25: Developing Community OT

Based on your score, you are currently developing your beliefs and skills about community practice and are still unsure about the challenges of community practice.

24–15: Emerging Community OT

Based on your score, you are interested in community practice but need to participate in skill-building activities.

Instructions: It is important to identify your practice approach for community practice. Conduct an analysis of the two types of frameworks for community practice discussed in the chapter: community-based occupational therapy practice and community-built occupational therapy practice. By identifying the pros and cons of each model for your practice setting, you can discover approaches and strategies from the frameworks that apply to your practice setting.

Community-Based Occupational Therapy Practice

Pros	Cons

Community-Built Occupational Therapy Practice

Pros	Cons

PROCESS WORKSHEET 1-3 ADVOCACY IN COMMUNITY PRACTICE

Instructions: Based on these case examples, describe how you would engage in advocacy related to community practice.

Case 1: You have received a grant from the state government to promote healthcare services in rural areas in your state. The grant is a 3-year grant with equal funding provided all three years. You receive notice that government priorities have changed and funding will not be provided for the third year of the grant. What do you do?

_____

_____

_____

_____

_____

Case 2: You are providing health education in a program on childhood obesity. You hear from the project director that if another grant is not secured, the program will dissolve. What do you do?

_____

_____

_____

_____

_____

_____

PROCESS WORKSHEET 1-4 **PROFESSIONAL DEVELOPMENT PLAN**

Instructions: Identify strategies for enhancing the roles and responsibilities of a community occupational therapy practitioner.

Example:

Roles/Responsibilities	Strategy for Skill Development
Advocacy	• Become a member of the state association legislative committee • Participate in OT monthly activities • Identify a mentor with advocacy experience

Your turn:

Roles/Responsibilities	Strategy for Skill Development
Advocacy	
Assessment skills	
Applying occupational therapy in the community context	
Consultancy	
Education	
Health promotion planning	
Networking	
Team skills	

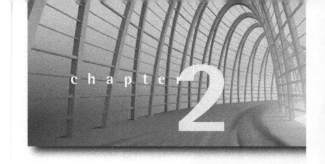

chapter 2

An Introduction to Program Development as a Foundation for Grant Writing

LEARNING OBJECTIVES

By the end of this chapter, the reader will be able to complete the following:
1. Describe program development within occupational therapy practice.
2. Analyze theoretical approaches to community-based practice in occupational therapy.
3. Distinguish different types of grants utilized in community-based program development.
4. Evaluate the role occupational therapy practitioners can play in program development and grant writing.

Key Terms

- Community assessment
- Enabling factors
- Evaluation plan
- Goal
- Impact evaluation
- Implementation plan
- Institutional review board (IRB)
- Mission statement
- Objective
- Outcome evaluation
- PRECEDE-PROCEED Model
- Predisposing factors
- Process evaluation
- Program development
- Reinforcing factors

Overview

This chapter provides an introduction to program development for occupational therapy practitioners. Grant proposals are simply a description of a program that is being proposed to address a problem or need; therefore, occupational therapy practitioners must have skills in program development to write successful grant proposals. This chapter outlines the basics of program development and how it integrates with writing grant proposals.

Introduction

Community practice is exciting because of its innovative and creative nature. Practice in community settings is challenging secondary to the many dynamics and constant change of the community context. Most community practice in occupational therapy is founded on program development models that provide a framework for consistent and solid practice. Program development and grant writing go hand in hand. Most grant proposals require the same components included in various models of program development. Therefore, prior to writing a grant proposal to support a program, occupational therapy practitioners must understand program development.

For many occupational therapy practitioners, the ability to develop a community program is innate because the process is not much different from the process used to design and implement treatment plans in traditional practice settings (Brownson, 2001). **Program development** incorporates many skills that occupational therapy practitioners already implement on a daily basis, including assessing needs, developing goals, facilitating intervention, and discharge planning. In program development, instead of focusing on the individual client, the practitioner focuses on groups or populations by applying the concepts of treatment planning to a larger context.

Program development can occur in any context of occupational therapy practice. However, program development has particular relevance to community practice and grant writing. In community settings, occupational therapy practice is focused on health promotion and education (Scaffa, 2001; Timmreck, 2003). By their nature, most community interventions focus on populations or groups of people (Edberg, 2007). Grants require a focus on developing a program that affects a problem or need among a group of people (Holtzclaw, Kenner, & Walden, 2009). All of these factors imply a relationship between program development and grant writing: Occupational therapy practitioners must have skills in program development to be successful in writing grant proposals to implement programs that are relevant and can effect changes in health behaviors in community settings.

Where Does the Occupational Therapy Practitioner Begin?

Community practice in occupational therapy begins with a program idea or recognition of a health issue that must be addressed (Fazio, 2008). Occupational therapy practitioners and community members might identify a need that represents either a gap in services or an issue that has gone unaddressed. Or perhaps the occupational therapy practitioner notices an issue while practicing in the traditional clinical setting and devises a program that can address the need in the community. For example, the practitioner may notice that many older adults are admitted to rehabilitation for hip fractures secondary to a fall. Questions begin to arise: How could occupational therapy prevent falls in older adults? What services could be

FIGURE 2–1   GRANT WRITING IS NESTED BOTH WITHIN PROGRAM DEVELOPMENT AND OCCUPATIONAL THERAPY PRACTICE.

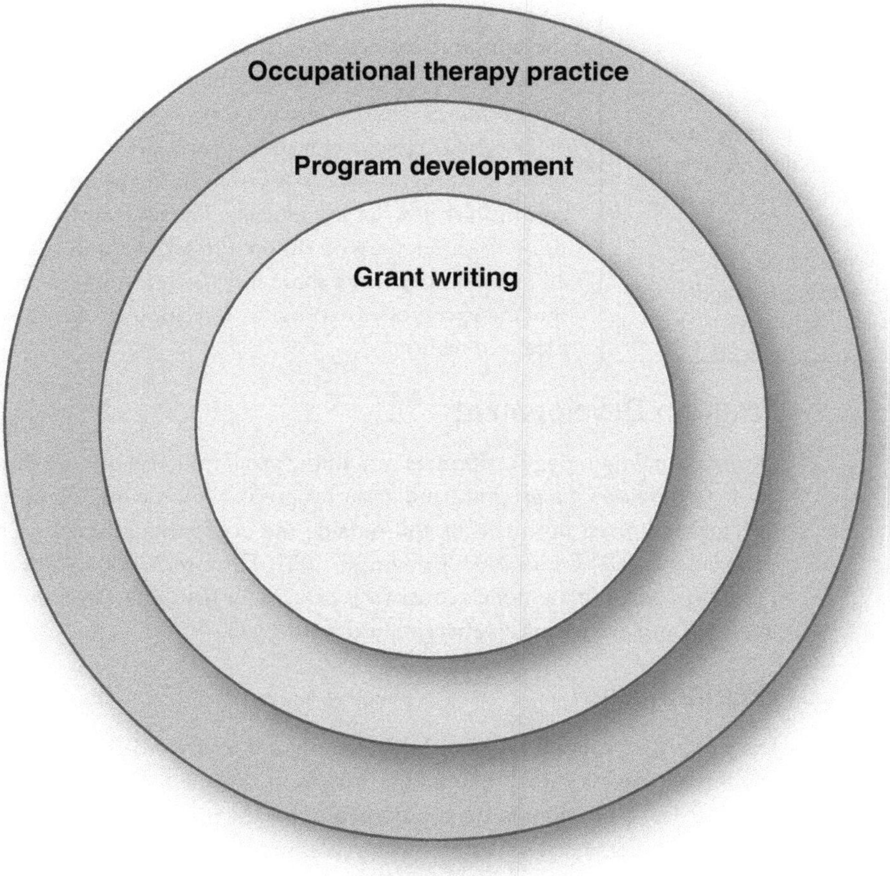

provided to help older adults prevent falls? What could an occupational therapy practitioner do here?

These questions lead the practitioner to explore the problem. What resources or programs address fall prevention in the community? How many older adults actually fall every year in the community? After discovering the staggering statistics and lack of programs addressing the problem, the occupational therapy practitioner starts to casually ask older adults how they fell and listens for the details. A trend starts to emerge in the reasons why older adults fall, and the practitioner begins to think about environmental modification and how this problem could be addressed through home safety assessments. Thus, the program idea is born.

An idea for community practice can develop as simply as in the preceding example, or it can grow from the community, which seeks an expert in occupation to facilitate healthy behavior change (Edberg, 2007). When an idea emerges like this, it leads the occupational therapy practitioner toward community practice, program development, and grant writing. Some practitioners have skills in these areas already, whereas others need to develop them.

The challenge in community practice is to translate the idea into a meaningful, successful community program. In a sense, community practice is a journey. The journey for each practitioner is different, with different obstacles and successes. Yet all journeys begin the same way, with a single step—an idea that then progresses to program development to transform the idea into reality.

> ## LET'S STOP AND THINK
>
> Think about a need or a problem you have noticed in your own community. Ask yourself the following questions: How could occupational therapy prevent this problem? What services could be provided to help address this problem? What could an occupational therapy practitioner do here?

Program Development

Occupational therapy practitioners can follow program development models as a guide to developing a program and grant proposal. Multiple models for program development exist both within and outside the occupational therapy literature (Braveman, 2001; Fazio, 2008; Brownson, 2001; Timmreck, 2003; Edberg, 2007). Program development models consist of a process for planning, developing, implementing, and evaluating an effective health program.

Preplanning

Developing a program requires organization and a forward-thinking approach, and it really begins with preplanning (Brownson, 2001; Edberg, 2007; Timmerick, 2003). Prior to developing the infrastructure for the program, occupational therapy practitioners need to engage in a preplanning process. Preplanning does not have to be complicated or detailed but should lay out the initial ideas and steps to achieve the overall program goal. It focuses on what will be accomplished through the program, resources needed, and the process required to achieve program success (Brownson, 2001).

> ### BEST PRACTICE HINT
>
> Initial preplanning does not have to be complicated or formal, but can be a simple brainstorming session about the problem or need and its impact on the community.

During preplanning, the occupational therapy practitioner evaluates the possibility and feasibility of an idea. Program development related to health promotion focuses on human behaviors and changing those behaviors for overall health and well-being of individuals and groups (Edberg, 2007). The complexity of health behaviors should be considered prior to engaging in program development. Occupational therapy practitioners need to consider the willingness of a community or group to change and the factors facilitating or impeding that change. Health behav-

TABLE 2-1 QUESTIONS TO ASK IN THE PLANNING STAGE
• What is the dominant community need(s)?
• Why should the need(s) be addressed?
• Does the community identify the proposed need(s) as important?
• Is the community ready to address the need(s)?
• What resources are required to address the need(s)?
• Who will help address the need(s)?
• What factors will impede meeting the need(s)?

TABLE 2-2 PREPLANNING STAGE EXAMPLE: FALL PREVENTION	
What is the dominant community need(s)?	• Older adults are experiencing falls, causing issues with quality of life and raising healthcare costs.
Why should the need(s) be addressed?	• Many falls may be preventable if community members are made aware.
	• Reducing falls reduces costs and increases quality of life for community members.
Does the community identify the proposed need(s) as important?	• The local older adult network has identified fall prevention as an important issue to address.
Is the community ready to address the need(s)?	• More formal assessment is needed to answer this question.
What resources are needed to address the need(s)?	• Funding
	• Programs to address the risk factors
	• Education of community members
Who will help address the need(s)?	• An interprofessional team including occupational therapy can address the need.
What factors will impede meeting the need(s)?	• Lack of buy-in by community members
	• Lack of funding

iors are influenced by individual factors, sociocultural factors, socioeconomic factors, political factors, and environmental factors (Edberg, 2007). People constantly interact with all of these aspects, which affect health choices and behaviors.

Developing a program is an intense and lofty process, and the occupational therapy practitioner should take time to thoroughly identify the issue or need that the program will address and consider the factors that will help the program be successful or that will be constant challenges. Worksheets at the end of this chapter can assist with initial program planning.

The Steps to Program Development

Program development is the vehicle for community practice in occupational therapy (Brownson, 2001). Program development includes planning, development of an intervention, and evaluation (Brownson, 2001). It is the "systematic efforts to achieve preplanned objectives such as changes in knowledge, attitudes, skills, and behaviors to maintain or improve function and/or health" (Brownson, 2001, p. 96).

This section discusses two models for program development to provide occupational therapy practitioners a foundation from which to understand program development from multiple perspectives. The first program development model was created by Grossman and Bortone (1986) and applied by Brent Braveman (2001) to occupational therapy practice in community settings. The second program development model is the PRECEDE-PROCEED Model, which is one of the best-known models in program development and can easily be applied in occupational therapy community practice.

Models of Program Development

Braveman (2001) applied the program development model developed by Grossman and Bortone (1986) to occupational therapy in community practice. This model includes four basic steps: (1) needs assessment, (2) program planning, (3) program implementation, and (4) program evaluation.

Needs Assessment

A needs assessment is simply an assessment of needs. In a clinical setting, occupational therapists conduct needs assessments on individual clients every day using the evaluation process. According to the Occupational Therapy Practice Framework (OTPF) (AOTA, 2008), evaluation focuses on "finding out what the client wants and needs to do, determining what the client can do and has done, and identifying those factors that act as supports or barriers to health and participation" (p. 649).

In a needs assessment for a group or community, the concept of the evaluation process is the same as stated earlier except that it has a broader focus. Regarding community needs assessment, the preceding OTPF statement would be reworded to state that evaluation focuses on finding out what the community or group wants and needs to do, determining what the community or group can do and has done, and identifying those factors that act as supports or barriers to health and participation.

According to Brownson (2001), a needs assessment is a "systematic set of procedures that serves to identify and describe specific areas of need and available resources in a given population" (p. 101). Needs assessments explore gaps in services and should also focus on exploration of resources that exist within a community (Timmreck, 2003). The purpose of a needs assessment is to gather information that will support the program and assist in establishing program goals (Brownson, 2001). Needs assessments can be done both formally and informally and are an essential component of the program development process (Timmreck, 2003).

In traditional practice settings, assessments are completed through chart reviews, patient interviews, and the initial evaluation process. In a **community assessment**, the occupational therapy practitioner explores the needs of the community related to health and wellness. Data and health statistics make a case for the importance of the program, and in grant funding they help the grant writer justify why the program is important enough to fund. Data collected in a needs assessment paint the picture of the community and build a foundation on which a program to address the identified needs can be built.

A needs assessment for a community includes demographic data and epidemiological data on the general health status of the community and its members. Data of this nature focus on both health and social indicators (Timmreck, 2003). Demographic data include information such as the average age of community members, gender, race, and socioeconomic status. Epidemiological data include health trends in a community. For example, if an occupational therapy practitioner plans to develop a program for fall prevention for older adults, the practitioner would collect data related to trends in falls such as the incidence and prevalence of falls, the impact of falls (for example, number of hospitalizations), and the social repercussions of falls (for example, anxiety felt by older adults, costs incurred by the healthcare industry secondary to falls, etc.).

Demographic and epidemiological data related to a community are not difficult to find. The Office of Minority Health, a division of the Department of Health and Human Services, provides information on national health trends among racial and ethnic groups. Practitioners can explore local and state health departments for health and social data. This information is usually readily available on health department websites. Sometimes community agencies have such data on file. Many nonprofits publish annual reports that include this sort of information about the population they serve.

BEST PRACTICE HINT

Ask local public health experts at the local health department or university to help you gather epidemiological data and health statistics.

If no accurate demographic or epidemiological information on the community exists, occupational therapy practitioners need to develop their own method for assessing needs, such as conducting surveys or interviews (Brownson, 2001; Timmreck, 2003). In most cases, grant proposals and program development will not require extensive surveys and the development of simple survey tools is adequate. However, extensive experience in research and a background in public health are most likely needed to gather conclusive epidemiological data. Consulting a public healthcare provider may prove beneficial in this case. Creative approaches and exploring local resources can facilitate this process. One strategy is to seek students in a public health program to assist in the needs assessment. Many students are required to conduct community projects to practice assessment skills.

Requests for proposals (RFPs) for a grant may require a needs assessment to be conducted as part of the program. RFPs may be very specific about what information to include in the needs assessment. In such cases, the grant writer must follow the grant guidelines and assess what is required. Most grants allow existing data to be used, but some may have specific guidelines for data use, such as specifying sources. Some aspects of needs assessments are outside of the model outlined by Grossman and Bortone (1986). A community assessment should focus on needs, strengths, and capacity of the community (Brownson, 2001). Assessing for capacity is very important in community practice to address chronic health issues and community health issues. In underserved communities where needs are high, a program must focus on community strengths to provide a basis for the program. For example, a community may hold strong cultural beliefs and be very collective when someone is ill. This is a strength that can be a great foundation for a community program for dealing with chronic illness. Programs based on cultural nuances will be more successful than those that neglect the community's culture. Because community needs assessments do not focus only on needs, hereafter needs assessments are referred to as community assessments.

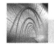

BEST PRACTICE HINT

Collect multiple types of data and information to help the grant writer tell the "story" of the community and its needs and capacities. A community assessment that includes multiple types of data can enhance any grant proposal.

Community assessments should include quantitative health data as well as the lived experience of the community collected using qualitative data methods. Strategies for collecting these data include case studies, interviews of community members, and focus groups of community members (Brownson, 2001; Timmreck, 2003). Including narrative in the executive report of the community assessment ties the story and lived experience to the assessment results. This information can be crucial when seeking outside funding or reporting to external funders. Furthermore, these data tell a story that can be useful for multiple reasons, including advocacy and raising funds from private donors.

The results of any type of assessment, whether quantitative or qualitative in nature, should be shared with the community. Practitioners can draft an executive report of these data and then share it with community members. When conducting any kind of data collection or analysis in a community, occupational therapy practitioners should recognize that the community owns the data and the data should be shared with the community for their benefit and use.

Prior to conducting any sort of community assessment, occupational therapy practitioners need to contact the local **institutional review board (IRB)** when applicable. An IRB is a panel of professionals and lay people that examines the safety of research conducted in clinical and community settings (Holtzclaw, Kenner, & Walden, 2009). Usually, academic institutions and hospitals have IRBs. Sometimes community organizations have IRBs that review local research projects. Individuals on the IRB are trained in research methods and the ethics of research. Approval from the IRB is not necessary if the data being collected derive from existing sources, for example, census data. Occupational therapy practitioners who plan on developing a survey or holding focus groups should seek IRB approval.

Community assessments are key to the success of community programs. Community assessments should be conducted to gather the community's perspective on needs and strengths. As the program begins to take shape, practitioners should refer back to the community assessment results to stay on track and develop a program that matches the community needs.

Program Planning

The program planning piece of the Grossman and Bortone (1986) model outlines multiple components including defining a focus, adopting a theoretical perspective, establishing goals and objectives, and developing referrals. This section discusses each component and applies it to community occupational therapy practice.

After the community assessment is complete, program development enters the planning stage. Planning the program should never be an isolated process; collaboration with the community is essential (Edberg, 2007). The occupational therapy practitioner needs time to draft or brainstorm ideas related to occupation but should always work with community members to ensure that these ideas mesh with community members' ideas. This activity aligns with Grossman and Bortone's (1986) first step of "defining a focus," which includes the prioritization of ideas. The community assessment will reveal a pattern of needs and provide the opportunity to identify which needs are priorities to the community.

Programs must have a focus to target and address community needs appropriately. A program should not attempt to be the answer to everything for everyone. Programs that attempt to address too much can confuse community members and strain program implementers. Programs that fail to address needs as promised can be damaging and promote distrust by community members (Kretzmann & McKnight, 1997).

As in traditional clinical practice, occupational therapy practitioners in community practice need to identify a frame of reference to guide their practice, the second task in Grossman and Bortone's (1986) program planning process. The frame of reference does not necessarily have to come from the

BEST PRACTICE HINT

If a program idea is in development, run the idea by community members to get a feel for buy-in and interest. This can be done formally through focus groups or town hall meetings or informally through networking.

field of occupational therapy. As discussed in Chapter 1, community-based practice and community-built practice provide frameworks for community practice, but many other theoretical frameworks based on community work in other disciplines can also guide occupational therapy practice. See Chapter 1 for a list of frames of references that can apply to community practice.

Adopting a frame of reference is not only important to program development and sound practice but also to grant writing. Many RFPs require a strong background and justification for a program. A strong frame of reference can assist in building a program's case. Some grantors require potential grantees to identify the frame of reference that guides the program and provide literature to support the use of the chosen frame of reference.

Grossman and Bortone (1986) recommend developing goals and objectives as the third part of the planning process in program development. Goals and objectives are necessary, and practitioners might find benefit in also developing a mission statement and vision statement as part of the planning process.

Companies and organizations use mission statements to guide employees in an overall plan and to make consumers aware of the purpose of the company. Yet the concept of a mission statement goes beyond simply educating workers and consumers and acts as the driving force or motivation behind decisions, actions, and the development of the entity. A **mission statement** is a written statement that "contains detailed information about the overall direction and purpose of the organization" (Timmreck, 2003, p. 31). Mission statements are not the same as goals because mission statements are not necessarily quantifiable (Timmreck, 2003).

> ### LET'S STOP AND THINK
>
> Identify some frames of reference discussed in Chapter 1 that might apply to one of your ideas for community program development.

Mission statements align with the concept of occupation, which is defined as "goal-directed pursuits that typically extend over time, have meaning to the performance, and involve multiple tasks" (Christiansen et al., 2005, p. 548). To create a mission statement, practitioners must focus on personal values, personal motivation, and what makes people get out of bed every day.

Mission statements are meant to embody the following:

- Purpose
- Personal values
- Future direction

Mission statements should also represent values of the program or organization (Timmreck, 2003). **Process Worksheet 2-4** at the end of this chapter provides assistance in developing and evaluating a mission statement.

Occupational therapy practitioners are familiar with goal and objective writing related to client treatment planning, but writing goals and objectives for a program can pose a challenge. Instead of focusing on the patient or client, in program development the goals and objectives are based on the program and the proposed out-

TABLE 2-3 DEVELOPING A MISSION STATEMENT	
Do some research.	Find mission statements of organizations that you admire or that you think are easy to understand.
Avoid emptiness.	Write a mission statement that encompasses personal and professional values. You should feel passionate about your mission, and that passion should be articulated to others through the mission statement.
Keep it short.	Mission statements should be brief snapshots to give others some insight into the purpose of the organization or program.
Write well.	Mission statements should be free of grammatical and syntax errors. These small issues can distract readers from understanding the mission. Write the mission statement in a clear and concise manner to make it easy to grasp.
Ask others.	Seek advice and feedback on the mission statement from peers and community members.
Do not settle.	A mission statement can be revised as the program evolves. Eventually, settle on a mission statement for sustainability.
Represent the program.	Ensure that the mission statement represents the services the program will provide.

Source: Voltz-Doll, J. D. (2008). Professional development: Growing as an occupational therapist. *Advance for Occupational Therapy Practitioners, 24*(5), 41–42.

comes of the program. In program development, a **goal** is defined as "a statement of a quantifiable desired future state or condition" (Timmreck, 2003). Goals are long term and future oriented (Brownson, 2001). **Objectives** facilitate goals being met and are measurable, short term, and usually contain a timeline for completion (Brownson, 2001; Timmreck, 2003). Goals and objectives are different but complement one another. Goals focus on general outcomes whereas objectives are specific and targeted toward the general goal. Goals do not have to be measurable but must indicate a tangible outcome.

Goals and objectives should plan for the following: program priorities, program outcomes, community priorities, and the evaluation plan. All goals and objectives should be related to the priorities of the program and tie in with all aspects of the program or grant. A program may have many outcomes, but it should have a defined focus and the outcomes of the program should be prioritized. Too many goals and objectives can make a program appear incoherent and disconnected and pose challenges to successful completion. Goals and objectives need to be outcomes based and measurable because this is crucial for evaluation and demonstrating the value of the program.

Goals and objectives should also be developed with the targeted population in mind and should be community-centered. They should align with community needs and wants to ensure that they can be successfully met. This concept follows the occupational therapy principle of client-centered practice applied to a program model (Brownson, 2001). Goals and objectives in a community-centered model facilitate community buy-in and program success.

BEST PRACTICE HINT

A typical grant proposal should have no more than three to five goals to be effective.

Practitioners can write program objectives using a variety of approaches, but all program objectives should contain the following three components:

- Behavioral statement
- Measurement of performance
- Condition statement

Another approach to drafting program objectives is the ABCD approach, as shown in **Table 2-4**.

Well-written objectives can also follow the rubric of SMART:

S = Specific
M = Measurable
A = Attainable
R = Relevant
T = Timely

All of these approaches provide frameworks for drafting program objectives that are measurable and relevant.

BEST PRACTICE HINT

Multiple approaches to writing goals exist. Choose the approach that fits best with the program you are developing and the grant proposal requirements.

Program goals and objectives need to be clear, concise, and accomplishable in an adequate time frame (Timmreck, 2003). This is especially true when developing a program in congruence with a grant proposal. Multiple individuals read grant proposals, and each individual needs to understand the program goals and objectives to buy in and support it.

Another essential component of program planning is to identify programmatic roles. In the planning stage, who will fill program roles and accomplish responsibilities need not be identified in detail, but practitioners should consider the potential roles and responsibilities required to make the program a success. Timelines and collaboration should also be discussed and preliminarily identified.

The next step in program planning is to establish referrals (Braveman, 2001; Grossman & Bortone, 1986). A key aspect of successful program implementation

FIGURE 2-2   PROGRAM OBJECTIVE

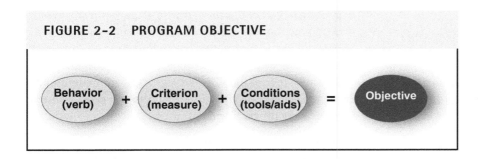

TABLE 2-4 COMPONENTS OF A LEARNING OBJECTIVE: THE ABCD MODEL

A = Audience	Who is the learner?
	Required for each learning objective
B = Behavior	Action verb
	Should follow hierarchical development (Bloom's Taxonomy)
C = Condition	Qualifier of the objective
D = Degree	Indicates acceptable level of achievement

is the recruitment of participants to the program. Obviously, without individuals using the program, the program will fail; therefore, participant recruitment and retention must be considered in the planning process. Practitioners must develop protocols and roles for each person involved in the program (Braveman, 2001). They outline how people will come to use or benefit from the program. When the program provides a service, the referral process identifies how people will be recruited to the program. Requirements or stipulations for admission to the program must be identified.

In some cases, this step may require developing a marketing plan to identify methods of recruitment. The marketing plan may be referred to as a community awareness campaign depending on the program and target audience. Whatever the title, practitioners need to consider the marketing of services during the planning stage. They should consider all necessary venues and use community resources such as partners, advisory boards, coalitions, and community members or participants. The marketing plan should take into account the services being provided, who will benefit from these services, and who needs to know about the services (Braveman, 2001). For example, a nonprofit that offers a health equipment recycling program provides used health equipment to individuals in need. The main

BEST PRACTICE HINT

If you are uncomfortable or unsure about marketing, find marketing experts or students in marketing to aid in the marketing process.

marketing targets of this program are social workers, physical therapy practitioners, and occupational therapy practitioners. These individuals refer many clients who cannot receive health equipment through insurance and can be a successful target audience for the program. Marketing and creating community awareness should be thoughtful processes because without customers the program will not succeed.

Program Implementation

When all the components of the program are planned out and fully designed, implementation can finally take place (Timmreck, 2003). At this point in program development, the program services are offered to those in need and the program will continue to grow and change.

Occupational therapy practitioners should develop an implementation plan to identify specifically how implementation will occur. According to Brownson (2001), an **implementation plan** "spells out the details of the program and specifies who is responsible for each procedure and activity" (p. 115). The details of who, what, when, where, and how for the program need to be finalized in the implementation plan (Brownson, 2001). As mentioned earlier, during the planning stages, specific individuals might not yet be in place, but when it is time for implementation, all staff should be identified and assigned clear roles and responsibilities.

Program implementation must be planned to stay on track and ensure that activities are completed (Timmreck, 2003). Many organizations now use strategic planning for program implementation. Strategic planning is a common method, and the program can hire facilitators with expertise in strategic planning to assist with the process.

Implementation planning should be completed in a group environment to promote communication among team members, especially if the program or project is new. Implementation planning provides an opportunity to clarify who will do what and when it will be done. Creating a document that outlines program activities ensures that all team members stay on track, communication flows smoothly, and the program goals and objectives are completed in an efficient manner. Implementation planning also allows the program team to plan and anticipate challenges in a proactive manner, which can affect program success (Timmreck, 2003).

Most grants require an implementation plan; however, implementation plans should not be limited to include only activities funded by a grant, especially if the program reaches outside the grant funding. The grant RFP will outline the requirements of the implementation plan. If one is not required, practitioners should still develop an implementation plan to ensure that program implementation goes smoothly and team members are informed about all activities and timelines.

Program Evaluation

All programs require an **evaluation plan**. Evaluation plans measure the effectiveness of a program (Brownson, 2001; Grossman & Bortone, 1986; Braveman, 2001). In an evaluation plan, practitioners must consider the design being used and the data to be collected. Evaluation plans demonstrate the outcomes of the program and should be designed to target the program's outcomes. Evaluation plans also help the program team be aware of their progress and the impact of the program. With this information, the team can modify processes if goals and objectives are not reached appropriately or in a timely manner.

Evaluation planning should be done consistently and should occur throughout the life of a program. Evaluation plans should not be used only when a grant proposal requires one because they are valuable in all programs and are truly necessary to implement an effective and thorough program. Evaluation planning will be discussed in detail in Chapter 10.

The PRECEDE-PROCEED Model

The **PRECEDE-PROCEED Model** is an approach to program development that entails both "a process of assessment and planning before putting a program in place (PRECEDE), followed by implementation and evaluation of the program (PROCEED)" (Edberg, 2007, p. 80). The model follows an ecological approach and comprehensively provides a structured framework for program development and implementation (Green & Kreuter, 1999). The purpose of the model is to help practitioners understand the complexity of a health problem and to focus on addressing the targeted need. The model is community focused.

The PRECEDE-PROCEED Model occurs in phases, moving from a broad focus to a narrow focus. The following subsections discuss each phase of the model and apply it to occupational therapy community practice.

Phase 1: Social Assessment and Situational Analysis

The purpose of the social assessment and situational analysis phase is to identify the community need or problem. In this phase, practitioners explore quality-of-life and social factors that affect health in a community. Practitioners can collect this information in multiple ways including talking to community leaders, arranging focus groups, exploring public health data, and mapping assets (Spence, 2002).

For example, in a community-based fall prevention program for older adults, in this phase, the practitioner would talk to older adults about how their lives have been affected by falls. The practitioner would see the impact on quality of life and the negative consequences of older adults not being able to age in place.

LET'S STOP AND THINK
Brainstorm ways in which you could engage in social assessment and situational analysis in a community occupational therapy role.

Phase 2: Epidemiologic Assessment

The epidemiologic assessment phase focuses on the extent of the health problem in the community. In this phase, practitioners explore who is affected by the health condition, how extensively the health condition permeates the community, and what trends surround the health condition (Edberg, 2007). Types of epidemiologic data collected during this phase include prevalence, incidence, and mortality rates. Practitioners can pull data from reliable sources such as the National Center for Health Statistics and the Centers for Disease Control and Prevention.

In the fall prevention program example, in this phase, the occupational therapy practitioner begins to explore the number of falls in older adults as reported by the Centers for Disease Control and Prevention and tries to gauge the prevalence of the problem. Other epidemiologic data such as healthcare costs and impact on perceived quality of life could also be explored here.

Phase 3: Behavioral and Environmental Assessment

In the behavioral and environmental assessment phase, practitioners identify risk factors related to behavior and environment. Behavioral risk factors relate specifically to people whereas environmental risk factors relate to external conditions.

At this stage, the occupational therapy practitioner in the example identifies which behaviors including judgment and decision making of older adults increase their falls. The practitioner would also identify the causes of falls such as throw rugs or improper assistive device use.

Phase 4: Educational and Ecological Assessment

The educational and ecological assessment explores which approaches can be used to effect behavioral change. Green and Kreuter (1999) identify several approaches to use in this phase including analysis of predisposing factors, enabling factors, and reinforcing factors. **Predisposing factors** are a group's knowledge, attitudes, beliefs, values, and perceptions. **Enabling factors** are the skills, resources, and barriers that either facilitate or inhibit a behavior. **Reinforcing factors** are the rewards people receive for engaging in a particular behavior.

During this phase, the occupational therapy practitioner conducts a focus group with older adults who have experienced a recent fall to explore their beliefs about why they have fallen, the value of aging in place, and the impact of the fear of falling. The practitioner also identifies issues of accessibility as a barrier to fall prevention and discusses quality of life for those who are able to prevent a fall.

Phase 5: Administrative and Policy Assessment

The administrative and policy assessment explores the support and infrastructure required to make the program a success. Supports and infrastructure include funding, established policies and procedures, and community involvement. During this phase, the focus is on the budget, space, timeline, and personnel. This phase is very practical and detailed.

In the example, the occupational therapy practitioner decides to develop a program around fall prevention through home safety modification and universal design. The practitioner begins to draft a program budget, explore reimbursement, develop policies and procedures, and find office space.

Phase 6: Implementation

In the implementation phase, the program is ready to implement with everything in place to make the program a success.

The occupational therapy practitioner begins working with older adult clients on home modification and developing spaces following universal design principles.

Phases 7–9: Evaluation

Phases 7 through 9 are grouped together because they all focus on program evaluation. Phase 7 focuses on **process evaluation**, which identifies whether the program was implemented as planned, goals were met, and the need was addressed. In other words, this phase looks at the quality of the program and whether the program meets established goals. Phase 8 focuses on **impact evaluation**, which explores the short-term impact or changes made by the program. Examples include changes in knowledge about a particular health topic. Phase 9 focuses on **outcome evaluation**, which explores the long-term impact of the program by identifying behavioral change, improved quality of life, and impact on the community need.

In these phases, the occupational therapy practitioner implements the evaluation plan for the fall prevention program, exploring how many people have been served, assessing knowledge about falls in older adults, and identifying whether falls have decreased secondary to the interventions.

The PRECEDE-PROCEED Model provides a comprehensive ecological approach to program development that occupational therapy practitioners can use in community practice settings to develop an efficient and effective health program. The model identifies specific phases for both development and implementation of a program.

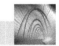

BEST PRACTICE HINT

Choose a program development model to follow, especially as a novice, to aid in ensuring that all the steps for developing a successful program are included.

Program Development and Grant Writing

As previously mentioned, program development and grant writing cannot be separated. Although grant proposals do not require all the components of program development, they include some. Therefore, these two processes integrate nicely, and learning one can aid in learning the other. In community practice, program development and grant writing are key skills required of occupational therapy practitioners. Rarely are community programs fully supported without external funding. Even if occupational therapy practitioners do not have to write grant proposals to support services, they undoubtedly will be part of the grant writing process by compiling data for a needs assessment or engaging in part of the evaluation process. Therefore, community practitioners must be informed about the grant process and act as an asset to a program or project in the community. Understanding both program development and grant writing can lay a foundation for community practice and beyond.

Conclusion

It is essential to remember that a grant proposal is the description of a community program and that program development principles are used to draft the grant proposal. By following the approaches to program development described in this chapter, practitioners can implement comprehensive community-centered programs that meet community needs and build on community capacity. Occupational therapy practitioners working in community settings can use their program development skills to draft successful grant proposals to support community practice.

Glossary

Community assessment (needs assessment) Finding out what the community or group wants and needs to do, determining what the community or group can do and has done, and identifying those factors that act as supports or barriers to health and participation

Enabling factors The skills, resources, and barriers that either facilitate or inhibit a behavior

Evaluation plan A plan to measure the effectiveness of a program

Goal "A statement of a quantifiable desired future state or condition" (Timmreck, 2003)

Impact evaluation Explores the short-term impact or changes made by the program

Implementation plan A plan that "spells out the details of the program and specifies who is responsible for each procedure and activity" (Brownson, 2001, p. 115)

Institutional review board (IRB) A panel of professionals and lay people who examine the safety of research being conducted both in clinical and community settings

Mission statement A written statement that "contains detailed information about the overall direction and purpose of the organization" (Timmreck, 2003, p. 31)

Objective An action or plan that facilitates goals being met and that is measurable, short term, and usually contains a timeline for completion

Outcome evaluation Explores the long-term impact of the program to identify behavior change, improved quality of life, and impact on the community need

PRECEDE-PROCEED Model An approach to program development that entails both "a process of assessment and planning before putting a program in place (PRECEDE), followed by implementation and evaluation of the program (PROCEED)" (Edberg, 2007, p. 80)

Predisposing factors A group's knowledge, attitudes, beliefs, values, and perceptions

Process evaluation Identifies whether the program was implemented as planned, goals were met, and the need was addressed

Program development Development of a program to meet or address a need or problem

Reinforcing factors The rewards people receive for engaging in a particular behavior

References

American Occupational Therapy Association. (2008). Occupational therapy practice framework: Domain and process, 2nd edition. *American Journal of Occupational Therapy, 62*(6), 625–683.

Braveman, B. (2001). Development of a community-based return to work program for people living with AIDS. *Occupational Therapy in Health Care, 13*(3–4), 113–131.

Brownson, C. A. (2001). Program development: Planning, implementation, and evaluation strategies. In M. Scaffa (Ed.), *Occupational therapy in community-based practice settings.* Philadelphia: F. A. Davis.

Edberg, M. (2007). *Essentials of health behavior: Social and behavior health in public health.* Sudbury, MA: Jones and Bartlett.

Fazio, L. (2008). *Developing occupation-centered programs for the community* (2nd ed.). Upper Saddle River, NJ: Prentice Hall.

Green, L. W., & Kreuter, M. W. (1999). *Health promotion planning: An educational and environmental approach* (3rd ed.). Mountain View, CA: Mayfield.

Grossman, J., & Bortone, J. (1986). Program development. In S. C. Robertson (Ed.), *Strategies, concepts, and opportunities for program development and evaluation* (pp. 91–99). Bethesda, MD: American Occupational Therapy Association.

Holtzclaw, B. J., Kenner, C., & Walden, M. (2009). *Grant writing handbook for nurses* (2nd ed.). Sudbury, MA: Jones and Bartlett.

Kretzmann, J. P., & McKnight, J. L. (1993). *Building communities from the inside out: A path toward finding and mobilizing a community's assets.* Skokie, IL: ACTA Publications.

Scaffa, M. (Ed.). (2001). *Occupational therapy in community-based practice settings.* Philadelphia: F. A. Davis.

Spence. C. (2002). Program development. Retrieved October 8, 2008, from http://oisse.creighton.edu/Learning%20Tools.aspx

Timmreck, T. C. (2003). *Planning, program development and evaluation* (2nd ed.). Sudbury, MA: Jones and Bartlett.

Voltz-Doll, J. D. (2008). Professional development: Growing as an occupational therapist. *Advance for Occupational Therapy Practitioners, 24*(5), 41–42.

PROCESS WORKSHEET 2-1 **PROGRAM PREPLANNING**

Instructions: Identify a community need and analyze its potential for program development.

Community Need: _____

What is the dominant community need(s)?	
Why should the need(s) be addressed?	
Does the community identify the proposed need(s) as important?	
Is the community ready to address the need(s)?	
What resources are needed to address the need(s)?	
Who will help address the need(s)?	
What factors will impede meeting the need(s)?	

PROCESS WORKSHEET 2-2 **PLANNING FOR THE PROGRAM**

Instructions: Prior to initiating formal program development, the occupational therapy practitioner must do some initial planning. This worksheet serves as tool for that planning process.

In each area, brainstorm what resources are needed to lead to the success of the program.

Area of Need	Resources Needed
Staff/Collaborators	
Funding	
Time	
Space/Facilities	
Experts/Consultants	
Advertising/Marketing	
Stakeholders	

PROCESS WORKSHEET 2-3 **EVALUATING HEALTH BEHAVIORS**

Instructions: Identify the health behavior to be addressed by the program idea brainstormed in Process Worksheet 2-1. Evaluate the factors affecting this health behavior. For each factor, identify how it affects the community or group for whom the program would be implemented. These factors demonstrate what will facilitate or inhibit health behavior change.

Factor	Community Profile
Health knowledge	
Biological factors (for example, genetics)	
Family structure	
Culture	
Social supports	
Socioeconomic status	
Education level	
Healthcare access	
Social stressors	
Health coverage	
Community health practices	
Environmental conditions	
Transportation	
Other: _____	
Other: _____	

PROCESS WORKSHEET 2-4 **EVALUATING THE MISSION STATEMENT**

After drafting the mission statement, step back and evaluate it. This worksheet will aid in the review process.

A mission statement should represent values of the program or organization. Analyze your mission statement using the following questions.

1. What core values does the mission statement represent?

2. Are these core values evident in the mission statement?

3. What future direction does this mission statement indicate for the program?

4. Do I feel inspired by this mission statement? Why or why not?

5. Other thoughts or comments:

PROCESS WORKSHEET 2-5 DEVELOPING A MARKETING PLAN

Instructions: Complete the worksheet to develop a marketing plan for the program or project.

What services will the organization provide?	Who will be served (i.e., who will benefit from the services)?	Who needs to know about the services (i.e., who will refer to the program)?

Once you determine the above, move on to this section:

What is the basic message that you would like to send to this market in regard to your service?	What is the best way of contacting your projected market (i.e., media, print, collab-oration, community partners, etc.)?	Identify chosen methods along with who will complete them and the date for completion.

PROCESS WORKSHEET 2-6 **PROGRAM IMPLEMENTATION PLAN**

Instructions: Complete the following table to develop a program implementation plan.

Goal	Objectives	Activities	Team Member	Timeline

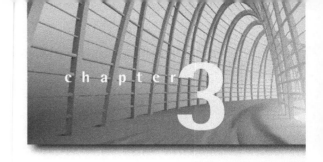

chapter 3

Bringing an Idea to Life: Foundations for Program Development and Grant Writing

LEARNING OBJECTIVES

By the end of this chapter, the reader will be able to complete the following:

1. Differentiate the roles of occupational therapy practitioners in community programs.
2. Brainstorm program ideas.
3. Analyze program ideas to explore the pros and cons of their implementation.

Key Terms

Administrator
Brainstorming
Consultant
Educator
Researcher
Strategic planning
SWOT analysis
Team

Overview

This chapter discusses how to bring an idea forth to examine its relevance for developing a program. This chapter also discusses team building and the role of the occupational therapy practitioner in program development and grant writing. Different models and approaches for developing a grant-funded program are introduced. All of these topics lay a foundation for developing relevant community programming.

Introduction

Occupational therapy (OT) practitioners are problem solvers. Daily, OT practitioners work in collaboration with clients to identify solutions to help clients complete activities of daily living despite their disabilities and functional challenges. Occupational therapy practitioners must be creative and recognize that the answer to one person's dilemma will not be the same for the next person. These skills transfer nicely to program development (Fazio, 2008). Often, for occupational therapy practitioners, program development is an attempt to tackle and solve an issue that affects a subset of the population. The purpose of programs is to put systems in place that address a health issue that affects many and that can be addressed collectively (Timmreck, 2003).

All programs and grant proposals begin with an idea—an idea that provides a potential solution to a community health issue. OT practitioners in community practice act as agents of change by developing programs that address needs and facilitate community members' engagement in healthy occupations, which can transform a community (Fazio, 2008). Program development is a key component of grant writing and community program development; the two are complementary and they share many of the same components. For example, in grant proposals grant writers outline many of the concepts and steps used in program development. Grant proposals should never drive program development, however, because programs should be based on community needs (Edberg, 2007; Fazio, 2008). Yet, a grant proposal cannot be written without program development.

In this chapter, the process of developing a program and writing a grant are discussed as well as the roles occupational therapy practitioners can play in community programs. Community programs require a collaborative approach and are never developed in isolation (Fazio, 2008). Before program development is begun, an idea needs to be formulated and planned. After the idea has been formalized, the team assisting with program development and implementation needs to be identified and recruited. Then, the program team must specify which model they will use to draft the grant proposal that will support the program. Each aspect of this process is discussed in this chapter.

Beginning with an Idea

Ideas are generated in many different ways. Occupational therapy practitioners and community members must dare to dream because an idea can transform into a program and be successful in facilitating positive change (Edberg, 2007). Needs are easy to identify, but creating solutions to address a health issue can be more challenging. More efficient methods to address needs may exist and can be implemented in a successful program (Fazio, 2008).

OT practitioners might recognize the importance of a program idea in conversation with others or by recognizing trends in the community (Fazio, 2008). Practitioners must move beyond simple discussion to identify how an idea can be transformed into a meaningful program. Formulating an idea is really one of the first steps to formulating a program, and many of the strategies discussed in this section can be used to develop the program and a grant proposal as well.

> ### TABLE 3-1 TIPS FOR BRAINSTORMING
>
> - Gather a group of 8 to12 people.
> - The brainstorming team should be diverse to gather diverse ideas.
> - A relaxed environment promotes easy generation of ideas.
> - The leader should define the problem.
> - A visual approach helps group members follow the brainstorming session (i.e., writing down ideas in front of the group where all can visualize).
> - Hold to a time limit (recommended is 25–30 minutes).
> - Hold to an idea limit (i.e., identify how many ideas the group wants).
> - Identify five key ideas from the brainstorm.
> - All ideas should be accepted with no criticism by other group members.
> - Identify top ideas with a scoring system.
>
> *Source:* Baumgartner, J. (2003). *The step by step guide to brainstorming.* Retrieved November 24, 2008, from http://www.jpb.com/creative/brainstorming.php

Brainstorming

Brainstorming is a key strategy for formulating a program idea (Bond, Belensky, & Weinstock, 2000). Practitioners can brainstorm to generate ideas and then brainstorm to determine a way to implement the ideas (Baumgartner, 2003). Brainstorming can be done either formally or informally. In more formal brainstorming, one individual may act as a facilitator who helps direct the session and assists the group in formalizing ideas (Baumgartner, 2006). In some cases, brainstorming occurs as a natural part of a discussion among peers or community members (Fazio, 2008). Bringing community members and professionals together to help develop an idea is also likely to enhance the idea's effectiveness as a program.

LET'S STOP AND THINK
Get into a small group. Think of a community that is meaningful to the group and a need that could be addressed in this community. Use brainstorming techniques to identify ideas for addressing the community need.

Another approach is to bring an idea forth to a group of community members for feedback and discussion. Brainstorming can occur in such a group. This approach ensures that the idea is not a response to a problem only the practitioner sees but one that the whole community can embrace. Collective interest is essential for a program to be successful. As an idea develops, a brainstorming or discussion session with community members and colleagues can help formulate the idea into a feasible program (Falk, 2006). This process can also begin to identify important aspects of the program such as time, space, and resources needed.

BEST PRACTICE HINT

Brainstorming can occur with multiple groups, including other healthcare professionals and community members, to get different ideas. Each population brings a unique perspective and ideas to the brainstorming process.

BEST PRACTICE HINT

Strategic planning is useful not only when beginning a program but should be used for ongoing program planning and implementation.

Strategic Planning

Another approach that brings ideas forth is **strategic planning**. For community programs, strategic planning can also occur when a program is already established and the program team wants to explore its future. It can be a formalized way to identify how an idea can be accomplished. Strategic planning aids an organization in defining its direction for a specified amount of time into the future by identifying strategies for attaining the identified goals (McNamara, 2008).

In some situations, communities already have organized efforts or programs ready to address new issues, and these can act as a foundation for strategic planning. A strategic plan includes the priorities of the team, measurable goals, and a timeline for completion of activities, and it should be easy for all team members to understand. The plan should be flexible and should evolve with the team (Foundation for Community Association Research, 2001).

Strategic planning not only identifies direction but ensures that a team is working toward the same goals. The team can participate in goal development and offer feedback to the organization (Alliance for Nonprofit Management, 2008). Strategic planning holds team members accountable to the goals and outcomes based on the program idea (Foundation for Community Association Research, 2001). It has many benefits beyond formulating an idea; it is one method occupational therapy practitioners can use to begin shaping an effective community program.

Explore Existing Programs

Once the idea has been formulated, the occupational therapy practitioner or team must conduct a literature review or an Internet search for similar programs (Timmreck, 2003). Exploring other programs can help the team understand challenges, successes, and potential funding streams. Also, practitioners must be knowledgeable about what similar programs exist so as not to reinvent the wheel. Practitioners should never assume that their idea is innovative and claim it so until they have researched other programs. It can be detrimental to a grant proposal to claim an idea's innovativeness if it is not innovative!

Practitioners can also use a literature review later in a grant proposal. Therefore, this step of conducting a literature review is valuable and can assist later in the process of program development and grant writing.

In addition to a literature review, to explore existing programs practitioners can contact program directors who run similar programs for help in developing an idea into a successful program. Practitioners can network and meet these individuals through state or national associations. OT practitioners can glean best practices and strategies for strengthening their program idea from other directors. In some cases, program directors are willing to share contact information of funders who have been responsive to their ideas and grant proposals. In other cases, program directors may provide copies of successful grant proposals that practitioners can use to see what has worked in the past. Furthermore, other program directors may identify which funding agencies *do not* fund certain types of programs; knowing which funders to avoid can be a timesaver. In the world of program development and grant writing, an invaluable resource is those who have been there, done that (Holtzclaw, Kenner, & Walden, 2009).

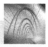

BEST PRACTICE HINT

Explore existing programs both in the literature and on government websites. Many government agencies that provide grant funding describe successful programs and best practices because grant funders require successful programs to disseminate their outcomes to the public.

Consult an Expert

Practitioners can consult experts in the program area (Lusky & Hayes, 2001). Experts may be individuals running similar programs, as previously discussed, or individuals who have conducted research on the idea. Experts do not have to be local and can be found in the literature, through networking, or by using listservs. OT practitioners can submit the idea to experts external to the program team to help determine the feasibility of the idea and identify resources that will be needed to transform the idea into a program or grant proposal (Falk, 2006).

BEST PRACTICE HINT

Experts in different practice areas can act as mentors by providing ongoing professional guidance and development. Be clear about your expectations of a mentor when contacting experts.

Ask the Community

As mentioned previously, it is easy to identify needs or issues in a community, but it may not be so easy to find solutions. OT practitioners should never forget the community! Community members may have relevant ideas on how to remedy problems and build on existing capacity. Practitioners can seek information from the community in many ways, including using surveys, community forums, town hall meetings, and focus groups. These efforts may tie into the community assessment (discussed later) and can provide valuable data for a grant proposal.

Be Creative!

Occupational therapy practitioners should be creative in exploring ideas for community programs (Fazio, 2008). Not only can creative strategies address community issues, but many grantors are looking for new, innovative ways to address community problems. An idea that might sound "out there" may be a potential solution that a grantor would be willing to fund.

Do Not Give Up

If an idea transforms into a program and is submitted as a grant proposal, rejection is common (Holtzclaw et al., 2009). Occupational therapy practitioners should not give up on a good idea simply because one grant funder did not support the idea— and rejection of a grant proposal does not mean an idea is invalid. A variety of reasons exist as to why a grant proposal might not be funded. Practitioners must remember this fact so that they do not compromise or discard good ideas after only one try.

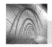

BEST PRACTICE HINT

If a grant proposal is rejected, always seek the feedback from grant reviewers to explore ways to improve the grant proposal. Also, ask for the opportunity to reapply in the next funding cycle. If this does not work, try exploring other funding agencies.

Transforming an Idea into a Program

When an idea has been identified, practitioners must figure out how the idea will translate into a viable program. At this point, there are many questions to consider. This process is often called the preplanning process because it occurs before any program development or assessment begins and while the program is still in the discussion stages (Brownson, 2001).

The best approach to begin is simply to examine the idea by asking who, what, when, where, and how questions. Answers to these questions help map out the idea and foster more formal discussion. Discussion of ideas can occur in groups or individually. Some questions practitioners should consider are the following: Who is the target audience of this program? What need(s) will this program address? When will the program begin? Where will the program be implemented? and How will this program be supported? (Ruhs, 2000).

Preplanning occurs in community programming and is important to ensure that an idea matches a community need. For example, a team working on an Indian reservation wanted to expand parent education about the health status of school children. Yearly school screenings examined the children's vision, hearing, oral health, body mass index, blood pressure, and type 2 diabetes risk. One day, the team brainstormed an idea to create a health report card that would be distributed to parents along with the children's school report cards. This report card would show the current year's and past years' screening results for each student. The team analyzed this idea using the who, what, when, where, and how process shown in **Table 3-3** (D. Parker, personal communication, October 2008). It took several years for the team to garner the resources to implement the idea, but the process came to fruition and is currently ongoing. The implementation of this idea led to future grant funds and enhanced programming allowing for ongoing community growth.

By using this approach, OT practitioners can begin to identify the feasibility of the idea as a program and explore what activities need to be done, resources garnered, and challenges faced. Engaging in preplanning ensures that the idea is well

---

TABLE 3-2 QUESTIONS TO CONSIDER IN PREPLANNING A PROGRAM

- Who is the target audience of this program?
- What need(s) will this program address?
- When will the program begin?
- Where will the program be implemented?
- How will this program be supported?

Source: Ruhs, B. (2000). *Successful grant writing tips and tactics.* Presented at the Massachusetts Department of Education Child Nutrition Programs.

TABLE 3-3 CASE EXAMPLE

Idea	Health report card to educate parents on children's health.
Who	Children and parents in the Native American community.
	The Diabetes Program staff who conducts the screenings will develop a health report card.
What	The health report card will aid in increasing parent education.
When	Distributed along with school health report cards.
Where	The health report cards will be compiled and stored by the school nurse and the diabetes program staff.
How	Assistance will be needed with compiling the data and putting them into the report cards.

---

thought out and helps practitioners avoid developing a program that will face many insurmountable obstacles and barriers.

If the idea seems feasible, occupational therapy practitioners can conduct a **SWOT analysis** (an analysis of strengths, weaknesses, opportunities, and threats) to examine the idea further. Process worksheets 3-6 and 3-7 provide instructors an example of SWOT Analysis. After engaging in preplanning, occupational therapy practitioners need to identify their role and form a team to begin to develop the program idea.

Exploring the Role of OT in Program Development and Grant Writing

Once an idea has been formulated and a program preplanned, occupational therapy practitioners must explore the role they will play in the program, such as providing direct practice or case management or consultation. In some cases, practitioners design and implement the program, and in others they are a component in a larger program. Whatever the approach, occupational therapy practitioners should assess their personal skills in program development and implementation and determine where they can fit most effectively in the program.

Other OT roles related to program development include administrator, consultant, educator, clinician, program developer, and researcher (Lemorie & Paul, 2001). Each role is discussed more fully in the following subsections.

Administrator

The role of **administrator** in the community can be complex. As a program administrator, the occupational therapy practitioner oversees the day-to-day activities that make the program work (Eggers, Munoz, Sciulli, & Crist, 2006). This role can include everything from managing staff and budgets, developing and maintaining policy and procedures, developing leadership, and conducting strategic planning (American Occupational Therapy Association [AOTA], 1993). Administrative duties in community practice are, in general, similar to administrative roles in traditional healthcare settings (Van Slyke, 2001). In some cases, the occupational therapy practitioner in administration may be referred to as a program director.

An example is a grant-funded program that included the development of a sensory room in a rural school to address sensory integration issues. The occupational therapy practitioner administered the program, appealed to the school staff for space, wrote the grant to get funding to buy the necessary supplies, drafted referrals and documentation forms, and educated the teachers on when to refer to the sensory room. The program was completely controlled by the occupational therapy practitioner and the practitioner oversaw all aspects of the program, from referrals to use of the sensory room and documentation.

Consultant

The occupational therapy practitioner in a consultant role can do a variety of activities. **Consultants** are usually considered to be experts in a certain area. OT practitioners' expertise may be as broad as understanding occupation or specific to a practice area (Fazio, 2008). In community practice, occupational therapy practitioners acting as consultants must understand organizational theory, be effective communicators, and be able to diagnose and problem solve issues that arise (Van Slyke, 2001; Epstein, 1985).

According to the American Occupational Therapy Association (AOTA, 1993), occupational therapy practitioners in the role of consultant should communicate professional expertise, assist in identifying and remediating problems, collaborate in the development of program outcomes, develop recommendations for the program, and assist the program in identifying resources. In community practice, the occupational therapy practitioner may consult on the program development and implementation, the evaluation, and clinical concerns (Scaffa, 2001, p. 14).

In consultative roles, the practitioner may simply consult on certain aspects of the program (Scott, 2003). For example, an occupational therapy practitioner may consult on a program geared to get youth interested in health careers. The practitioner may suggest resources, activities, and individuals who can discuss the occupational therapy profession. In this role, the occupational therapy practitioner helps the program identify ways to educate the youth participants appropriately by providing expertise on the field of occupational therapy.

Another aspect of consultation is assisting with program evaluation and sustainability plans. OT practitioners may be able to assist in the evaluation process by collecting data or helping with data analysis. They might also suggest milieus for data dissemination. OT consultants can provide feedback on program sustainability by identifying which services are reimbursable. These simple roles can really enhance a program.

Occupational therapy practitioners may find themselves fulfilling the role of consultant in unique ways, such as becoming a member of a task force, board of directors, or advisory board. In such a role, practitioners are asked to use their expertise to guide a program by providing feedback on the entire program (Fazio, 2008). For example, an occupational therapy practitioner may find it useful to join a home safety task force that is focused on tackling issues related to fall prevention and home safety for older adults. Or by being a member of an advisory board, the practitioner may be able to provide advice to a program that promotes well-being.

Sometimes, consultation is not necessary for long periods of time and acting as consultant may be periodic rather than constant (Scaffa, 2001). Many consultants work on a contract basis and outline their services in the contract. The sky is the limit on the kinds of programs for which occupational therapy practitioners can provide consultation; program team members and practitioners must figure out the specifics of the consultation role as part of the development process.

Educator

By the nature of practice, occupational therapy practitioners are **educators**; community practice is no exception. According to the American Occupational Therapy Association (AOTA, 1993), the role of an occupational therapy educator includes developing and providing "educational offerings or training related to occupational therapy to consumer, peer, and community individuals or groups" (p. 1090). The role of educator in community may be very simple, such as when the practitioner provides educational seminars to community members. Educational activities can be scheduled for local support organizations such as the local chapter of the Alzheimer's Association or the Amyotrophic Lateral Sclerosis Foundation. Education can also reach beyond these boundaries.

An example of the role of education in community program development is a program developed for faith communities. This program provided intensive training for lay people in faith communities to complete home safety checks in the homes of older parishioners. The purpose of the program was to help connect the faith community members to one another and ensure that older parishioners could maintain living in their homes and be involved in the faith community. The occupational therapy practitioner in this program developed all the training materials including a training manual, a training presentation, case studies, and other educational materials. These materials were then used to implement the program. The focus of this program was educational and the actual action of completing the home safety checks was done by those being trained (Voltz, 2003, 2005).

Clinician

In some cases, occupational therapy practitioners may find themselves providing traditional clinical services in a community practice model (Van Slyke, 2001). For example, an occupational therapist may perform home safety assessments in an assisted living facility as part of an overall fall prevention education program. Although the practitioner provides direct clinical services, the services fit into a broader community program. Another example is a practitioner providing developmental screenings as part of a community-wide initiative to address fetal alcohol syndrome. Again, the practitioner provides clinical services but in the context of a greater community program. The clinical role in the community will vary with the context of the program.

Program Developer

OT practitioners can also develop the programs in a community setting. A multitude of examples exist of occupational therapy practitioners developing and implementing community programming. Eggers, Munoz, Sciulli, and Crist (2006) discuss an occupational therapist who, by "providing opportunities for incarcerated men and women to engage in occupations that support adaptive patterns of functioning both in and outside the county jail" (p. 21), acted as program developer in a jail setting. Braveman (2001) describes an occupational therapy practitioner who developed a program for individuals diagnosed with AIDS. Because of their expertise in occupation, there is no limit to the types of programs occupational therapy practitioners can develop (Fazio, 2008).

Researcher

According to AOTA (1993), an occupational therapy **researcher** should perform "scholarly work of the profession including examining, developing, refining, and evaluating the profession's body of knowledge, theoretical base, and philosophical foundations" (p. 1097). Research should not be excluded from community practice. In the role of researcher, practitioners can participate in designing research studies, collecting data, analyzing data, and disseminating results. Occupational therapy practitioners can play a role in community research including community-based participatory research (Minkler et al., 2008).

Occupational therapy practitioners can play a multitude of roles in the community (Lemorie & Paul, 2001). Identifying the role the practitioner will play in a community program is an important piece of program development. In communities that are not aware of the field of occupational therapy and its role in community settings, OT practitioners may need to educate community members to help define the practitioner's role in programming (Miller & Nelson, 2004). One way to educate community members is to describe the skills occupational therapy practitioners possess to work in communities.

Program Development as a Skill

Program development is a skill that comes very naturally for some occupational therapy practitioners and one that must be cultured in others. OT practitioners develop programs daily in traditional practice settings, so these skills can be transferred to the community context. For example, when a practitioner works with an individual client, the practitioner assesses the client's needs and then develops a plan or program to help the person address those needs. The practitioner builds on existing abilities and utilizes the environment to enhance the person's performance. These same principles apply to community program development.

BEST PRACTICE HINT

Explore the poster presentations at the AOTA Annual Conference for many examples of occupational therapy practitioners who have developed successful community programs.

To develop program development skills occupational therapy practitioners must see themselves as program developers. For many, the process of developing and implementing a program and/or writing a grant proposal sounds intimidating and impossible. However, there are many successful occupational therapy programs in community practice. Practitioners simply need to search the literature or attend the American Occupational Therapy Association annual conference to witness the success of OT in community practice. Being a successful community practitioner is believing program development is possible and the community context is an appropriate place in which to practice.

Chapter 1 discussed the skills required of a practitioner for practicing in the community. To be successful in the community, occupational therapy practitioners need to alter their thinking from the traditional model of practice. According to Lemorie and Paul (2001), "practicing in the community requires occupational therapists to acquire new skills, fill new roles, and use a client-centered approach to treatment." Yet, many of the skills from traditional practice *can* transfer to community practice. Program development requires an occupational therapy practitioner to think using

TABLE 3-4 TRADITIONAL PRACTICE VERSUS COMMUNITY PROGRAM DEVELOPMENT	
Traditional Practice	**Community Practice**
Evaluation	Community assessment
Drafting a treatment plan	Program planning
Occupational therapy intervention	Program implementation
Ongoing patient evaluation and documentation	Program evaluation
Discharge planning	Sustainability planning
Documentation	Dissemination plan

a systems approach instead of the traditional individual patient model (Fazio, 2008). **Table 3-4** compares the traditional practice model and the community practice model.

Specific skills promote success among occupational therapy practitioners working in community practice. These key skills are identified in the occupational therapy literature as flexibility, ability to communicate clearly, desire, openness, organization, and client-centeredness.

Community practice, by its nature, is unpredictable, which can be a challenge for some practitioners. This unpredictability requires practitioners to exhibit flexibility in both the program development and grant writing processes. Miller and Nelson (2004) discovered the unpredictable nature of community practice when they placed occupational therapy students in community settings for a Level I fieldwork experience. In Miller and Nelson's study of students in community settings, successful program development occurred when the process was mentored by faculty with prior experience in program development and grant writing. Faculty were able to assist students in reflecting and could make suggestions for modification to aid the students in maintaining flexibility throughout program development and grant writing.

For some practitioners, the unpredictable nature of community practice is a welcome difference from practice in the reimbursement-driven healthcare industry. Simply, it is important to recognize that being flexible is a necessary skill in community practice and program development because activities never go exactly as planned. By being flexible, practitioners can listen to others and search for solutions in an effective and community-centered way. Flexibility might not come easily to all practitioners, and mentorship can aid in ensuring a practitioner is adaptable to the community and its needs when engaged in program development and grant writing.

Occupational therapy practitioners in community settings also need to have strong communication skills (Lemorie & Paul, 2001). Practitioners need both verbal and written communication skills to be successful. Depending on their role, OT practitioners must be able to communicate with diverse individuals, openly discuss community needs and programmatic challenges, and deal with the issues that arise in groups and with partnerships. Being able to communicate across different groups is important to ensure that quality program implementation occurs. Communication is essential when educating others, including community members and funding agencies, about the program. Furthermore, in grant proposals occupational therapy practitioners must be able to articulate a program idea clearly in written form.

A desire and passion for community practice are required to be successful (Grady, 1994). Having the heart for community practice is essential and carries a practitioner through the tough times. The timing and pace of community work are drastically different from traditional clinical practice, with change occurring slowly (Kretzmann & McKnight, 1993). Occupational therapy practitioners often have to "stick it out"

for long periods of time to witness change, and this can be difficult for some (Jensen & Royeen, 2001). Furthermore, with passion and desire the practitioner can be open. Openness is an important characteristic in times of change and for understanding the community. Practitioners have to be open to the community's—not the practitioner's—desires and needs. Openness aids in maintaining strong communication and flexibility as described earlier.

A community can be a group of people who have been marginalized or who are struggling to make a change. It is important that the focus of programs be on what the community wants and needs (Kretzmann & McKnight, 1993). Using a client-centered approach can ensure that programs developed and grants written fit with the desires of the community (Lemorie & Paul, 2001). Some research in occupational therapy states that practitioners who lack a client-centered approach are engaging in a "professional failure" (Lemorie & Paul, 2001). Using client-centered practice principles in community practice ensures that change occurs when the community is ready and values the approaches proposed by the community to address a problem (Law, 1998).

Last, but not least, a core skill of any practitioner working in communities is organization (Munoz, Provident, & Hansen, 2004). Program development and grant writing require significant thought, preparation, and organization. When working in community practice, the practitioner is also called upon to engage in community assessment, gather evaluation data, and facilitate community change. By being organized, practitioners can ensure that a program is developed efficiently; organization also increases the program's likelihood of success. Because there is no one right way to develop a program or

BEST PRACTICE HINT

Keep a journal of the activities and ideas that have and have not been successful. Recognize lessons learned and best practices as a form of ongoing professional development and to ensure future successful program implementation.

write a grant proposal, practitioners must follow the organizational methods that work best for them and that meet community needs. Practitioners can develop best practices with experience and based on the nature of the community.

Creating the Program Team

If an idea appears strong enough to move into the program development phase, it is important to create a strong team for program development and grant writing. Because of its complicated nature, community practice cannot be done in isolation, so community programs require a team approach (Fazio, 2008). A **team** is "two or more individuals with a high degree of interdependence geared toward the achievement of a goal or the completion of a task" (West & White, 2008). Together, team members make decisions, solve problems, develop a focus, and accomplish outcomes. Program development and grant writing are not done in isolation and require the collaboration of a team (Holtzclaw, Kenner & Walden, 2009). Furthermore, a team approach provides different perspectives, enhances success and sustainability, and expands expertise and resources (Ruhs, 2000).

Teams require time to develop. The team life cycle generally goes through four predictable phases: forming, storming, norming, and performing. In the forming stage, team members get to know one another and establish goals for the team. They begin to explore which tasks they will undertake as a team. In the storming stage, team members voice their opinions about the team and its proposed tasks. Dysfunction can occur at this stage as team members negotiate goals and team member roles. However, this negotiation process is normal for a successful and effective team. The norming stage is when team members agree on the expectations of the team and its members. Trust begins to develop and team member roles are clearly defined. In the performing stage, the team achieves goals successfully and effectively. Team members work together toward the team's goals without conflict (Blue et al., 2008).

In general, grant writers identify the need for a team "to be assembled quickly in response to a request for proposal (RFP) to brainstorm and write the application and to ensure complete accuracy" (Wurmser, 2006, p. 38). Teams should be assembled prior to the actual writing and program development processes; preferably, the team is ready to go when an RFP is a match. The multiple eyes and minds of team members expand the grant search and can share tasks during the grant writing process.

For a program to be successful, the team has to be able to work together in a collaborative, cooperative fashion (Holtz-

---

LET'S STOP AND THINK

Recall a team you have been a member of and describe how the group went through each stage of forming, storming, norming, and performing.

BEST PRACTICE HINT

Be prepared for team challenges in which disagreements occur. Team-building activities, such as time to reflect on the team's progress, can aid in ensuring that the team continues to be effective.

TABLE 3-5 LIFE CYCLE OF TEAM DEVELOPMENT	
Stage	**Process**
Forming	• Team members get to know one another.
	• Establish goals and tasks for team.
Storming	• Team members begin to voice opinions.
	• Dysfunction can occur with arguments about goals or team member roles.
Norming	• Agreement is achieved on the team expectations.
	• Trust develops.
	• Team roles become clearly understood.
Performing	• Team completes tasks.
	• Team members share leadership.
	• Tasks are completed effectively and efficiently.

Source: Blue, A. V., Hamm, T. L., Harrison, D. S., Howell, D. W., Lancaster, C. J., Smith, T. G., et al. (2008). *Team skills handbook.* Charleston: Medical University of South Carolina.

claw et al., 2009; Blue et al., 2008). Members of the team need to be chosen carefully. The expertise and contribution of each team member must be thoroughly defined and discussed. Furthermore, the amount of time each team member will spend on the program must be clearly defined in the grant proposal. To some granting agencies, particularly for research-based grants, the expertise and experience of the team affect whether the program receives funding. In such cases, the members of the team need to be considered for their experience, which can enhance a grant proposal (Holtzclaw et al., 2009).

In community practice, teams can include occupational therapy practitioners, other experts, and community partners. The process and strategies for building community partnerships are discussed later in this book. Occupational therapy practitioners should recognize early in the process the importance of including community members on the program team, both for development and grant writing (Holtzclaw et al., 2009).

Key activities of a team include communication, decision making, delegation, and problem solving (White & West, 2008). To design and implement a community program successfully these activities should be collectively accomplished in the collaborative model of the team. Yet working in a team is challenging. According to Patrick Lencioni (2002), author of

BEST PRACTICE HINT

Treat community team members the same as other team members. Provide them with role expectations and define the purpose of the team for them.

The Five Dysfunctions of a Team, teams become dysfunctional when there is an absence of trust, fear of conflict, lack of commitment, and inattention to results. These factors can destroy a team, which ultimately destroys a program or the ability to address a community need. The team should be aware of these dysfunctions and develop plans to remedy them as they arise.

Teams are different for each program. Some key aspects to consider when building a team are structure and development. A collaborative and cooperative team can lead to success, ensuring that the program gets up and running and grant proposals are submitted on time. When building a team, practitioners must identify who needs to be involved and when these individuals need to be involved (Brooks, 2006). In some cases, pulling in people too late can be detrimental to the team and ultimately the planning process.

BEST PRACTICE HINT

Review group process protocols to aid in team development.

Next, the team should collectively define its purpose and vision for the program (Blue et al., 2008). During this process, team members communicate and begin to build trust with one another. Team members should also take time individually to identify what each member brings to the group. This activity also helps to build trust as well as aids in delegation of activities later. As discussed earlier, group process is an important component of a team's development (Cole, 2005).

In a team or group setting, power is shared. When working in community practice, this is an especially important principle to emphasize. On teams that include educated healthcare professionals, community members may feel inadequate, which can decrease their active participation. This situation should be avoided if possible by helping each team member recognize their ability to contribute and what they can contribute (Israel, Eng, Schulz, & Parker, 2005). Teams should also celebrate together. Taking the time to celebrate is crucial to ensuring ongoing commitment from team members and for members to feel rewarded for their participation.

Prior to engaging in the grant writing process, members of the team need to have a good understanding of the group's mission and the purpose of the grant funding (Holtzclaw et al., 2009). To foster understanding, the program must be

LET'S STOP AND THINK

Reflect upon why team building is so crucial to successful program development and grant writing.

fleshed out so that all team members fully understand and comprehend it. Involving experts in the grant writing process either for drafting portions of the grant or for consultation on best practices to include in the grant is valuable. It is essential that these individuals fully understand the program ideas so that they fully support and provide for the program during implementation.

Teams need ongoing development and care, especially if members of the team change (Holtzclaw et al., 2009). Group dynamics always come with challenges, but overcoming these challenges is possible. The processes of the team, including communication, decision making, and problem solving, need to be clearly defined. As a team changes and develops, team members must revisit the purpose of the team frequently to ensure success and effective outcomes (Blue et al., 2008).

Where Do Grants Fit In?

Many community programs need a financial jumpstart and grants can provide it. Similar to interesting an investor or getting a loan for a business, grants can provide the initial financial startup money for a program. Many types of grants are available to support community programming (Nelson & McNulty, 2005). The specifics of finding and writing a grant proposal are discussed in greater detail later in this book. It is important to acknowledge during the preplanning phase of a community program that grants can be a viable option for transitioning an idea into a successfully developed program.

Conclusion

This chapter discusses the process of turning an idea into a program and the skills required of occupational therapy practitioners to be successful in implementing programs based on an idea. Practitioners must fully evaluate an idea prior to jumping into program development and must ensure that all the right questions are asked to evaluate the idea fully. Just as it takes a village to raise a child, it takes a group of talented people to develop and implement a successful program. The skills and roles of the occupational therapy practitioner in the program development process are unique to community practice but mirror many of the skills of traditional practice.

Glossary

Administrator The person who oversees the day-to-day activities that make the program work

Brainstorming A process for generating ideas

Consultant An expert in a certain area who provides assistance to a program or group

Educator A role that includes developing and providing "educational offerings or training related to occupational therapy to consumer, peer, and community individuals or groups" (AOTA, 1993, p. 1090)

Researcher A person who performs "scholarly work of the profession including examining, developing, refining, and evaluating the profession's body of knowledge, theoretical base, and philosophical foundations" (AOTA, 1993, p. 1097)

Strategic planning A form of planning that aids an organization in defining its direction for the next year or so by identifying strategies for attaining identified goals

SWOT analysis An analysis that examines the strengths, weaknesses, opportunities, and threats of an idea, team, or organization

Team "Two or more individuals with a high degree of interdependence geared toward the achievement of a goal or the completion of a task" (White & West, 2008).

References

Alliance for Nonprofit Management. (2008). Strategic planning. Retrieved November 24, 2008, from http://www.allianceonline.org/FAQ/strategic_planning

American Occupational Therapy Association. (1993). Occupational therapy roles. *American Journal of Occupational Therapy, 47*(12), 1087–1099.

Baumgartner, J. (2003). *The step by step guide to brainstorming.* Retrieved November 24, 2008, from http://www.jpb.com/creative/brainstorming.php

Blue, A. V., Hamm, T. L., Harrison, D. S., Howell, D. W., Lancaster, C. J., Smith, T. G., et al. (2008). *Team skills handbook.* Charleston: Medical University of South Carolina.

Bond, L. A., Belensky, M. F., & Weinstock, J. S. (2000). The Listening Partners Program: An initiative toward feminist community psychology in action. *American Journal of Community Psychology, 28*(5), 697–730.

Braveman, B. (2001). Development of a community-based return to work program for people living with AIDS. *Occupational Therapy in Health Care, 13*(3–4), 113–131.

Brooks, D. M. (2006). *Grant writing made easy.* Presentation at the E-Tech Conference, Columbus, OH.

Brownson, C. A. (2001) Program development: Planning, implementation, and evaluation strategies. In M. Scaffa (Ed.), *Occupational therapy in community-based practice settings.* Philadelphia: F. A. Davis.

Cole, M. B. (2005). *Group dynamics in occupational therapy: The theoretical basis and practice application of group intervention* (3rd ed.). Thorofare, NJ: Slack.

Edberg, M. (2007). *Essentials of health behavior: Social and behavior health in public health.* Sudbury, MA: Jones and Bartlett.

Eggers, M., Munoz, J. P., Sciulli, J., & Crist, P. A. (2006). The community reintegration project: Occupational therapy at work in a county jail. *Occupational Therapy in Health Care, 20*(1), 17–37.

Epstein, C. F. (1985). The occupational therapy consultant in adult day care programs. *Gerontology Special Interest Section Newsletter, 8,* 3–4.

Falk, G. W. (2006). Turning an idea into a grant. *Gastrointestinal Endoscopy, 64*(6), S11–S13.

Fazio, L. (2008). *Developing occupation-centered programs for the community* (2nd ed.). Upper Saddle River, NJ: Prentice Hall.

Foundation for Community Association Research. (2001). *Best practices: Strategic planning.* Alexandria, VA: Author.

Grady, A. P. (1994). Building inclusive community: A challenge for occupational therapy. *American Journal of Occupational Therapy, 49,* 300–310.

Holtzclaw, B. J., Kenner, C., & Walden, M. (2009). *Grant writing handbook for nurses* (2nd ed.). Sudbury, MA: Jones and Bartlett.

Israel, B. A., Eng, E., Schulz, A. J., & Parker, E. A. (2005). Introduction to method in community-based participatory research for health. In B. A. Israel, E. Eng, A. J. Schulz, & E. A. Parker (Eds.), *Methods in community-based participatory research for health.* San Francisco: Jossey-Bass.

Jensen, G. M., & Royeen, C. B. (2001). Analysis of academic–community partnerships using the integration matrix. *Journal of Allied Health, 30,* 168–175.

Kretzmann, J. P., & McKnight, J. L. (1993). *Building communities from the inside out: A path toward finding and mobilizing a community's assets.* Skokie, IL: ACTA Publications.

Law, M. (1998). *Client-centered occupational therapy.* Thorofare, NJ: Slack.

Lemorie, L., & Paul, S. (2001). Professional expertise of community-based occupational therapists. *Occupational Therapy in Health Care, 13*(3/4), 33–50.

Lencioni, P. (2002). *The five dysfunctions of a team: A leadership fable.* San Francisco: Jossey-Bass.

Lusky, M. B., & Hayes, R. L. (2001). Collaborative consultation and program evaluation. *Journal of Counseling & Development, 79*(1), 26–38.

McNamara, C. (2008). Strategic planning (in nonprofit or for-profit organizations). Retrieved online November 24, 2008, from http://www.managementhelp.org/plan_dec/str_plan/str_plan.htm

Miller, B. K., & Nelson, D. (2004). Constructing a program development proposal for community-based practice: A valuable learning experience for occupational therapy students. *Occupational Therapy in Health Care, 18*(1/2), 137–150.

Minkler, M., Hammel, J., Gill, C. J., Magasi, S., Vasquez, V. B., Bristo, M., et al. (2008). Community-based participatory research in disability and long-term care policy: A case study. *Journal of Disability Policy Studies, 19,* 114–126.

Munoz, J. P., Provident, I. M., & Hansen, A. M. (2004). Educating for community-based practice: A collaborative strategy. *Occupational Therapy in Health Care, 18*(1/2), 151–169.

Nelson, L. E., & McNulty, S. (2005). Beyond the box: Strategies for emerging community practice. *Home and Community Health Special Interest Section Newsletter, 12*(4), 1–3.

Ruhs, B. (2000). *Successful grant writing tips and tactics.* Presented at the Massachusetts Department of Education Child Nutrition Programs.

Scaffa, M. (Ed.). (2001). *Occupational therapy in community-based practice settings.* Philadelphia: F. A. Davis.

Scott, J. B. (2003). Keeping older adults on the road: The role of occupational therapists and other aging specialists. *Generations, 27*(2), 39–43.

Timmreck, T. C. (2003). *Planning, program development, and evaluation* (2nd ed.). Sudbury, MA: Jones and Bartlett.

Van Slyke, N. (2001). Adult day care programs. In M. Scaffa (Ed.), *Occupational therapy in community-based practice settings* (pp. 163–172). Philadelphia: F. A. Davis.

Voltz, J. D. (2003). *Project CHERISH training manual.* Unpublished document.

Voltz, J. D. (2005). Health ministry: A role for occupational therapy. *Advance for Occupational Therapy Practitioners, 21*(5), 40–41.

West, V. T., & White, A. (2008). An introduction to teamwork [PowerPoint presentation]. Retrieved November 24, 2008, from http://academicdepartments.musc.edu/ collaborative_care/publications/index.htm

Wurmser, T. (2006). Advance your nursing career with philanthropy and grant writing. *Nursing Manager, 37*(3), 35–39.

PROCESS WORKSHEET 3-1 **ANALYZING A PROGRAM IDEA**

Got an idea for a program? Use this worksheet to analyze the idea to determine whether it will work as a successful program.

Instructions: Complete this form to analyze the quality of a program idea.

Idea	
What? Describe the idea.	
Who? Who is the target population? Who will this program serve?	
When? When would this idea be implemented?	
Where? Where would this idea occur?	
How? How can this happen? How will it be funded?	

PROCESS WORKSHEET 3-2 **FORMING A TEAM**

Instructions: Use this worksheet to analyze how to form the team. Identify individuals who might be good for the team.

Name	Characteristic/Strengths for the Team

PROCESS WORKSHEET 3-3 **BUILDING A TEAM**

Instructions: Use this worksheet to identify and build your team. Answer the following questions to identify the strengths of the team. Share this worksheet with all members of the team so that everyone is aware of what each member can contribute.

1. Identify collective mission and vision for the team.

2. Identify the strengths of the team.

3. Identify the expertise of those on the team.

PROCESS WORKSHEET 3-4 **THE ROLE OF THE OCCUPATIONAL THERAPY PRACTITIONER**

Instructions: Use this worksheet to determine the role of the occupational therapy practitioner.

For each role, identify your strengths and weaknesses. Identify which roles you could play for the program in each category.

Role	Strengths	Weaknesses	Potential Activities of OT Practitioner
Administrator			
Consultant			
Educator			
Clinician			
Program developer			
Research			

PROCESS WORKSHEET 3-5 **GRANT WRITING PLANNING TEAM TASK WORKSHEET**
Instructions: For each section, identify which member of the team will complete the task.

Task	Team Member
Collect demographic data	
Conduct needs and assets assessment	
Draft statement of need	
Draft background/literature review	
Draft and collect support letters	
Draft budget and justification	
Write goals and objectives	
Draft implementation plan	
Draft sustainability plan	
Develop evaluation plan	
Collect biosketches	
Compile appendix	
Develop logic model	
Review grant proposal	
Seek necessary signatures of grant team and others as needed	
Communicate with community partner(s)	
Collate grant sections into one flowing document	
Draft abstract	
Draft and submit institutional review board (IRB) application	
Other: _____	

PROCESS WORKSHEET 3-6 **SWOT ANALYSIS**

Instructions: Analyze a program idea using the SWOT analysis format. SWOT = Strengths, Weaknesses, Opportunities, Threats. From this analysis, the team can explore the feasibility of the program idea.

Strengths	Weaknesses
Opportunities	**Threats**

PROCESS WORKSHEET 3-7 SWOT ANALYSIS EXAMPLE

Program Idea: Use the Wii Fit to engage youth who struggle with obesity to increase their activity tolerance

Strengths	Weaknesses
Interactive	Cost
Can use unique activities for each child by creating a unique Mii to monitor progress	Monitor student's use
	Self-esteem related to obesity
Team building	
Increase physical activity	
Opportunities	**Threats**
Would engage students in physical activity	Update when technology becomes too outdated
School is supportive of idea	
Students indicate interest in participation	Establishing ongoing funding to support program

According to this analysis, the idea has many strengths. If funding can be garnered and staff can monitor the youth, this idea should be feasible.

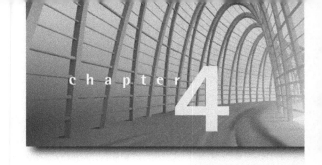

Finding a Grant That Fits

LEARNING OBJECTIVES

By the end of this chapter, the reader will be able to complete the following:
1. Compare and contrast types of grants appropriate for community-based programs.
2. Engage in a search of grants based on interest topics.
3. Evaluate a request for proposals to determine a strong programmatic match.

Overview

This chapter presents a comprehensive introduction to all the basics of grant writing. Grants use unique terminology, and an occupational therapy (OT) practitioner must have a unique set of skills to complete a grant proposal. The presumption of this chapter is that the OT practitioner can act as a grant writer for developing community programs. This chapter introduces terminology and principles required for grant writing in a context relevant to occupational therapy practitioners. The chapter focuses on the basics for finding a request for proposals (RFP) that fits with the program idea.

85

Key Terms

Cash match
Catalog of Federal
    Domestic Assistance
    (CFDA) number
Co-investigator
Collaborative grant
    model
Community
    foundation
Consultative grant
    model
Cooperative grant
    model
Corporate foundation
Demonstration grant
Educational grant
Fellowship
Foundation
Funding cycle
Grant eligibility
Grantee
Grantors
Individual foundation
Individual grant model
Operating foundations
Peer review panel
Planning grant
Principal investigator
    (PI)
Program officer
Request for application
    (RFA)
Request for proposals
    (RFP)
Research grant
Subcontract grant
    model
Training grant

Introduction

Grant writing in occupational therapy requires unique skills, and practitioners can easily slide into the role of grant writer or act as part of a grant writing team. Occupational therapy practitioners must be able to describe a program in the format prescribed by the grant funder. Although it is not the only approach, Brownson (1998) suggests grant writing as a method for funding community practice. Occupational therapy practitioners who plan to write a grant need to understand terminology common to grants, procedures required for grant writing, and the skills needed to implement the program if funding is granted (Holtzclaw, Kenner, & Walden, 2009). Basic skills required for successful grant writing include the ability to decipher different types of grants, the ability to search and find a grant RFP appropriate to a program's goals, and the ability to write a grant proposal according to the grant guidelines.

The Language of Grants

Grants have their own language and terminology that both grantors and grantees use. It is important for occupational therapy practitioners to know and understand this terminology when reading RFPs, communicating with program officers of grant agencies, and speaking with other grant writers.

Request for proposals (RFP) is a common grant-related term. An RFP is the call or request that granting agencies make public to encourage programs or organizations to apply for funds. RFPs outline the grant application requirements, due dates, amount of funding, and program requirements. Some granting agencies refer to an RFP as a **request for application (RFA)**. Both RFPs and RFAs have the same meaning and purpose, which is to encourage organizations to apply for funds.

Agencies that provide grant money are called **grantors** while agencies receiving grant awards are referred to as **grantees**. Most grant agencies or grantors have a designated individual, known as the **program officer**, available to answer questions about RFPs and program requirements, whereas the grantee organization's person in charge of the grant program is called the **principal investigator (PI)**. The program officer is the main contact the principal investigator has with the granting agency. Ultimately, the principal investigator is in charge of managing the grant, including the programmatic portions and the budget (Holtzclaw et al., 2009). The PI is the main liaison between the program and the grantor.

Grants are often reviewed by an anonymous team of individuals who will select which programs receive funding. These individuals form a **peer review panel**. The **funding cycle** indicates when the grant application is due. Funding cycles may occur more than once depending on the grant. Funding cycles can be annual or can occur multiple times a year.

TABLE 4-1 BASIC GRANT TERMINOLOGY	
Term	**Definition**
Co-investigators	Team members listed in the grant proposal who help with the program implementation and grant goals/objectives
Funding cycle	Date when the grant proposal is due
Grantee	Person, program, or project receiving the grant money
Grantor	Agency providing the grant funds
Peer review panel	Individuals at funding agency who review and rate the grant proposal
Principal investigator (PI)	Program director of a grant project
Program officer or project director	Employee of funding agency who provides guidance and technical assistance to individuals seeking funding
Request for proposals (RFP)	A notice of a grant opportunity

Types of Grants

Many types of grants exist. The phrase *type of grant* refers to the type of program the grant will fund. Examples include research grants, educational grants, training grants, planning grants, and demonstration grants. Each type of grant funds different types of programs, and requirements for the grant proposal vary according to the grant type.

Research grants fund research projects including everything from bench research in a laboratory to community-based participatory research. For research grants, the grant writer must define the research question, the research design, data collection methods, data analysis methods, sample size, and the need for the proposed research (Holtzclaw et al., 2009). Health research grants come from many funding agencies, the most prominent of which is the National Institutes of Health (NIH) (Reif-Lehrer, 2005).

An example of a research grant in occupational therapy is the one awarded by the Substance Abuse and Mental Health Services Administration (SAMHSA) to a community-based participatory research project that focused on suicide prevention for at-risk adolescents using sensory integration approaches. In this program, sensory rooms were set up in two schools and training was provided to staff and students on the use of the sensory room to reduce stress and modulate the nervous system. The intervention was analyzed to determine whether sensory integration techniques, including use of the sensory room, could reduce stress and increase individual coping strategies to reduce the number of suicide attempts (Anderson, Penn, Grandgenett, & Doll, 2007).

For research grants, approval of research by an institutional review board (IRB) is necessary. IRBs exist within academic institutions, hospitals, and in some community settings. The role of the IRB is to act as a protecting body for research participants (Holtzclaw et al., 2009). An example of a community IRB is a tribal IRB that is organized and run by tribal communities. This IRB focuses on evaluation of research in the Native American community. Each institutional review board maintains guidelines and application procedures for research. Researchers must contact the IRB and follow all proper procedures to secure approval prior to implementing a research project.

Educational grants focus on providing education for a group of people. In an educational grant proposal, the grant writer recommends implementing an educational program on a specific topic for a specific group. For example, the *A Heart for Health: The Health Report Card Project* used a report card as a model for educating a local African American community about health disparities and the health status of community members. Educational events were coordinated based on a community needs assessment conducted by a local emergency services organization that provides food, emergency funds for utilities, and clothing. Through the community assessment, community members expressed a desire to learn more about their own health status and reported that there was little access to health maintenance services. One of the objectives of this project was to provide primary care assessments (hypertension checks and education, diabetes screenings, skin cancer screenings, osteoporosis screenings, drug information, healthy walking approaches, cholesterol checks, calcium and vitamin D counseling, etc.) to a minimum of 40 community members at a local community health fair. The grant project maximized resources by using trained health professions students to implement the health screenings under licensed supervision. At the health fair, each community participant received a health report card and health education on each screening to assist him or her in tracking health status and understanding basic health maintenance. The health fairs were followed up with educational sessions based on the areas of need including diabetes and hypertension management. The overall goal, which aligned with an educational grant, was to "promote health education and empower a predominantly African American community to become more aware of their health status" (Voltz, Ryan Haddad, Hohnstein, & Martens Stricklett, 2007).

Training grants are focused on developing and implementing a specific type of training for a specific population. The Health Resources and Services Administration (HRSA) is a federal agency that has historically provided training grants for interprofessional training in rural areas (HRSA Advisory Committee on Interdisciplinary, Community-Based Linkages, 2008). The Office of Interprofessional Scholarship, Service and Education (OISSE) in the Creighton University School of

Pharmacy and Health Professions received a series of four such training grants from HRSA (Cochran et al., 2006). The focus of the training grew out of a partnership with two tribal communities that sought rehabilitation services. Through these training grants, students were placed on interprofessional teams and immersed in the community for a short-term intensive health-related experience. The team of students completed case studies, worked with Indian Health Service employees, and explored the culture (Jensen & Royeen, 2001, 2002; Barrett, 2002; Jensen, Ryan Haddad, Coppard, & Cochran, 2002; Jensen, Coppard, & Cochran, 2001; Royeen & Jensen, 1997).

Planning grants are grants that provide funding for program planning or for planning a project (Gitlin & Lyons, 1996). When grantors offer a planning grant, they usually offer a subsequent demonstration grant or further funding if the planning is successful. Planning grants are rare because most granting agencies expect planning to occur prior to applying for funding. Some grants allow time in the grant implementation for planning, but the requirements for planning and amount of time are usually outlined and grantees must comply to receive full funding.

Demonstration grants are provided to fund programming directly. According to Gitlin and Lyons (1996), demonstration grants "provide support to projects that evaluate a model program, set of services or methodology" (p. 6). Demonstration grants fund program implementation and usually fund programs that have demonstrated success or that use evidence-based approaches. Many demonstration grants fund programs related to health and human services (Gitlin & Lyons, 1996, 2004).

A grant titled *What's in Your Future? A Health Education and Health Professions Program for Community Youth* is an example of a demonstration grant. This grant proposal used evidence from pediatric obesity prevention programs and health professions minority recruitment data to implement a program at a parochial school serving low-income African American students. Physical education was offered only one day a week at the school, and the students had little exposure to health careers. The goals of this project were twofold: (1) engage children in physical activity to increase learning as suggested by research, and (2) engage health professions students as role models for a minority underserved population to educate the children implicitly about health careers. To justify the grant funding, the grant writing team described how research has shown that a lack of physical activity among children in school can affect learning (Veugelers & Fitzgerald, 2005; Kavey et al., 2003; Schmitz & Jeffrey, 2000). Furthermore, the grant writing team cited data about minority students not being exposed to health careers. The proposed program integrated health professions career education in primary school (Cohen, Gabriel, & Terrell, 2002) and provided monthly interactive educational sessions on the health professions to actively engage and teach the students about health. The program culminated with a health

> **LET'S STOP AND THINK**
>
> Which type of grant is most useful for occupational therapy practitioners? Why do you think this type is the best suited for occupational therapy practitioners?

TABLE 4-2 TYPES OF GRANTS	
Type of Grant	**Description**
Demonstration grant	A grant that provides funding specifically for program implementation
Educational grant	A grant proposal that implements a program of education for a population or group on a specific topic
Planning grant	A grant proposal that outlines how a team will plan a program or project
Research grant	A grant proposal that uses scientific inquiry to carry out a research project. Funds are sought to support the research implementation.
Training grant	A grant proposal that focuses on training groups

fair that family members were invited to attend (Begley, Doll, Martens Stricklett, & Ryan Haddad, 2008). The purpose of the grant was to implement the program to address the community need and grant funds supported the supplies needed for program implementation.

Different types of grants require different roles and responsibilities to be fulfilled. Practitioners must consider these roles and responsibilities during preplanning and the grant writing process. Typically, for research-based grants, the roles that need to be filled are principal investigator, co-investigators, coordinator, consultants, data collector, data entry person, and statistician. For a community-based or demonstration grant, typical roles include principal investigator, coordinator, funding specialist, statistical expert, and data collector. In the case of a community-based organization, the PI commonly is the executive director of the organization. In academic institutions, garnering grants links to promotion and tenure (Holtzclaw et al., 2009).

In many cases, roles can be covered by more than one person and may not be supported by the grant. Depending on the institution, individuals may already be in place to help with statistics or maintaining the budget, and this does not affect the grant proposal other than their assistance with the program must be mentioned. Sometimes the responsibilities of these individuals can be included in the in-kind aspects of the budget.

The credentials of the principal investigator can affect a program's worthiness for funding. Some grants specify the required qualifications of the primary investigator (PI). For example, to be eligible to receive funding from the National Insti-

BEST PRACTICE HINT

Not all roles exist for every grant program. Determine which roles are crucial to the implementation of your program.

TABLE 4-3 ROLES/RESPONSIBILITIES FOR A RESEARCH-BASED GRANT MODEL

Role	Responsibilities
Principal investigator (PI)	• Manages project and staff • Ensures project goals are met • Oversees funding and grant reporting
Co-investigator (Co-I)	• Has expertise in a specific area and is responsible for a particular aspect of the grant project
Grant coordinator	• Is responsible for day-to-day management of the grant activities • Not all grants have a grant coordinator.
Consultants	• If needed, outside persons who help ensure that objectives that might not fit the PI's expertise are met • Typically hired in the area of program evaluation
Data collector	• Collects necessary data to demonstrate goals are being met • Collates reports based on outcomes and evaluation plan
Data entry person	• Enters data into databases and other grant tracking systems
Statistician	• Analyzes the data gathered based on the grant project

Source: Gitlin, L. N., & Lyons, K. J. (2004). *Successful grant writing: Strategies for health and human service professionals.* New York: Springer.

tutes of Health (NIH), primary investigators must have a demonstrated history of research and publication (Reif-Leher, 2005). At times, OT practitioners will find it necessary to be strategic about who is listed as the primary or lead investigator on the grant proposal. For example, some grants require that a PI must have published in a certain area of the professional literature. In such cases, regardless of how excellent the proposal is, it would be rejected if the PI cannot identify a scholarly article that he or she published in the specified area of practice.

LET'S STOP AND THINK

What grant roles are best suited for occupational therapy practitioners? Why do you think these roles are a best fit?

TABLE 4-4 ROLES/RESPONSIBILITIES FOR A COMMUNITY-BASED GRANT MODEL	
Role	**Responsibilities**
Principal investigator (PI)	• Manages project and staff
	• Ensures project goals are met
	• Oversees funding and grant reporting
Coordinator	• Is responsible for day-to-day management of the grant activities
	• Not all grants have a grant coordinator or will pay for a coordinator, but a centralized coordinator is necessary for community programs to be a success.
Funding specialist	• Is responsible for managing the grant budget and paperwork associated with the grant budget
Statistical expert	• Is responsible for analyzing outcomes data collected as part of the grant
	• May assist with the evaluation plan or other grant-related data
Data collector	• Is responsible for collecting outcomes data related to the project/program

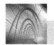

BEST PRACTICE HINT

Program directors can provide advice on choosing an appropriate PI. Ask them to help in the decision-making process to ensure that the best match is chosen, both for the grantor and grantee.

Currently, some funding agencies allow those applying for grants to designate more than one PI. However, it is common practice to allow only one PI, and then list other grant support staff as **co-investigators** (Holtzclaw et al., 2009). Again, these decisions need to be made in the grant planning process. The roles of each individual are outlined in the grant proposal. Some grant funders request that an abbreviated résumé for each investigator and staff be included in the proposal. The federal government uses a standardized form for submitting this information, but grant writers should review the RFP for specifics on this aspect of the grant (Ward, 2006).

Grant Models

A team can follow one of several different grant models. The grant model determines who will be needed on the grant team and what roles and responsibilities each team member will play. Determining the model and structure of the grant is an important part of the planning process because, for example, some funding agencies look for specific qualifications of the primary investigator and other grant team members. Knowing the requirements for the grant team upfront helps ensure that team members who fit the program and meet the grant requirements are chosen to participate.

Choosing an appropriate grant model can help the team determine which tasks each team member is responsible for and who will lead the team to the program's fruition. The first type of grant model is the **individual grant model** with a single principal investigator. This is a traditional model for academic research or educational grants. Although it is important to understand this model, OT practitioners will rarely, if ever, use it for grants, which by their very nature require collaboration to address the community needs (Gitlin & Lyons, 2004).

The **consultative grant model** is similar to the individual model but includes a single principal investigator with co-investigators to support the program. Experts usually act as consultants, providing feedback on the program as it is implemented. An example of an expert consultant is an external evaluator who is hired and paid by the grant money to complete the grant evaluation plan but who is not directly involved in the program implementation (Gitlin & Lyons, 2004). Depending on the community and the program, this model could be appropriate for community programs or clinical programs.

The **cooperative grant model** includes more than one principal investigator or is a grant that is submitted by more than one institution. In this model, a community coalition might partner with a university to apply for a grant. The **collaborative grant model** involves a team approach with multiple investigators who each have a specific assigned role in program implementation. This model is commonly used in community-based participatory research projects and fits well with community practice (Gitlin & Lyons, 2004).

BEST PRACTICE HINT

If grant writing and implementation are new practice skills for you, act as a consultant on a grant program so that you can learn about grants. As a consultant for a program, you may have the opportunity to learn through reporting and implementation.

Finally, some grants follow a **subcontract model**. In this model, one institution acts as the primary investigator but subcontracts another institution to carry out certain aspects of the grant program. Examples include when a community coalition contracts out evaluation services and when one agency applies for the grant but subcontracts services from a partner agency (Gitlin & Lyons, 2004).

Determining the grant model and the team of individuals to implement the program is very important and should be considered early in the grant development process. Practitioners must consider the following when determining a grant model:

1. Identify whether the RFP specifies a grant model to follow.
2. Identify whether certain credentials or accomplishments are required of the PI.

TABLE 4-5 GRANT MODELS

Grant Structure	Description
Collaborative model	• A team approach with multiple investigators each of whom has a specific role related to the grant project
Consultative model	• Includes a single investigator with possible co-investigators • Includes expert consultants who provide feedback on the grant project
Cooperative model	• Could have more than one investigator OR • Includes an agreement between more than one institution • Usually includes work groups focused on certain aspects of the project
Individual model	• Includes a single investigator • Can occur with research or educational grants • Typically a traditional academic model
Subcontract model	• A situation in which one institution acts as the primary investigator and subcontracts funding to another institution to carry out certain aspects of the grant

Source: Gitlin, L. N., & Lyons, K. J. (2004). *Successful grant writing: Strategies for health and human service professionals.* New York: Springer.

3. Identify the roles needed for the grant project.
4. Identify potential members of the grant team. Be strategic in this process and build a team that will strengthen the grant proposal.
5. Brainstorm the roles and responsibilities of each grant team member.
6. Research consultants or experts needed for the grant project.
7. Collect résumés or curriculum vitae from the grant team members.

By following these steps, practitioners can ensure that the grant proposal is thoroughly constructed and the team of individuals involved will achieve program success.

Grant Eligibility

After determining the type and model of the grant to apply for, practitioners next should determine **grant eligibility**. All grants have eligibility requirements outlined in the RFP that specify who can apply for the grant. Occupational therapy practitioners must closely review eligibility requirements when searching through RFPs prior to moving forward with a proposal.

Eligibility requirements differ based on the type of program to be funded. For example, to be eligible for health-related funding agencies commonly have to have nonprofit 501(c)3 status and be public institutions, private organizations, or federally recognized tribal governments (Grants.gov, 2008c). Or they have to be a public or private institution, such as a university, public or parochial school, or hospital. Also, grants from the federal government often are available to local and state governments and only specific types of agencies.

Individuals are rarely eligible for grants. However, **fellowships** provide funding for individuals to complete special projects for an organization. Fellowships available to healthcare professionals often focus on career development and research training (Holtzclaw et al., 2009). One example is the National Institutes of Health (NIH) fellowships for postdoctoral healthcare professionals.

Sometimes, eligibility requirements can change. For example, during his presidency, President George H. W. Bush expanded the designation by the federal government of fundable community agencies to include faith communities such as churches and other religiously affiliated organizations (Perry, 2008). With this legislation, more types of agencies became eligible for federal grants, opening up the doors for faith-based organizations. Unfortunately, the change in eligibility requirements increased competition for grants by allowing more agencies to apply for the same funding opportunities.

BEST PRACTICE HINT

If questions arise about the eligibility requirements, the program team should contact the project director to discuss eligibility prior to applying for the grant funds.

Granting agencies identify specifically who can and cannot apply for a grant in the RFP. Eligibility is based on the program to be funded and the mission and priorities of the granting agency. Grant agencies are allowed to determine what makes an organization eligible to apply for funding. For example, grantors can specify that funds are available only to minority organizations, federally recognized tribes, or organizations with a budget under a certain specified number. Other eligibility requirements can relate to the principal investigator. For example, for grants submitted to the NIH, PIs must demonstrate a record of research and publication (Reif-Lehrer, 2005).

Eligibility requirements can be very specific. Practitioners should review them thoroughly to ensure that there is a match between the applicant and the granting agency. Program directors at the granting agency are available to discuss eligibility requirements in case questions arise.

Grants from the federal government have a section specifically dedicated to eligibility requirements that outlines which organizations qualify to apply for the grant. Foundations that offer grant funding often use eligibility quizzes to determine eligibility. Potential grantees must complete the quizzes prior to submitting a grant application, and in some instances, they must complete the eligibility quizzes prior to accessing the RFP. Eligibility quizzes usually ask about an organization's

BEST PRACTICE HINT

When reading RFPs, explore the eligibility requirements early to make sure the organization is eligible.

operating budget and tax identification information (i.e., their non-profit status). If the grantee organization is denied but still considers itself or the program eligible, a representative of the grant team should contact the project director or foundation director immediately. If the grant team ignores eligibility requirements, the grant proposal may be removed from the review process.

Basic Principles of Grant Funding

A successful grant proposal requires an innovative idea, a well-written proposal, and a match between an idea and a funder (Reif-Lehrer, 2005). Grants are also affected by external factors including trends, economics, and relationships. Grant writers must understand the complexities that affect grant writing and funding to navigate successfully through grant applications. Understanding some basic principles and trends related to grants can help make the grant writing process simpler and less time consuming.

Principle 1: Grants Are Trendy

In a sense, the grant writing sector is a community unto itself. The grant writing world is dynamic and transforms and changes according to trends and needs. For example, after September 11, 2001, many grant RFPs were developed focusing on Homeland Security (U.S. Department of Homeland Security, 2008). Prior to this event, funding in this area was very small, if not nonexistent. However, the event of 9/11 forced many to identify homeland security as a need and funding was set aside to support programs focused on this national need. Grants follow the social and cultural needs of society.

RFPs are developed and issued based on the concerns and problems in the world at large. If a health issue arises or a group of people is in need, money is often set aside

BEST PRACTICE HINT

To discover the latest grant trends, explore the websites of major foundations such as the Robert Wood Johnson Foundation to see which current important health topics are receiving funding.

by both the government and foundations to meet this need. Another example of the ebb and flow of grant funding availability is in regard to childhood obesity, which is developing into a national problem. Large foundations, such as the Robert Wood Johnson Foundation, have set aside significant amounts of money to support community leaders who desire to address this issue (Robert Wood Johnson Foundation, 2008).

Recognition of the trendiness of grants is important, especially in the grant search process. Developing a program that aligns with a trend increases the likelihood that more funding will be available and the grant writer will have multiple agencies from which to choose to submit a proposal.

Principle 2: Grants Come in All Shapes and Sizes

Grants are diverse and can provide funding in large or small amounts. For example, grant funding can start as small as $500 or can amass to more than a million dollars. Whereas some grants are targeted to fund the implementation of a program, other grants provide support or infrastructure for new programs or enhance existing programs. For example, a grant titled *Engaging Students: The Community as Classroom* provided funding to support ongoing research on the impact of service learning for occupational therapy students. The grant money went to support the research by purchasing resources and research-related computer software (Doll & Flecky, 2008); however, no funds from the grant supported the community-related programming.

For beginning grant writers, proposals for smaller amounts of funding tend to be less demanding to draft and can get a program started. If the grant writer is creative and thoughtful, small amounts of funding can make a large impact and at times can be just what a program needs. For example, the *A Heart for Health: The Health Report Card Project* received only $500 of funding but was able to use the funds to provide primary health screenings for more than 100 individuals in an underserved community. The grant writer was also able to garner donations, maximizing the funding to provide needed services (Voltz et al., 2007).

To implement far-reaching health programs large amounts of funding are needed. In most cases, as the amount of funding offered increases, the grant proposal requirements become more intense, detailed, and stringent (Holtzclaw et al., 2009).

Principle 3: Grants Are Not Really Free Money

With grant funding comes responsibility. Grantors expect outcomes from grantees and may be very specific in what is required of the funded project. For every grant, the grantee must document information as outlined by the funder and provide reports based on a timeline established by the funder. The grant writer needs to understand all the reporting and outcome requirements thoroughly to build these components into the grant proposal and program to ensure that the funded program meets the funder's requirements.

Not following the requirements can lead to consequences such as not receiving subsequent years' funding or having to give money back to the funder. If a grantee is required to return money to the grantor, this consequence is not only viewed as disgraceful but can give the grantee a reputation that prevents other funding agencies from granting it funding in the future.

Principle 4: Grants Pay for All Kinds of Things

Grants are very diverse, and this can be of great benefit when a practitioner or an organization is looking for program funding. Grants are available to fund everything from research to technology to building a baseball field! Requests for proposals specifically outline what a grant will fund. There are many options for programs that simply need supplies or community members looking to fund something specific.

For example, the Nebraska Native American Public Health Act provides funding for a community wellness center for a Native American community in the state of Nebraska (Cross & Voltz, 2005). The grant money provides funding for running the building that contains the wellness center and for necessary equipment. The grant does not provide funding to support the programs implemented by the wellness center but funds the infrastructure required to offer wellness programming in the community.

Principle 5: Grants Are Not Forever

Grant funding does not last forever, so when planning a grant, practitioners must consider sustainability (Holtzclaw et al., 2009; Ward, 2006). Although this is a basic principle of program development, grant writers may not recognize its importance (Timmreck, 2003; Edberg, 2007). Grants are temporary and are not meant to fund a program for the duration of its existence. Furthermore, grant funders' priorities change, and community programs should be community-centered and developed to address community needs—not be based on the latest grant funding available. Because grant funding priorities change and because grants are competitive and have a finite life span, a grant should not be the only source of financial support for a program.

BEST PRACTICE HINT

Because grants do not last forever, it is best not to develop a program just to receive grant funding, but instead to develop a meaningful and sustainable program. In other words, do not rely on receiving grant funds as a way to sustain a program.

Usually, a grant is a way to kick-start a program that will ultimately be sustainable even after the funding period ends. In reality, a program might not be able to achieve the goal of sustainability because funding may not be enough or last long enough. Planning for sustainability in the early stages—even before searching for a grant—can help a project or program succeed in the long term (Holtzclaw et al., 2009). Practitioners must be aware of the importance of sustainability and the temporality of grants so that they can ensure that a program avoids being completely dependent on grant funding for success. Program sustainability will be discussed in detail in Chapter 11.

Principle 6: Grants Are Not Guaranteed

Applying for a grant is a risk. In most cases, grants are competitive. Many programs apply for the same funding and only so many awards are given (Reif-Lehrer, 2005; Ward, 2006; Holtzclaw et al., 2009). As a rule, grant writers should never rely on only one grant source. Smart grant writers explore and apply to several sources over time to ensure some funding is received. Practitioners must also be aware that the amount of the grant award may differ from the amount requested. A grant proposal is simply that: a *proposal* for funding (Holtzclaw et al., 2009). At their discretion, grant funders can change the award amount and will expect the grant writer to modify the program accordingly.

For example, a small nonprofit community agency partnered with a university to request funding to provide primary health services to family caregivers in a grant program titled *Caring for the Caregiver: An Outreach Program for Caregivers.* Although the program was awarded funds, the federal granting agency reduced the budget by $1,000 and requested that the grant writer adjust both the budget and activities. The granting agency provided a time period for revision and resubmission of the proposal. After adjustments were made, the agency resubmitted the proposal with the new plan and was approved by the grant agency prior to receiving the funding (Ryan-Haddad, Koenig, & Voltz, 2007).

BEST PRACTICE HINT

RFPs often identify how many awards will be given away, which can hint about the competition for funds. Use this information to gain some insight into the opportunities for receiving funds. For example, if a funding agency plans to award money to only one program, the chances of your program receiving funding are lessened.

Grant funding agencies might also ask grant writers to amend a program in the submitted grant proposal. In the case of the *A Heart for Health: The Health Report Card Project,* a program targeted at bringing primary health care services and health education to older adults in an African American community, the funding agency asked the grantee to expand the age range for services to include not only older adults but also adults over the age of 30 because many chronic diseases affect African Americans at an earlier age. Then, the funders approved the project and awarded the money. In the final report, the grant writer had to address how to integrate individuals older than 30 into the project (Voltz et al., 2007).

In rare cases, grantees may not receive the full amount of funding awarded. For many grant programs that are more than one year in length, the funding is provided to the grantee each year. In cases where a federal initiative is changed, grantees may not receive funding for completion of a project. This occurrence is very rare but could possibly occur. In such cases, the grant team must have a plan for sustainability that can be put into place quickly to maintain the program.

In other cases, awards from government agencies may be pending federal approval. Therefore, the RFP may be made available and applications accepted, but funding may or may not be federally approved, which means that the federal government did not allocate the proposed funds to the granting agency in the requested amount or with the priorities submitted by the government agency. If the money is not allocated by the government, no money will be granted to any proposals submitted. If funding for a grant is pending, the details and timeline for its approval are described in the RFP. Overall, grant writers should be prepared at all times for funding to change or even cease.

Principle 7: Grant Requirements Vary Widely

Although the federal government has made some attempts to make grants from federal agencies more universal through the implementation of Grants.gov, a clearinghouse for federal grants, overall grant requirements are widely different (Grants.gov, 2008a). As previously discussed, grantors can create very specific requirements for a project or program. Each granting agency has the discretion to identify eligibility requirements based on the organization's priorities.

Grant requirements are not only widely different in regard to eligibility but also in regard to the application process. Each granting agency has specific requirements for what needs to be included in a grant proposal. The request for proposals outlines all the required components for each grant proposal.

Principle 8: Collaboration Is Key

Grant writing is a very active process. When writing a grant , the grant writer cannot work in isolation (Holtzclaw et al., 2009). The grant writer has to be in touch with community needs and capture those needs in the proposal. Furthermore, when working with communities, capacity building is a strategy for ensuring success and sustainability, so knowledge of and relationships with the community assist grant writers in capturing this aspect in the proposal and project (Chaskin, Brown, Ventakesh, & Vidal, 2001).

BEST PRACTICE HINT

If you are involved in a coalition or with an agency, document this partnership with memorandums of understanding or contracts, which can later aid in applying for grant funding.

Many individuals are needed to assist in project implementation and evaluation of health programs (Cochran et al., 2007). The current trend for grants funding community health includes documentation of collaboration, including memorandums of understanding, evidence of community collaboration through formation of a community coalition, and letters of support (Community Anti-Drug Coalitions of American, 1999). Successful programs rely on collaborative work, which ultimately strengthens a grant proposal and the subsequent program (Ingersoll & Eberhard, 1999).

Principle 9: If Funding Is Not Received, It Is Not the End of the World

One of the most frustrating aspects of grant writing is that much work is put forth with no guarantee of funding! Receiving a denial of funding is disappointing, especially for first-time grant writers who have a good idea that they consider worthy of funding. Because of the competition for grant funding, there is an increased likelihood that many proposed programs go unfunded. Rejection is the reality of grant writing, and even experienced grant writers receive rejections. According to Holtzclaw, Kenner, and Walden (2009), "Submissions at the federal level often take three to four submissions of the same grant before it is actually funded" (p. 112).

Inevitably, every grant writer faces rejection; yet, no unfunded grant proposal is worthless—it should be reviewed for future use. Options include exploring other funding streams or resubmission. When a grant proposal is rejected, grant writers should always call the project director and request the review. In most cases, especially for federal grants, the project director can send the actual comments made by the reviewers. Many federal grant proposals are ranked based on a numbering system, and reviewers draft comments along with the number ranking.

Grant writers can use feedback and suggestions for future revisions. In some cases, the program director or reviewers might advise grant writers to resubmit with suggested revisions for the next funding cycle or when a new RFP is released. Reading reviewer comments is important because the suggested changes can be minor and require little work to revise for resubmission (Holtzclaw et al., 2009). In any case, rejected grant proposals can fit the priorities of another agency or be used as a framework for a future grant proposal.

> **LET'S STOP AND THINK**
>
> What have you learned about grants so far? Did this change your thinking about grant writing? If so, which of your thoughts changed?

Grant proposals and all the requirements that go with them do not follow a simple protocol. However, the principles discussed here are common to most grants and can be used as strategies for the beginning grant writer to explore and understand prior to engaging in the grant planning and writing process.

Searching for Grants

Finding a grant RFP that matches and fits with a health program can be tedious and overwhelming but gets easier with experience. Grant writers can find grants in many ways such as by conducting grant searches, using list-servs, and by word of mouth. Prior to searching for a grant, grant writers must identify exactly what the funding would support and how the funding would affect the program. If salary support is needed, the search must be for a larger grant, usually one for more than $50,000 (Holtzclaw et al., 2009). Although a definitive amount need not be determined prior to conducting a search, the grant writer should decide on a ball-park figure to aid in searching for an appropriate RFP. Occupational therapy practitioners should plan to explore multiple avenues and spend some time at it.

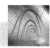

> **BEST PRACTICE HINT**
>
> When searching for grants, use all avenues possible to maximize opportunities for finding funds.

Funding Agencies

Many types of agencies award grants, but typically there are two main sources for grant funding: government agencies and foundations. Other sources that can provide funding are professional societies and associations, which focus on priorities related to their members (Holtzclaw et al., 2009). For example, the World Federation of Occupational Therapists provides grants for specific OT projects.

Foundation Grants

Foundations are private not-for-profit agencies that have funds or an endowment that they can use to support community programs. According to Camarena (2000), a foundation is "a non-profit, nongovernmental organization with a principal fund or endowment of its own, managed by its trustees or directors, established to maintain or aid charitable activities serving the common good" (p. 29). Foundations have a targeted topic or topics that they choose to support, or they might support any significant programs in a geographic area. In other words, foundations support a wide variety of initiatives including everything from the arts to health care.

Foundations can be local, national, or international. Some foundations serve only a city or county whereas others address national or international initiatives. The amount of funding that foundations provide for projects varies widely. Some foundations provide large amounts of money while others provide small amounts of funds for local projects. Foundations are often managed by a board of directors that may help in the development of RFPs and participate in the grant reviewing process, or the board simply might provide the agency with direction as to what to fund.

There are two main types of foundations: corporate and individual. **Corporate foundations** generally donate a portion of corporate profits to a foundation created by the corporation. Some examples include the Pepsi Foundation and the Wal-Mart Foundation. There are many more out there, including both national and local corporate foundations. **Individual foundations** are foundations created with money donated by a family. Probably the most well known individual foundation is the Bill and Melinda Gates Foundation. In this case, the family contributes money to the start-up of the foundation and may seek donations to continue its existence (Camarena, 2000).

Although less popular, two other types of foundations exist: community foundations and operating foundations. **Community foundations** are public foundations that support a local community and that accept donations to support their programs. **Operating foundations** are foundations that exist for supporting a service or research but that award very few grants.

Foundations hold 501(c)3 nonprofit status. This means that they do not make a profit, but they are different from typical nonprofit organizations that provide specific interventions. In the case of foundations, their intervention is to provide funding to other nonprofits. Some foundations even accept donations and sponsor campaigns to raise money to support the programs that they will, in turn, support through grant funding.

Corporate (and individual) foundations do not necessarily fund only the initiatives of their own companies, so grant writers should not exclude these agencies from a search based solely on the name of the foundation. For example, PepsiCo supplies grants to communities in which it does business that

BEST PRACTICE HINT

In the search process, include all options—regardless of foundation name—based on eligibility requirements.

TABLE 4-6 TYPES OF FOUNDATIONS

Type of Foundation	Description
Community foundations	A public foundation that supports a local community and accepts donations to support its programs
Corporate foundations	A foundation with an endowment from a corporation
Family foundations	A foundation started and run by a family
Operating foundations	A foundation that exists for supporting a service or research but that gives very few grants

support education, health and wellness, diversity and inclusion, and thought leadership. The Gates Foundation does not distribute computers but supports numerous humanitarian programs ranging from sustainable agricultural development to global health challenges.

Foundation grants often have less restrictive requirements for the grant proposal and subsequent program. Foundation grant proposals are often shorter in length. However, it can be challenging to draft a proposal following the guidelines that expresses the breadth of a program (Holtzclaw et al., 2009).

BEST PRACTICE HINT

For the novice grant writer, a small foundation providing funds is a good place to start in the grant writing process. These proposals are often simpler to draft and provide more flexibility than government grants do.

Government Grants

Government grants are awarded by governmental agencies at a variety of levels including federal, state, and local. Local grants are awarded by local government entities such as the mayor's office. State grants are awarded by state governmental agencies. An example is a grant awarded by the state Department of Health. These grants depend on the initiatives of the government including policies and issues of the time.

Federal grants are those grants awarded directly by the federal government and managed by a federal agency. According to Grants.gov (2008b), a federal grant is "an award of financial assistance from a federal agency to a recipient to carry out a public purpose of support or stimulation authorized by a law of the United States." Federal grants are allotted funding based on federal initiatives. Overall, there are 26 federal agencies that award grants. Federal grants can be found in two ways. Many federal agencies list grant RFPs on their websites. However, the best way to search for federal funding is by using Grants.gov.

BEST PRACTICE HINT

Explore both government agency websites and Grants.gov to maximize the grant search.

TABLE 4-7 FEDERAL GRANTMAKING AGENCIES

Agency	Description
Agency for International Development	• "Provides economic and humanitarian assistance in more than 100 countries to ensure a better future for us all" (Grants.gov, 2008b)
Corporation for National and Community Service	• Focuses on service and volunteerism • Programs include AmeriCorp and Senior Corp
Department of Agriculture	• Focuses on anti-hunger and food safety
Department of Commerce	• Focuses on trade
Department of Defense	• Focuses on peacekeeping, homeland security, and humanitarian efforts
Department of Education	• Promotes excellence in education
Department of Energy	• Advances "national, economic and energy security in the U.S." (Grants.gov, 2008b)
Department of Health and Human Services	• Focuses on health
Department of Homeland Security	• Focuses on prevention of terrorism
Department of Housing and Urban Development	• Focuses on home ownership and affordable housing
Department of the Interior	• Focuses on preservation of cultural heritage of U.S. communities including those of Native Americans
Department of Justice	• Focuses on public safety, crime control, fair and just treatment for all
Department of Labor	• Focuses on work environments
Department of State	• "Strives to create a more secure, democratic and prosperous world for the benefit of the American people and the international community" (Grants.gov, 2008b)
Department of Transportation	• Focuses on transportation systems and infrastructure
Department of the Treasury	• Focuses on economics and financial systems
Department of Veterans Affairs	• Focuses on veterans' benefits
Environmental Protection Agency	• Focuses on the environment and environmental health
Institute of Museum and Library Services	• Supports nation's libraries and museums • Focuses on cultural preservation
National Aeronautics and Space Administration	• Focuses on space exploration
National Archives and Records Administration	• Focuses on government record keeping
National Endowment for the Arts	• Focuses on bringing the arts to all Americans
National Endowment for the Humanities	• "Dedicated to supporting research, education, preservation and public programs in the humanities" (Grants.gov, 2008b)
National Science Foundation	• Focuses on the progress of science
Small Business Administration	• Focuses on small businesses
Social Security Administration	• Manages the Social Security System

TABLE 4-8 FEDERAL GRANT CATEGORIES

- Agriculture
- Arts
- Business and Commerce
- Community Development
- Disaster Prevention and Relief
- Education
- Employment, Labor, and Training
- Energy
- Environmental Quality
- Food and Nutrition
- Health
- Housing
- Humanities
- Information and Statistics
- Law, Justice, and Legal Services
- Natural Resources
- Regional Development
- Science and Technology
- Social Services and Income Security
- Transportation

Grants.gov is a centralized website on which all federal agencies can post their RFPs. The federal government has attempted to streamline its grantmaking through the Grants.gov website. Grants.gov was established as part of the 2002 Fiscal Management Agenda proposed by the president (Grants.gov, 2008a). The federal government has divided grants into 21 categories. Each grant must fit into one of the 21 categories, and grants can fit into more than one category.

Other Funding Avenues

In larger institutions, opportunities might arise for what is called an "internal grant." Internal grants are grants offered by an institution to individuals or groups in the institution to implement a project or program. This model is typical in academic institutions. These grants are usually small amounts to assist in research or program development. The funding topics, resources, and requirements for these types of grants are outlined by the internal agency awarding the funding and can be as varied as other RFPs.

BEST PRACTICE HINT

Internal grants are viable options for the novice grant writer. Those providing the grant funding may even assist with the grant writing process.

Tips and Strategies for Finding the Just-Right Grant

As mentioned, finding an appropriate RFP can be challenging. However, the following tips and strategies can make the search process more effective and purposeful:

1. *Explore all avenues.* Strategic grant writers are always exploring and reading RFPs and are strongly networked to find the right RFPs applicable to their

program. Occupational therapy practitioners in an academic setting can utilize the grants administration office or can team up with other academicians with expertise and experience in grant writing.

Informing community members can also lead to some hidden expertise or exposure to an unknown resource. Never forget that the best resources may be right in the community itself. A community member may be connected to a board member of a local foundation. Relationships can be a strong factor in gaining funding from a local agency.

2. *Develop key terms.* Searching a grant database can be overwhelming. Develop a list of key terms that you can use in search engines. These key terms will reduce the number of hits, making the search process more effective and less time consuming.

3. *Explore specific agencies or foundations.* Explore local corporations that may have foundations that support local programs. Also, national agencies sometimes offer grants. For example, the American Diabetes Association (ADA) offers grant funding for diabetes-related projects and RFPs are located directly on the ADA website.

4. *Get to know the neighborhood.* Many communities have foundations that fund projects within the community. These may be family foundations or even corporate foundations. Many corporations fund initiatives where they run their businesses. Some corporations that provide funding nationally may also focus on certain communities. These guidelines will be outlined on the foundation website, in the RFP, or they will be available from the project director.

5. *Get to know the agency or foundation.* Many agencies and foundations have extensive websites that describe their initiatives and priorities. Every grant writer should fully explore the agency to understand its mission and priorities to ensure that the proposed grant program will be a match. Grant writers should always review eligibility requirements to determine whether an idea is a fit with the agency.

6. *Explore what has been funded.* Explore what foundations and agencies have funded prior. You can find this information on funding agency websites or through discussion with the project director. In most cases, agencies and foundations want to fund novel ideas. Exploring previously funded programs also provides insight into the priorities of the agency. Reviewing previously funded programs also provides insight into programs funded in the geographic area and for similar organizations. Successful grant writers take the time to do this research because it can save time and effort.

7. *Note the funding cycle.* RFPs outline the funding cycle. The funding cycle is when the grant is awarded and how long the program will have to be implemented. Funding cycles on grants vary widely. Most common funding cycles last for a year, but different models exists. Some grants provide funding over

multiple years, but sometimes funding is reduced with each year. This approach is often used to promote sustainability of the program and to avoid continued reliance on grant funds for implementation.

8. *Go with what you know.* Grants are available through affiliations. For example, grants are provided to groups connected with specific religious denominations. Organizations can qualify for grant funding based on affiliations including religious, professional, ethnic, or geographic location.

9. *Network, network, network.* Sometimes the easiest way to receive funding is through relationships. Grant writers seeking funding for a program should let others know about the program and the funding amount desired. Contacting foundations and networking with other grant writers can lead to opportunities. Occupational therapy practitioners may need to attend community meetings or join a coalition to develop professional relationships. Relationships and networking can lead to opportunities.

   For example, an occupational therapist providing services pro bono at a local parochial school needed money for supplies and told the principal that services were limited because of a lack of therapy equipment. The school principal did not have funding for the supplies but encouraged the practitioner to attend the school's Parent–Teacher Association (PTA) meetings. After attending two meetings and sharing his concerns regarding the therapy program, the occupational therapist was awarded a small grant from the PTA to pay for supplies including *Handwriting Without Tears.* All the occupational therapist was asked to do was to draft a short request. Through service provision, the parents had already seen the benefits of his service and wanted to support his ongoing services (Kathman, personal communication, December 22, 2008). This example demonstrates the importance of networking, especially for community programming.

10. *Consider what is needed.* If a large amount of funding is needed, do not waste time exploring small funding sources. Targeting a specific amount can decrease the requirement to read a full RFP. Instead, the grant writer can scroll through the RFP to the award amount to help filter which RFPs are a good fit.

11. *Be patient.* Reading RFPs can be a time-consuming process. Many times, upon reading an RFP, a grant writer will think that it is a perfect match for a program except for one small factor that does not fit or qualify. When searching for grants, the occupational therapy practitioner has to be patient. The right grant is out there for any program. One trap many people fall into is modifying their program or project to fit an RFP. The danger in this is that it might no longer be the program the community needs, so practitioners must be careful to avoid this trap.

12. *Use the Internet.* The Internet is the best place to search for grants. There are many resources and Internet databases that you can use to find grants such

TABLE 4-9 GRANT SEARCH DATABASES	
Type of Grant	**Website**
Federal grants	http://www.Grants.gov
Foundation grants	http://www.foundationcenter.org

as Grants.gov. Many foundations have their own websites that offer information about eligibility, funding priorities, funding cycles, and previously funded projects. Practitioners can find specific foundations by searching for specific names on the Internet. Foundationcenter.org provides details on foundation RFPs. Another strategy is simply to explore by using Google or another search engine by typing in keywords.

13. *Become a member of relevant listservs.* Listservs are one method for finding out about grants that can be a significant time-saver in the grant search process. Grants.gov, the federal government's website resource, offers a listserv that sends out recent RFPs. Anyone can sign up for this on the Grants.gov website. Most listservs are free to join, and although they lead to an increase in e-mail volume, it is well worth it. Because RFPs are always being released and initiatives transforming, a grant writer must stay in the know, and listservs are one way to do this. It also helps practitioners keep their eyes open for opportunities instead of having to engage in a comprehensive search.

14. *Use the grant office, if applicable.* In academic settings, practitioners can contact the grants office located on campus. Not only do most grants offices assist with the grant submission, they also assist with the search. Some grants offices maintain profiles on faculty members and will send RFPs that fit with the faculty members' profiles. Some grants offices will assist in searching if keywords are provided to them. Grant offices may use listservs and send grant RFPs as they arise. There are also many resources available at the grants office including information on foundations and what other projects have been funded within the institution. One smart step in the grant search process is to contact the grants office to explore what services they offer and to make good use of them.

15. *Stay positive!* Searching for grants can be a drawn-out and time-consuming process. But chances are a match will be found. The best strategy is for practitioners not to give up and to keep looking for the right fit.

These strategies can aid any grant writer, whether novice or experienced, in easing the RFP search process. After finding RFPs, the next step is to learn to read them in a way that helps determine whether the RFP is a viable match to fund a program.

How to Read an RFP

A request for proposals (RFP) is simply a solicitation to apply for funding for a program. For those without prior experience, reading an RFP can be like reading a document in a foreign language. However, there are key strategies and aspects of an RFP to look for when searching for RFPs to support a program. Just like grants, RFPs come in all shapes and sizes. Federal RFPs are very lengthy and detailed in their requirements. Federal RFPs target a very specific type of program to fund and have to follow government regulations for formatting.

RFPs from other sources can be very short and open-ended, allowing a lot of flexibility in proposals. This is more typical of foundations, but some foundation requirements are also quite lengthy. Because requirements vary across RFPs, the grant writer needs to read the RFP in its entirety, whether large or small.

Although no RFP is the same, the RFPs posted on Grants.gov follow a similar format. Understanding this format can increase the speed and efficiency of the search process. On Grants.gov, search results list grant titles and the name of the granting agency awarding the funds. By clicking the title of an RFP, practitioners can see a brief synopsis of the RFP. This brief synopsis provides basic information such as the following: type of notice, funding opportunity number, date the RFP was posted online, proposal due dates, funding category, number of awards, total funding to be awarded, award ceiling and floor, the **Catalog of Federal Domestic Assistance (CFDA) number**, and whether the grant requires cost sharing or a match. The synopsis also provides information related to eligibility, the agency providing funding, and a link to the full request for proposals.

BEST PRACTICE HINT

Always read the entire RFP, especially if you are pursuing it as a funding source. Getting to know the grant requirements is crucial to writing a grant proposal that matches the requirements appropriately.

Grant Searching Strategies

Just as there is no universal protocol for RFPs, there is no protocol or exact science to searching for grants. However, certain strategies can increase search efficiency. By knowing which aspects of the RFP are essential to review, practitioners can eliminate funding opportunities that do not fit with a program. Strategies for increasing efficiency and effectiveness in searching for an RFP include reviewing key components of the RFP such as eligibility, number of awards, and budget requirements.

Read, and Read Again

Experienced grant writers advise that after finding an RFP that fits the program idea, practitioners should read and reread it. The RFP contains the instructions and guidelines for drafting for the grant proposal and also provides insight into

TABLE 4–10 COMPONENTS OF A GRANT SYNOPSIS ON GRANTS.GOV

Information	Description
Document type	Identifies the type of notice (grant notice, modification of grant notice, etc.)
Funding opportunity number	Government number assigned to the grant RFP
Posted date	Date grant opportunity was posted on Grants.gov
Closing date for applications	Due date for grant proposal
Category of funding activity	Governmental grant category (e.g., health)
Expected number of awards	The number of programs that will be funded
Award ceiling	The highest amount of funding that will be offered to a program
Award floor	The lowest amount of funding that will be offered to a program
CFDA number	Government Catalog of Federal Domestic Assistance number
Cost sharing or matching requirement	Whether the grant requires a cost share or matching to be provided by the agency

what specifically will receive funding. Grant writing is extremely competitive and the RFP provides hints and strategies for receiving the funding. Ultimately, funders want to provide funding to programs that will succeed. In other words, they want to make a good investment. Some RFPs are very long (for example, exceeding 50 pages) and can be time consuming to read, but every component of the RFP is important. One mistake in following the guidelines can lead to rejection of a proposal.

Explore Eligibility

Eligibility is important to consider when reading and reviewing RFPs. Eligibility requirements signify whether a grant is a fit for a program. A key strategy of successful grant writers is to learn to read between the lines of an RFP for hints and strategies that can increase or decrease opportunities for receiving funding. Although it sounds negative, many successful grant writers read grant RFPs with an eye for why their proposal might be rejected. They read the exclusion criteria closely to prevent them from engaging in work related to a proposal that is not eligible. Obviously, if the organization or the program is not eligible, there is no point in moving forward with the proposal—or even finishing reading the RFP.

Discover the Number of Projects Funded

Another piece of information that experienced grant writers look for is the number of projects being funded. If the number is one or two, the grant writer must consider whether applying is worth the time and effort. Grant writing takes time and resources, which must be weighed against the likelihood of funding. Grants that offer a low number of awards but that have a high number of proposals submitted might not be worth the effort. It is important to be strategic when determining the right grant to apply for. Although these efforts sound negative, having a critical eye when reading an RFP can save time and resources.

Writing a grant is never a waste of time because it is a learning process, and even if the program does not receive funding, a basis has been developed that could be used in the future. However, it is also important to maintain a strategic focus when applying for grants to be sure they fit appropriately with the program.

Review Budget Requirements

Always review the budget requirements in an RFP. Budget guidelines can be very specific in what is paid for and what is not paid for. Be sure to read this section in detail. Look for challenges in the budget including major components of need that would not be covered by the grant, such as not paying for food or for travel. Some grants outline few budget exclusions while others have many. Some grants outline specific requirements of the budget such as travel expenses for grant trainings.

Other grants may have requirements such as matching. Matching funds may be quantified as in-kind or sometimes require a cash match. A **cash match** means that the organization, if funded, must match the grant budget based on a certain percentage. For some organizations, coming up with a cash match is difficult. For example, one RFP required a university–community partnership to contribute a 20% cash match for funding technology for a healthy Internet cafe. The community and university were unable to identify a donor and were therefore unable to submit the written proposal (Goulet et al., 2007).

BEST PRACTICE HINT

Grant reviewers usually critique budgets very intensely, so make sure the budget follows the RFP requirements exactly.

When reviewing the budget, practitioners must evaluate whether the budget requirements are too restrictive to the program or simply not feasible. If finding a donor to provide a cash match is impossible, the RFP is not a good match. By reviewing the budget requirements to ensure a match, practitioners take a strategic approach to reviewing RFPs. Submitting a grant proposal that does not follow the budget guidelines can result in the proposal being thrown out of the pool, so it is important to take the time to review these requirements early in the process.

Finding the Right Fit

Searching for an RFP can be an intense process, and knowing how to read and filter RFPs is an essential skill. The focus of reading RFPs should be to find one that fits a program and to filter out those that do not fit. At times, it may seem easier to change the program to fit the funding. But in cases where a community program really stands to make a difference, making changes to the program for the sake of a grant application may not allow the program to remain community driven. Receiving funding for an unsuccessful program benefits no one, so this is an important fact practitioners must keep in mind while searching for RFPs.

Seek Clarification

It is important to understand the requirements of an RFP because simple errors, such as leaving something out or not following proper application guidelines, can cause a grant proposal to be thrown out and not even reviewed. If anything in an RFP is confusing, practitioners should contact the project director for clarification. In rare cases, the project director will not want to be contacted and most often specifies this fact in the grant guidelines. However, most project directors are available by phone and/or e-mail and their contact information is either listed in the RFP or on the website of the funder.

Prior to contacting the project director, practitioners should draft a list of questions to ask to ensure that all questions are asked at one time if possible. Even though program project directors are available to answer questions, it is wise not to waste their time. It is best to plan ahead for conversations with project directors; practitioners should be prepared to describe the program, the organization seeking the funding, and have a list of questions to ask. Practitioners must always act professional by addressing project director using their formal name either in e-mail messages or by phone.

BEST PRACTICE HINT

When contacting program directors, always be prepared. Document what the program director says so that you can share this information with the entire grant proposal writing team.

Sometimes grant agencies provide training regarding grants. Training may be face to face or may take place in the form of a webinar. Attending such events, if practitioners are planning to submit a proposal to the agency, is always wise. Not only does participating in such training clear up any confusion or questions about the RFP, but it also allows practitioners to network with the agency. Sometimes showing an interest or making an investment in the funding organization can lead to funding opportunities. If the principal investigator of the program cannot attend the training, someone on the grant writing team should plan to attend and take notes for the team. If no one on the grant writing team can attend the training opportunities, the PI should contact the program officer to seek an individual training or to discuss ways to learn what was provided in the training.

Contacting the project director to clear up questions is a strategic move. For example, in one case, a team was ready to begin writing the grant proposal when they noticed one small area of confusion in the RFP. Upon contacting the project director, the team discovered that the funding was available only to agencies with undergraduate programs in the health sciences. This fact was not made explicitly clear in the RFP but was important to know. There is no point in putting all the work into a grant proposal just to go unfunded or even unreviewed because of a minor confusion. Always ask!

Before Beginning to Write . . .

Once practitioners find the right RFP, read it thoroughly, and determine it to be a match, they have several other tasks to complete before beginning to write the proposal. These include planning ahead, building a team, and reading the RFP many more times! These tasks are covered later in this book.

The grant writing team should plan and schedule times to write. The best approach is to schedule actual blocks of time to engage in the grant writing process. This includes time for conducting the literature review, collating background data, drafting and getting letters of support signed, drafting the budget, and actually writing the grant. When writing a grant, it is best that practitioners follow well-known strategies used by scholars, including "write what you know," setting up an environment in which to write, and developing a writing process.

BEST PRACTICE HINT

Know your team and their writing abilities. For example, if a team member is proficient with numbers, ask this individual to do the budget. Use the resources of your team members effectively.

Conclusion

Even though not explicitly stated, grant writing and program development can be considered married. Besides bench research grants, for any kind of grant that focuses on addressing a need, a program needs to be developed. Grant proposals include most of the components that are also used in program development: understanding community, identifying a need, identifying a potential solution to address the need, conducting a community assessment, drafting an evaluation plan, and implementing a program (Timmreck, 2003).

As discussed in previous chapters, the premise of this book is that grant writing and program development cannot be separated when discussing occupational therapy practice in community settings. Therefore, occupational therapy practitioners must have basic skills in program development as well as grant writing to be successful in community practice. This chapter covers the basic terminology, principles of, and strategies for finding a grant that fits a program. Occupational therapy practitioners can use all these skills and strategies to be successful in the grant writing process for community practice.

Glossary

Cash match A grant budget requiring the organization, if funded, to match the grant budget based on a certain percentage

Catalog of Federal Domestic Assistance (CFDA) number Government Catalog of Federal Domestic Assistance number assigned to every RFP listed on Grants.gov

Co-investigator Team member listed in the grant proposal who helps with the program implementation and grant goals/objectives

Collaborative grant model A grant proposal that involves a team approach with multiple investigators that each have a specific assigned role in the program implementation

Community foundation A public foundation that supports a local community and accepts donations to support its programs

Consultative grant model A grant proposal that includes a single principal investigator with co-investigators to support the program and experts who act as consultants and provide feedback on the program as it is implemented

Cooperative grant model A grant proposal that includes more than one principal investigator or that is submitted by more than one institution

Corporate foundation A foundation that generally donates a portion of corporate profits to a foundation created by the corporation

Demonstration grant A grant that directly funds programming

Educational grant A grant that focuses on education for a group of people in which the grant writer proposes to implement an educational program focused on a specific topic

Fellowship Funding for a special project completed by an individual for an organization

Foundation A private not-for-profit agency with funds or an endowment to support community programs

Funding cycle Indicates when the grant application is due

Grant eligibility The categories or requirements of an organization to be eligible to apply for grant funding

Grantee Person, program, or project receiving the grant money

Grantors Agencies that provide grant money

Individual foundation A foundation created with money donated by a family

Individual grant model A grant proposal that includes a single principal investigator and that occurs in a traditional academic model with either research or educational grants

Operating foundations A foundation model that exists for supporting a service or research but that gives very few grants

Peer review panel Anonymous team of individuals that reviews the grant proposals and selects which programs receive funding

Planning grant A grant that provides funding for planning the program

Principal investigator (PI) Person in charge of the grant program and a member of the team drafting the proposal

Program officer The main contact for the grant program, who is available to answer questions about RFPs and program requirements

Request for application (RFA) Another name for an RFP; the call or request that granting agencies make public encouraging application for funds. RFPs outline the grant application requirements, due dates, amount of funding, and program requirements.

Request for proposals (RFP) The call or request that granting agencies make public encouraging application for funds. RFPs outline the grant application requirements, due dates, amount of funding, and program requirements.

Research grant A grant that funds research projects that describe a defined research question, research design, data collection, data analysis, sample size, and the need for the proposed research

Subcontract grant model A grant proposal for which one institution acts as the primary investigator with funding subcontracted to another institution to carry out certain aspects of the grant

Training grant A grant focused on developing and implementing a specific type of training for a specific population

References

Anderson, J., Penn, J., Grandgenett, N., & Doll, J. D. (2007). *Omaha Nation Community Response Team—Project Hope*. Garrett Lee Smith Memorial Act State and Tribal Youth Suicide Prevention Grant Program, Substance Abuse and Mental Health Services Administration, $500,000.

Barrett, K. (2002). Facilitating culturally integrated behaviors among allied health students. *Journal of Allied Health, 31*, 93–98.

Begley, K., Doll J. D., Martens Stricklett, K., & Ryan Haddad, A. (2008). *What's in your future? A health education and health professions program for community youth*. Grant provided by the Omaha Urban Area Health Education Center.

Brownson, C. A. (1998). Funding community practice: Stage 1. *American Journal of Occupational Therapy, 52*, 60–64.

Camarena, J. (2000). A wealth of information on foundations and the grant seeking process. *Computers in Libraries, 20*(5), 26–31.

Chaskin, R. J., Brown, P., Ventakesh, S., & Vidal, A. (2001). *Building community capacity*. New York: Walter de Gruyter.

Cochran, T. M., Jensen, G. M., Gale, J. R., Voltz, J. D., Coppard, B. M., Ryan-Haddad, A., et al. (2006, May). *Practice and educational innovation: Revision of rehabilitation roles to extend scarce resources in a rural community*. National Rural Health Conference, Reno, NV.

Cochran, T. M., Goulet, C., Coppard, B. M., Ryan Haddad, A., Wilken, M., & Voltz, J. D. (2007) *Leadership in rural health interprofessional education and practice: Challenges, opportunities...a moral imperative?* Center for Health Policy and Ethics Roundtable, Omaha, NE.

Cohen, J. J., Gabriel, B. A., & Terrell, C. (2002). The case for diversity in the health care workforce. *Health Affairs, 21*(5), 90–102.

Community Anti-Drug Coalitions of American. (1999). *Coalitions 101: Getting started*. Washington DC: Author.

Cross, P., & Voltz, J. D. (2005). *Four Hills of Life Wellness Center Nebraska Native American public health grant*. Nebraska Health and Human Services.

Doll, J. D., & Flecky, K. (2008). *Engaging students: The community as classroom*. Internal grant from the Creighton University Office of Academic Excellence and Assessment.

Edberg, M. (2007). *Essentials of health behavior: Social and behavior health in public health*. Sudbury, MA: Jones and Bartlett.

Gitlin, L. N., & Lyons, K. J. (1996). *Successful grant writing: Strategies for health and human service professionals*. New York: Springer.

Gitlin, L. N., & Lyons, K. J. (2004). *Successful grant writing: Strategies for health and human service professionals*. New York: Springer.

Goulet, C., Cochran, T. M., Voltz, J. D., Wilken, M., Parker, D., & Ryan Haddad, A. (2007). The healthy internet café. Unsubmitted grant to the Department of Agriculture.

Grants.gov. (2008a). About Grants.gov. Retrieved October 14, 2008, from http://grants.gov/aboutgrants/about_grants_gov.jsp

Grants.gov. (2008b). Agencies that provide grants. Retrieved October 14, 2008, from http://grants.gov/aboutgrants/agencies_that_provide_grants.jsp

Grants.gov. (2008c). Who is eligible for a grant? Retrieved October 14, 2008, from http://www.grants.gov/aboutgrants/eligibility.jsp

Health Resources and Services Administration Advisory Committee on Interdisciplinary, Community-Based Linkages. (2008). *Healthcare workforce issues in rural America.* Retrieved October 14, 2008, from http://bhpr.hrsa.gov/interdisciplinary/acicbl/0708 minutes.htm

Holtzclaw, B. J., Kenner, C., & Walden, M. (2009). *Grant writing handbook for nurses* (2nd ed.). Sudbury, MA: Jones and Bartlett.

Ingersoll, G. L., & Eberhard, D. (1999). Grants management skills keep funded projects on target. *Nursing Economics, 17,* 131–141.

Jensen, G. M., Coppard, B. M., & Cochran, T. M. (2001). *Dreamcatchers and the common good: Allied health leadership in generational health and ethics.* Health Resources and Services Administration Allied Health Grant.

Jensen, G. M., & Royeen, C. B. (2001). Analysis of academic-community partnerships using the integration matrix. *Journal of Allied Health, 30,* 168–175.

Jensen, G. M., & Royeen, C. B. (2002). Improved rural access to care: Dimensions of best practice. *Journal of Interprofessional Care, 16,* 117–128.

Jensen, G. M., Ryan Haddad, A., Cochran, T. M., & Coppard, B. M. (2002). *Circles of learning: Community and clinic as interdisciplinary classroom.* Health Resources and Services Administration Quentin N. Burdick Rural Interdisciplinary Training Grant.

Kavey, R. W., Daniels, S. R., Lauer, R. M., Atkins, D. L., Hayman, L. L., & Taubert, K. (2003). American Heart Association guidelines for primary prevention of atherosclerotic cardiovascular disease beginning in childhood. *Journal of Pediatrics, 142*(4), 368–372.

Perry, S. (2008). President Bush calls "faith-based" grant effort "bigger than politics." *Chronicle of Philanthropy.* Retrieved October 10, 2008, from http://philanthropy.com/news/updates/5054/president-bush-calls-faith-based-grant-effort-bigger-than-politics

Reif-Lehrer, L. (2005). *Grant application writer's handbook* (4th ed.). Sudbury, MA: Jones and Bartlett.

Robert Wood Johnson Foundation. (2008). What we fund. Retrieved October 14, 2008, from http://www.rwjf.org/childhoodobesity/approach.jsp

Royeen, C. B., & Jensen, G. M. (1997). *Building community: Collaborative interdisciplinary training among occupational and physical therapists with Native Americans in rural Nebraska.* Health Resources and Services Administration Allied Health Grant.

Ryan Haddad, A., Koenig, P., & Voltz, J. D. (2007). *Caring for the caregiver: An outreach program for caregivers.* Take Action: Healthy People, Places, and Practices in Communities Project. United States Office of Disease Prevention and Health Promotion.

Schmitz, M., & Jeffrey, R. (2000). Public health interventions for the prevention and treatment of obesity. *Medical Clinics of North America, 84*(2), 491–512.

Timmreck, T. C. (2003). *Planning, program development, and evaluation* (2nd ed.). Sudbury, MA: Jones and Bartlett.

U.S. Department of Homeland Security. (2008). Programs. Retrieved October 14, 2008, from http://www.ojp.usdoj.gov/odp/grants_programs.htm

Veugelers, P. J., & Fitzgerald, A. L. (2005). Effectiveness of school programs in preventing childhood obesity: A multilevel comparison. *American Journal of Public Health, 95*(3), 432–435.

Voltz, J. D., Ryan Haddad, A., Hohnstein, S., & Martens Stricklett, K. (2007). *A heart for health: The Health Report Card project.* Nebraska Minority Public Health Association, $500.

Ward, D. (2006). *Writing grant proposals that win* (3rd ed.). Sudbury, MA: Jones and Bartlett.

PROCESS WORKSHEET 4-1 WHAT DO I NEED?

Instructions: Prior to searching for a grant, it is important to consider what is needed to fund the components of the program. This worksheet outlines some potential needs of a typical community program. Complete this worksheet to help begin to determine what is needed. Remember that this is just a beginning brainstorming session to come up with an approximate amount of funding needed for the program.

Funding Needed?

Items Needed for Program	Y	N	Approximate Amount of Funding Needed
Staff salary			
Staff benefits			
Office supplies			
Capital expenses (supplies over $500 such as computers, copier)			
Mileage (use the federal rate)			
Travel expenses			
Therapy supplies			
PR/marketing materials			
Educational supplies			
Internet			
Phone			
Rent			
Other: _____			
Other: _____			

PROCESS WORKSHEET 4-2 **GRANT SEARCH WORKSHEET**

Instructions: Complete this worksheet prior to engaging in a grant search to aid in the process.

Name of Project/Program: _____

Identify key terms:

_____   _____

_____   _____

_____   _____

Basic Project Goals/Objectives:

1. _____

2. _____

3. _____

4. _____

5. _____

Funding amount desired: _____

Key Project/Program Items Needing Funding:

_____   _____

_____   _____

_____   _____

Key Personnel Needing Funding:

_____   _____

_____   _____

_____   _____

PROCESS WORKSHEET 4-3 **RFP ANALYSIS**

Instructions: When reviewing an RFP, use this worksheet to pull out components and apply these concepts to the program.

What to Look For	Analysis
What are the funders looking to fund?	
Identify some key words used in the RFP	
Identify the funding amount	
What is the population the RFP would like to serve? Why do you think this population is significant?	
Is there an evaluation plan required? If so, describe.	
What role would OT have in this grant proposal?	
What is unique about this RFP? Are there any unique requirements?	
Review the budget requirements. Is there anything the grant will not pay for?	
Any other observations?	

PROCESS WORKSHEET 4-4 **REFLECTION: A STEP TO TAKE BEFORE BEGINNING TO WRITE THE GRANT**

Date: _____

Instructions: A short reflection before the writing process begins can help the grant writer or grant writing team ensure that it is ready to embark on the journey of grant writing. These questions are meant to help the grant writer think and consider the grant writing process in preparation for writing. This activity is simply meant to engage the grant writer in reflective practice and ensure that the grant writing process has been well thought out. This reflection can be completed individually or as a group. One suggestion is to have individuals of a grant writing team complete the reflection independently and then come together for discussion.

1. Am I ready to embark on the grant writing process?

2. What strategies can I employ during the grant writing process to ensure success?

3. My fears about writing this grant include . . .

4. What can I do to alleviate my fears?

5. What else do I need to get started?

6. What am I most looking forward to in the grant writing process?

PROCESS WORKSHEET 4-5 GRANT WRITING PLANNING SCHEDULE

Instructions: Use this worksheet to plan the grant writing process. Have team members identify their task(s) for the grant writing team, describe their grant writing process, and identify a deadline for completion of their portion. Be sure to check the RFP deadline to ensure compliance.

Team Member	Task(s)	Grant Writing Process	Deadline to Grant Team

PROCESS WORKSHEET 4-6 **DEVELOPING THE GRANT TEAM**

Instructions: Use this worksheet to identify the grant team.

Name of Grant Project: _____

Grant Model Used: _____

Identify the person responsible for each role. Remember that one person may fill multiple roles depending on the RFP guidelines.

Role	Person Responsible	Qualifications	Contact Information
Principal investigator (PI)			
Co-investigator			
Coordinator			
Funding specialist			
Statistical expert			
Data collector			
Other: _____			
Other: _____			
Other: _____			

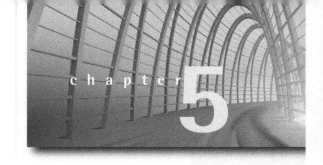

Tips and Strategies for Writing a Successful Grant Proposal

LEARNING OBJECTIVES

By the end of this chapter, the reader will be able to complete the following:

1. Discuss strategies for writing a successful grant proposal for community health programs.
2. Engage in critical self-reflection of grant writing skills.

Key Terms

Grant review
Grant submission
Data Universal
Numbering System
(DUNS) number

Overview

This chapter provides strategies and tips for grant writers who focus on grant writing for community practice. Practitioners can use the information in this chapter to strengthen a grant proposal and increase the likelihood of writing a successful proposal.

Introduction

Grant writing is a unique skill that requires a specific type of writing. Grant proposals need to be written clearly so that reviewers who have never visited a community or experienced a program can understand what is being proposed. A good perspective for understanding grant writing is to approach the task like an artist: The grant writer paints a picture for grant reviewers that

TABLE 5-1 BASIC COMPONENTS OF A GRANT PROPOSAL
• Description of problem
• Outcomes for addressing the problem
• Approach to the problem
• Team members in charge of activity implementation
• How the outcomes will be measured
Source: Markin, K. M. (2006). How to write an outreach grant proposal. *Chronicle of Higher Education.* Retrieved July 21, 2008, from http://chronicle.com/jobs/news/2006/09/2006091501c.htm

draws on the passion and desire of the reviewers so that they will be more likely to support the community program.

Through experience, occupational therapy practitioners can easily see health issues that can be addressed with a variety of community-based or community-built programs. Earlier chapters discuss the processes of program development. To a funder, a successful program is only as good as the grant writer behind it. The grant writer's challenge is to convince the funder that an idea is worth supporting financially (Bordage & Dawson, 2003). In a way, grant writing and grant funding are a gamble for the grant writer and the funder because there is no guarantee of a successful outcome.

According to Lusk (2004), a grant proposal should be "thought of as a sales pitch, a request for dollars for a product" (p. 367). Grant proposals always must be very clear and concise, providing the reviewer with a clear picture of the program and the proposed outcomes (Inouye & Fiellin, 2005). According to Markin (2006) and as outlined in Table 5-1, there are five basic components to a grant focused on community programming including a problem description, the outcomes for addressing such a problem, the approach to the problem, the team members in charge of activity implementation, and how the outcomes will be measured. Using these basic tenets lays the groundwork for a successful grant proposal.

BEST PRACTICE HINT

A poorly written grant proposal reflects poorly on a program. Ask others to review the proposal to ensure that writing quality is sufficient.

The Basics of Writing a Grant Proposal

Grants are not written in the same way in which a typical paper is written. Grant proposals require a distinct technical style, and some writers find it challenging to alter their writing style for grant proposals. Proposals are written in a straightforward manner and describe exactly what is proposed, what activities the program entails, and when those activities will be completed (Dahlen, 2001). Proposals must be succinct and to the point so that reviewers can read them easily. Grant writers must always consider the writing guidelines outlined in the request for proposals (RFP) and follow these guidelines in detail (Bordage & Dawson, 2003). By following the format of the RFP and using the titles and categories of information discussed in the RFP, grant writers can align the grant proposal with the RFP and facilitate an efficient review process. Following this format clearly identifies how the grant proposal complements the initiatives of the funding agency. Not following the RFP guidelines will lead to a poor review or to the proposal being rejected for review.

In most cases, grant narratives have a page number limit that the grant writer should follow strictly. Grants longer than the page limit are usually discarded and do not even reach reviewers. Writers who are wordy and include too much in a grant proposal require a good editor. Editors need to be able to help the grant writer be more succinct but not lose the point of the proposal. Collaborating with a good editor can be a great way to ensure that the proposal follows the guidelines and is well written.

Grants should never be written in the first or second person and should always be checked for spelling and grammatical errors (Bordage & Dawson, 2003). Grant writers need to use simple language that is easy to read and understand. However, using simple language can be a challenge in occupational therapy, and grant reviewers may be unfamiliar with occupational therapy terminology and practice. In such cases, grant writers may need to use portions of the narrative to define and describe treatment approaches. The grant writer must judge and consider the reviewers' level of understanding. When writing grants, it is best to avoid assumptions. But, for example, if your organization is applying for a grant from the American Occupational Therapy Foundation, you could assume the reviewers understand occupational therapy terminology. Consider whether the use of jargon is appropriate. If jargon is required, evaluate whether the jargon needs to be defined or explained to help reviewers understand the proposed program (Inouye & Fiellin, 2005).

Grant writers also need to follow the referencing style required by the grantor (Bordage & Dawson, 2003; Holtzclaw, Kenner, & Walden, 2009). If the reference guidelines are not listed, the grant writer should contact the project director or use a style with which they are familiar. At this point, grant writers should use their best judgment. If the grant is a small amount from a foundation, the likelihood of a preference for citations is small. However, for funding agencies such as the National Institutes of Health or the Robert Wood Johnson Foundation, specific guidelines for referencing are identified in the RFP. Some requests for proposals allow reference lists to be included in an appendix, but others require it be counted in the total page numbers of the narrative section.

BEST PRACTICE HINT

When writing a grant, grant writers need to consider the knowledge and expertise of the reviewers so that they write a grant that uses terminology the reviewers understand.

As mentioned, grant writers should always avoid making assumptions in grant proposals. In most cases, the grant reviewers do not know the community or the

TABLE 5-2 GRANT WRITING TIPS
• Be succinct
• Be detailed but not wordy
• Never write in the first or second person
• Follow citation requirements of grantor
• Check for spelling and grammatical errors
• Follow RFP page limit guidelines

proposed program. The grant proposal must be written in a way that describes all the details of the community and program based on the level of the reviewers' understanding. Again, grant writers must use their best judgment. If the grant application is to a local community foundation, the grant reviewers likely understand the needs of the community. For federal grant applications, it is less likely that any of the reviewers know and understand the community. Based on the funding agency and reviewers, the grant writer decides how much detail and description to include. In general, grant writers should avoid blanket statements and, instead, always be specific about activities and outcomes. Vagueness in a proposal can come off as disorganization or a lack of sureness about the proposed program.

If resubmitting a proposal that has been rejected by another agency, the grant writing team must be sure to modify the proposal to meet the requirements of the new agency. Although it is perfectly acceptable to submit a proposal for an idea that was rejected by another agency, the grant writing team needs to conduct a thorough review and ensure that the revised proposal follows the guidelines of the new RFP.

Grant proposals require a delicate balance: Grant writers must describe the problem, the proposed programmatic solution, and the proposed outcomes in detail; however, too many details can distract reviewers from the purpose of the proposal. Grant writers need to be strategic in what to include in the grant proposal. When justifying the need, the grant writer should only use statistics and facts that support the proposal and not use facts simply to include references. A grant proposal should target the specific need but not necessarily try to describe every detail of the community.

BEST PRACTICE HINT

Rework rejected grant proposals and send them to alternate funding agencies.

General Tips for Writing a Successful Grant Proposal

The writing style used in grant proposals is very basic compared to scholarly or theoretical writing. Successful grant proposals are clear and objective in laying out the plans of the program (Bordage & Dawson, 2003). A grant writer must succinctly articulate not only the goals, objectives, activities, and outcomes but also the organization and management of the project. These aspects include important factors such as how the program participants will be recruited, where activities will take place, and who will complete the public relations activities for the program. For most grant proposals, these details need to be included in the proposal. For some grant proposals, the details of the program need not be written out but can be demonstrated with an organizational chart (Markin, 2006).

Grant writers employ a variety of techniques and strategies to increase the likelihood of a grant being funded. These techniques and strategies are common to the world of grant writing. To be successful at grant writing, the occupational therapy practitioner should take the following strategies into account when writing a grant proposal:

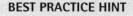

BEST PRACTICE HINT

Let others know how they can help collect necessary documentation such as support letters, biosketches, and other needed documents.

1. *Plan ahead.* Part of writing a successful grant proposal is being prepared to write it when the request for proposals (RFP) is released. An example of planning ahead includes having a file containing demographic data for the community. Portions of an existing grant proposal can be modified and reused when a new RFP with a similar focus is released. Grant writers can draft and have on file letters of support or memorandums of understanding from partnering or supporting agencies. Gathering biosketches or curricula vitae of all potential members of the grant proposal team ahead of time saves time and increases the efficiency of the grant writing process once an RFP has been released.

   Grant writers should consider spending anywhere from 3 to 6 months planning and writing a grant proposal (Davidson, 2005; Falk, 2006). Some grants may require more planning time than others, and according to one authority, 9 months of planning should occur to develop a National Institutes of Health (NIH) grant application (Davidson, 2005). If the grant proposal requires application to the institutional review board (IRB), the time needed for approval of research must be taken into account (Falk, 2006; Gitlin & Lyons, 1996; Barnard, 2002).

   Planning ahead also applies later on in the grant writing process. A successful grant writer is always prepared for last-minute challenges such as difficulty uploading an electronic application or retrieving necessary signatures from the grants office. Grant writers must allow time for these challenges so that they can remain calm and not allow these disturbances to keep them from submitting the grant on time.

2. *Always use the grant RFP language.* The request for proposals provides insight into how the grant should be written. By using the language used in the RFP, grant writers can demonstrate a knowledge and understanding of what the fun-

der proposes. Furthermore, the language used in the RFP is often the language understood by the reviewers. This tip can lead to the approval of a project because reviewers require less time to understand the basis of the program.

3. *Be in contact with the grant program manager.* Unless stated in the request for proposals or on the funder's website, it is accepted and most of the time expected for grant writers to contact the program manager, sometimes referred to as the grant project director (Inouye & Fiellin, 2005). Grant writers can ask the program manager whether a program has the potential for funding or about anything that is unclear in the RFP. Asking these simple questions can help avoid errors in the grant proposal. If questions arise, grant writers should contact program managers early in the grant writing process to ensure that the grant proposal follows all RFP guidelines appropriately. Many program managers are available by phone or e-mail. The benefit of e-mail communication is that it documents the answers to questions asked. However, if a question arises, it is better to have it addressed no matter what the form of communication. Grant writers recognize that, although program managers are helpful in answering questions related to the RFP, these individuals have little to no impact on the review and approval process (Inouye & Fiellin, 2005).

4. *Support ideas with evidence-based literature and appropriate data.* Grant proposals require background support and literature along with demographic and epidemiological data to profile the population to be served by the project or program. Proposals should include the latest evidence-based literature and statistics to support the background or statement of need for the project (Inouye & Fiellin, 2005; Barnard, 2002; Bordage & Dawson, 2003).

5. *Choose a theoretical approach.* Some funding agencies require the grantee to identify a theoretical approach to the program. Whether required or not, identifying a theoretical approach or approaches strengthens a proposal. Grant proposals can use theoretical approaches in two ways: Theories can be used as a framework for the program. In other words, the program is based on the theoretical framework. Or the grant proposal can implement and, in a sense, test the viability of the theory. If using a specific theoretical approach, the grant writer must discuss and define the approach to be used in the grant proposal. The writer can include this discussion in the background portion of the grant proposal and should include complementary literature to support the approach's relevance to the proposed program.

Grant writers must clearly explain and link the theoretical approach to the purpose and outcomes of the proposed program (Colwell, Bliss, Engberg, & Moore, 2005). Although a theoretical approach can be used to strengthen the proposal, if the theory is controversial or unknown to the reviewers, it might be beneficial to leave it out.

6. *Describe the program's novelty* (Falk, 2006). Many grantees are seeking new ideas to solve community problems. If an idea is novel, then a description of its importance and innovation is important (Dahlen, 2001). Reviewers may read multiple proposals. When your program contains a unique idea, it can stick out from a crowd. Extrapolating on why the program is unique and innovative is very important because of the competitive nature of grants.

   To ensure that an idea is novel, the grant writer needs to conduct research, such as a literature review, to explore other programs. Innovation does not mean the idea is complicated, and a completely new idea can be a twist on an existing idea. For example, a proposed idea may be utilized in a program for a population that has never attempted anything like it before, or a program may be modified to account for community cultural beliefs. In a grant, the program should always be described thoroughly, and innovativeness should not be claimed without clear explanation of how it fits into the program.

   A grant writer should keep in mind the economic context of the times. In difficult economic times, granting agencies may fund innovative ideas or may focus on funding previously successful projects to maintain them. The occupational therapy practitioner can explore RFPs or talk to program managers to determine the focus of the funds.

7. *Tie the program to the bigger picture.* Although a program may be focused on a certain population or community, it is important to tie the program to the larger picture. One strategy is to tie the grant proposal to national initiatives (Holtzclaw et al., 2009). For health, it is easy to tie to federal documents like Healthy People 2020, which outlines goals and objectives related to the health of the U.S. population (U.S. Health and Human Services, 2008). Relating to documents such as these can strengthen a proposal.

   Tying the program to larger initiatives explores the possibility of applying the program, if successful, to other communities and populations. Many funders look for programs that can be replicated to address public health issues.

8. *Seek out a mentor* (Davidson, 2005). Grant writing is not a solo process. Successful grant writers seek out experts and mentors to assist in all stages of the grant writing process (Inouye & Fiellin, 2005). Occupational therapy practitioners writing grants should find mentors who have had success with grants and implementing successful programs. These individuals can provide invaluable insight along the way.

   Beyond having a mentor, a grant writer may want a support system to assist in the grant writing process. Consultants and experts can help with drafting portions of the grant proposal or assist in reviewing proposal drafts (Inouye & Fiellin, 2005; Holtzclaw et al., 2009). Successful grant writers often employ a support system during the grant writing process.

9. *Recruit a reviewer.* Sometimes the grant writing process can be so consuming, the grant writer loses context. In this instance, the grant writer has written so much that he or she loses objectivity. Having a neutral eye that can provide constructive feedback on the project or the written proposal can assist in clarifying aspects of the project or the grant. It is crucial to have others review the grant, whether along the way or before submitting the final proposal (Holtzclaw et al., 2009).

10. *Be cognizant of the deadline.* A grant writer must always be cognizant of the grant deadline. In the grant writing process, it seems that no matter how much the grant writer plans ahead, there still never seems to be enough time!

    Depending on the setting, certain procedures and policies might require additional time (Dahlen, 2001). For example, in academic institutions a grant proposal may need to be reviewed and approved by multiple parties prior to its submission. The grant writer must plan time for these procedures in the grant writing process. Failure to follow institutional procedures can lead to the inability to submit a proposal after a lot of hard work.

    Once some requests for proposals are released, there is not a lot of time in which to complete the proposal. Federal grant agencies are especially known for releasing RFPs with little turnaround time. Grant writers need to be organized and plan carefully because most federal proposals include a narrative of around 25 pages, which takes time to draft.

11. *Create a schedule for grant planning and writing.* Communication with all parties involved is a necessity at all points in the grant writing process. Scheduling meetings ahead of time for review and setting aside time for writing can ensure that the grant is written in a timely and collaborative manner. Creating a schedule and scheduling meetings prior to grant submission ensures that all aspects of the grant are thoroughly reviewed and ready to submit.

12. *Plan ahead for challenges* (Davidson, 2005). The federal government has instituted electronic submissions, and many other grantors are now moving to this format. Successful grant writers do not let challenges in technology prevent submission of the grant. Most grantors are not flexible with deadlines. If the grant is to be mailed, successful grant writers ensure that the application is mailed in a timely manner using features such as delivery confirmation so that the grant writer knows the grant proposal reached its destination. These details may seem insignificant but are factors that can mean the difference between getting funded or not.

Strategies for Maximizing Funding

Anyone can write a grant. However, grant writers can use specific strategies to maximize their chances of receiving funding. Beyond following general guidelines as previously discussed, including certain factors in a grant proposal can increase or decrease a program's likelihood of receiving funds. The following strategies can strengthen any proposal.

Strategy 1: Integrate a Strong Team

Community grants are never completed independently because collective change requires commitment and the strengths of many (Holtzclaw et al., 2009). Building a collaborative team of community stakeholders and others in the community who can affect the proposed program is an important step in completing a successful grant proposal. A thriving team includes individuals who have a commitment to the community and who have demonstrated a track record of success and also people who can work well with a diverse team. Roles and responsibilities will vary based on the grant, and there are multiple models to follow when approaching a community grant. In Chapter 3, different grant models and team building strategies are discussed. Grant writers increase their likelihood of funding if the grant proposal discusses the strengths and expertise of the team members, identifying the skills and strengths each team member brings to the program.

> **LET'S STOP AND THINK**
>
> Think back to the grant models discussed in Chapter 3. Describe as many as you can remember.

Strategy 2: Demonstrate a Track Record

For some granting agencies, particularly the National Institutes of Health (NIH), an established track record of the principal investigator and the grant team can determine whether a proposal receives funding (Barnard, 2002). In the case of NIH grants, the grant team must have a demonstrated successful record of prior grant acquisition, research, and publications. Although these factors do not guarantee funding, a demonstrated successful record is taken into account by grant reviewers.

When identifying members of the program team, prior successes and accomplishments are important to consider. For funding agencies, such as NIH, the requirements of an established record of success is well known and understood by researchers applying for funds. However, in any grant proposal, establishing a track record of success is important. Several strategies can be utilized to demonstrate a track record for a community grant proposal.

One strategy is to identify how the grant team has worked together previously. Grant writers essentially need to "sell" their idea to funders, so it makes sense that funders are more likely to fund groups that have demonstrated success and have an established relationship with the community.

Another strategy is to integrate data from pilot studies or community surveys. Data of this nature demonstrate an existing infrastructure and knowledge of the community. Discussion of existing collaboration and partnerships is important to demonstrate that relationships within the community have been previously established. In this discussion, the grant writer should identify how long the community

---

TABLE 5-3 DEMONSTRATING A TRACK RECORD IN A GRANT PROPOSAL

- Prior record of success with grant acquisition
- Established community partners
- Established community initiatives
- Team success
- Demonstration of community knowledge
- Community involvement

---

partnership or the team has worked together to address community problems (Jensen & Royeen, 2001). Identifying specific programs and collaborative activities can also be used to strengthen a proposal. Examples of items to discuss include formal community agreements, collaboratively developed programs, cross-training, and shared grant funding (Jensen & Royeen, 2001).

Another method for demonstrating a track record is to discuss the project team members' involvement in the community even if in a different capacity than proposed in the current program. The grant writer should be creative and be honest about community involvement and past experience. Examples include active engagement in a community coalition, on a community advisory board, or in volunteerism with local agencies. Overall, identifying a track record lets funders know that this program has a strong chance for success if funded because of the established infrastructure.

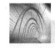

BEST PRACTICE HINT

Maintain a record of participation in community activities that can be used later in grant applications to demonstrate commitment and knowledge of the community.

Strategy 3: Go Interprofessional

In any health-related projects, forming an interprofessional team establishes a comprehensive view of a health problem and a collective team of experts who can address the issue. An interprofessional team also offers more services by utilizing the expertise of each person involved (Mu, Chao, Jensen, & Royeen, 2004). In a grant proposal, using the perspectives and expertise of multiple professionals demonstrates that the grant team views the issues and proposed program comprehensively.

Strategy 4: Identify the Outcome

Ultimately, grantors "want to see their money make a difference" (Markin, 2006). The focus of any grant proposal should be on the outcomes of the program. Outcomes identify the specific differences or changes the program will make if it is implemented. The bottom line for grant funders is to have their funding implement positive change in health behaviors or specifically affect some health issue. Rarely do funders provide money simply to provide services.

Grant writers should be specific about the proposed outcome, but also realistic. A grant proposal should identify how the proposed program is going to make a difference and why it is significant to fund over other programs. The proposal must outline any new knowledge that will be an outcome of the project, whether it be research or simply best practices, and how it can be applied. Successful grant writers discuss how the proposed outcomes will contribute to the local community being served and beyond (Beitz & Bliss, 2005).

Strategy 5: Identify Resources

Funders provide money to proposals that sound like they will be successful. Remember, a grant reviewer has only the proposal with which to determine whether the program is worth the risk of supporting (Inouye & Fiellin, 2005). Therefore, a strong grant proposal identifies a need and strategies for addressing that need and also names resources that will enhance the program's success (Falk, 2006).

Resources include assets the organization receiving funding can offer to the program such as space or equipment. Other resources include a strong team and established partnerships, as previously discussed. Identifying resources is as important as identifying needs to demonstrate that funding will not go to waste. Funders want to know what strengths and resources can enhance the program. A successful grant writer includes a thorough discussion of resources in the grant proposal.

Strategy 6: Be Prepared for Rejection

Every grant writer gets rejected, even if he or she has a successful track record. A grant proposal can be well written and include all the components of success and still be rejected. Grants writers should always seek feedback from the reviewers as to why the proposal was rejected and reflect on what could be done differently the next time (Holtzclaw et al., 2009). Sometimes rejection is simply a result of the number of proposals submitted or because the program does not exactly fit with the organization's priorities. In any case, finding out the reasons for the rejection is important so that the grant writer can learn which strategies worked and which need to be revised.

As discussed in previous chapters, grants are trendy and reviewers can be fickle. Grant writers should employ every strategy possible to increase the likelihood of funding, but accept rejection with dignity.

Mistakes to Avoid

In the grant world, small errors can prevent an application from being reviewed and accepted. For example, one grant writer mailed a grant proposal to a funding

---

TABLE 5-4 NIH COMMON GRANTEE MISTAKES

- Lack of strong rationale
- Too much proposed
- Unclear goals
- Uncertain about future directions
- Too much background data
- Poor design
- Proposal unrealistic

Source: National Institutes of Health. (2005). Common mistakes in NIH applications. Retrieved July 18, 2008, from http://www.ninds.nih.gov/funding/grantwriting_mistakes.htm

---

agency using overnight delivery. When the grant writer called the agency to confirm receipt, she received an angry reply from the project director emphasizing that he could not spend time signing for overnighted packages (K. Begley, personal communication). In this situation, the grant was sent back to the grant writer unopened and obviously unreviewed.

Grant writers can make a plethora of mistakes in the grant writing process. Some of them are thematic in nature, while others are procedural, such as not following the request for proposals guidelines. The National Institutes of Health (NIH, 2005) outlines common mistakes made by grant writers that cause a grant to go unfunded and sometimes unreviewed. For example, mistakes made in NIH proposals include lack of a strong rationale to support the proposed program, too many ideas proposed for one program, unclear goals, lack of explanation of future direction if funded, too much background data included in the proposal, poor research or program design, and an unrealistic proposal. Other grant writing mistakes discussed in the literature include wordiness in the proposal, errors in the budget, grammatical errors, use of jargon, the proposal does not match funder's objectives, the budget justification does not match with the budget, inappropriate statistics are included unrelated to establishing the need, and submission after due date (Ward, 2002; Egan, 2006).

Grant writers should be aware of these common mistakes and plan to avoid them. A grant proposal should be focused and should not try to solve all of the community's problems. Grantors want to provide funding to feasible projects. To avoid mistakes, grant writers need to be strategic and write a proposal that describes a targeted and well-developed program idea. To avoid mistakes, grant writers should review the grant proposal carefully. Peer review can also help. Grant writers should never let a small mistake in following the guidelines or writing mechanics be a barrier to funding a need.

Submitting the Grant

Once a grant proposal is complete, the submission process begins. To determine the submission process, the grant writer must review the grant agency submission guidelines. The submission process can be time consuming, so the grant writer must be prepared, allowing time for troubleshooting. Grant writers should never wait until the last minute to submit. For example, a power outage could prevent a grant from being submitted on time. The grant writer needs to review and understand submission procedures prior to the day the grant needs to be submitted.

Some foundations have online applications that require the entire application be submitted online. For such foundations, the grant writer should draft the grant proposal in a word processing program, and then copy and paste the components into the online form. By following this process, the grant writer ensures that the applying agency retains a copy of the proposal and can check spelling and grammatical errors easily in the word processing document.

Federal agencies have also transitioned to online submission (Holtzclaw et al., 2009). The online application process can be very time consuming, especially the first time, and requires specific software. Although the process may be similar across federal agencies, specific paperwork requirements are outlined in each grant's submission guidelines. Grant writers must follow these procedures strictly to ensure that the application is received. Applying agencies also are required to have a data universal numbering system, or a DUNS, number. The DUNs number is a governmental number assigned to an agency. Organizations apply for a DUNS number through the federal government. Applying organizations also must complete required forms prior to **grant submission**, such as specific budget worksheets. Grant writers must review all included documents prior to submission to ensure that all the forms are completed correctly. If the forms are not completed correctly, the online submission will fail.

Because the requirements for online grant submission are always changing, grant writers must be sure to review the submission guidelines and review Grants.gov for the latest steps to completing this process. In some cases, especially in federal grants, the submission process is so complicated that it may require training.

BEST PRACTICE HINT

Prior to submitting a proposal participate in an online webinar or organizational training on the federal requirements for uploading grants.

Others granting agencies require the grant proposal to be mailed in. In many instances, funders require copies of the proposal for each reviewer. Grant writers should not miss this little detail! Sending an inappropriate number of copies can hamper the review process. Again, submission details are outlined in the submission guidelines. Due dates are also important to review. In some cases, a grant is due in the project director's hands on a certain date, and in other cases, the grant simply must be postmarked by a certain date. Grants writers should choose a mailing procedure that guarantees arrival of the proposal. Taking care of these minute details can ensure that the grant proposal arrives in a timely and appropriate fashion. As discussed previously, minute errors can cause a grant proposal not to be submitted or reviewed.

The Review Process

Once a grant has been submitted to a funding agency, it can take as little as a few weeks to almost a year to hear back about the status of the funding (Gitlin & Lyons, 1996). Grant reviewers are usually volunteers who donate their time to reviewing grant applications for funding agencies. Most RFPs will identify when the funding announcements will be released, but agencies do not always follow these guidelines strictly.

If the grant is funded, the agency receiving funding will receive an announcement letter informing it of the amount of funding received (Holtzclaw et al., 2009).

BEST PRACTICE HINT

If a grant proposal is rejected and returned without reviewer feedback, the principal investigator should contact the project director to seek this information.

The grant team must be cognizant that grants are proposals and that sometimes the amount of funding requested is not the amount of money granted. In other cases, the grantor may require modifications to the proposal prior to final approval. Often, in cases where modifications are required, the applying agency is allowed a certain amount of time to revise the budget and activities to match with the allocated funding. When changes are required, the budget often needs to be resubmitted to the funding agency for approval. The grant writer should always be prepared for the chance to revise and must follow the appropriate guidelines for the revisions (Holtzclaw et al., 2009).

Many review panels use a numbering system to rank proposals, and whether the proposal is funded or not, the proposal will be returned with a ranking (Gitlin & Lyons, 1996; Holtzclaw et al., 2009). In some grant requests for proposals, the points are distributed differently for different sections. Grant writers should become familiar with the grant sections and the points allocated to each section. These points are directly tied to the ranking system. The rankings inform grantees where their proposal fits in among all the other applicants (Holtzclaw et al., 2009).

If a ranking is not provided, then often reviewers' comments are provided. When a grant is not funded, the ranking and comments are of utmost importance because they provide the grant writer with feedback on the proposal and provide a learning experience for any grant writer, experienced or not. Furthermore, the reviewers may indicate that the grant writer has an opportunity for resubmission. Resubmission usually occurs under the conditions that the components on which the reviewers commented will be revised or clarified.

When receiving a rejection, grant writers need to relax and recognize that all grant writers have been rejected at some time (Holtzclaw et al., 2009). Reading the reviewers' comments after working so hard on a grant proposal can be challenging.

Grant reviews often identify weak areas or areas that lack clarity in a grant proposal. The best approach is to take the comments as food for thought that can be applied to the next grant proposal. If the comments do not make sense or the reason for not receiving funding is unclear, the grant writer should contact the agency and seek further feedback. Most agencies do not mind clarifying or discussing strategies for a possible resubmission.

Conclusion

Writing a grant proposal takes a unique skill set and requires a specific writing style and a strategic approach. The submission and review process are also important components in the grant writing process. Ultimately, becoming a good grant writer requires practice, and everyone receives rejection at some point. Following the guidelines outlined in this chapter and avoiding common mistakes can aid in writing a successful grant proposal that will support a community program.

Glossary

Data Universal Numbering System (DUNS) number A governmental number assigned to an agency; organizations apply for a DUNS number through the federal government
Grant review A process in which a submitted grant proposal is reviewed and ranked by a peer review panel. This peer review panel is organized by the funding agency
Grant submission The process by which a grant writer submits a grant outlined in the RFP

References

Barnard, J. (2002). Keys to writing a competitive grant. *Journal of Pediatric Gastroenterology and Nutrition, 35*, 107–110.

Beitz, J. M., & Bliss, D. Z. (2005). Preparing a successful grant proposal. Part 1: Developing research aims and the significance of the project. *Journal of Wound, Ostomy, and Continence Nursing, 32*(1), 16–18.

Bordage, G., & Dawson, B. (2003). Experimental study design and grant writing in eight steps and 28 questions. *Medical Education, 37*, 376–385.

Colwell, J. C., Bliss, D. Z., Engberg, S., & Moore, K. N. (2005). Preparing a grant proposal—part 5: Organization and revision. *Journal of Wound, Ostomy, and Continence Nursing, 32*(5), 291–293.

Dahlen, R. (2001). Fundamentals of grant writing: Lessons learned from the process. *Nurse Education, 26*(2), 54–56.

Davidson, N. O. (2005). Grant writing and academic survival: What the fellow needs to know. *Gastrointestinal Endoscopy, 61*(6), 726–727.

Egan, K. (2006). Top 10 grantwriting mistakes. Retrieved October 21, 2008, from http://www.nsls.info/articles/detail.aspx?articleID=49

Falk, G. W. (2006). Turning an idea into a grant. *Gastrointestinal Endoscopy, 64*(6), S11–S13.

Gitlin, L. N., & Lyons, K. J. (1996). *Successful grant writing: Strategies for health and human service professionals*. New York: Springer.

Holtzclaw, B. J., Kenner, C., & Walden, M. (2009). *Grant writing handbook for nurses* (2nd ed.). Sudbury, MA: Jones and Bartlett.

Inouye, S. K., & Fiellin, D. A. (2005). An evidence-based guide to writing grant proposals for clinical research. *Annals of Internal Medicine, 142*, 274–282.

Jensen, G. M., & Royeen, C. B. (2001). Analysis of academic-community partnerships using the integration matrix. *Journal of Allied Health, 30*, 168–175.

Lusk, S. L. (2004). Developing an outstanding grant application. *Western Journal of Nursing Research, 26*(3), 367–373.

Markin, K. M. (2006). How to write an outreach grant proposal. *Chronicle of Higher Education.* Retrieved July 21, 2008, from http://chronicle.com/jobs/news/2006/09/20060 91501c.htm

Mu, K., Chao, C. C., Jensen, G. M., & Royeen, C. (2004). Effects of interprofessional, rural training on students' perceptions on interprofessional health care services. *Journal of Allied Health, 33*(2), 125–131.

National Institutes of Health. (2005). Common mistakes in NIH applications. Retrieved July 18, 2008, from http://www.ninds.nih.gov/funding/grantwriting_mistakes.htm

Non-Profit Guides. (2008). Guidelines for grant writing. Retrieved July 18, 2008, from http://www.npguides.org/guide/index.html

U.S. Health and Human Services. (2008). Healthy People 2020: The road ahead. Retrieved October 21, 2008, from http://www.healthypeople.gov/hp2020/

Van Sant, S. (2003). Successful grant writing strategies. *Leadership, 32*(4), 16–19.

Ward, D. (2002). The top 10 grant-writing mistakes. *Principal, 81*(5), 47.

PROCESS WORKSHEET 5-1 **GRANT CRITIQUE**

Instructions: Use this form to critique a grant proposal. This form can be used by the grant writer or a reviewer.

Criteria	Y	N	Comments
Does the title represent the proposal?			
Does the abstract describe the program?			
Is the purpose of the program clear in the proposal?			
Is the problem statement or question clear and specific?			
Is the problem statement supported well?			
Is the program innovative?			
Does the program make a significant community impact?			
Does the grant include measurable goals and objectives?			
Is the evaluation program appropriate?			
Is the program or project feasible?			
Is the sustainability plan appropriate?			
Is the budget appropriate?			
Are proposed costs reasonable?			
Do the references follow the RFP guidelines?			
Are the appendices appropriate?			

PROCESS WORKSHEET 5-2 **PLANNING WORKSHEET**

Instructions: Find an RFP and then identify each component of the grant to assist in planning for the grant writing process.

1. Identify page number limit: _____

2. Identify grant due date: _____

3. Identify referencing style: _____

4. Describe the reviewers: _____

    a. Based on the review panel, what jargon should you avoid:

        i.   _____

        ii.   _____

        iii.   _____

5. Identify language used in the request for proposals:

    _____

6. Questions for project director:

    _____

    _____

7. Identify theoretical approaches:

    _____

8. Describe program's novelty:

    _____

    _____

9. Identify national initiatives that relate to program:

    _____

10. Identify mentors or peer reviewers:

    _____

11. Other important information:

    _____

    _____

PROCESS WORKSHEET 5-3 **GRANT PREPARATION CHECKLIST**

Instructions: Use this worksheet to develop and maintain a grant proposal timeline for successful completion and submission.

Item	Targeted Completion Date	Completed
Letters of support		
Memorandum of understanding		
Grant team members selected		
Biosketches of team members		
Grant paperwork		
Grant mailing/submission		
Other: _____		
Other: _____		
Other: _____		

PROCESS WORKSHEET 5-4 **ANALYZING YOUR TRACK RECORD**

Instructions: Use this worksheet to identify your established track record to include in a grant proposal.

Category	Description
Publications	
Presentations	
Community partners	
Community participation	
Prior grants received	
Community surveys	
Community trainings	
Other: _____	
Other: _____	

Perform a SWOT analysis of your program. SWOT stands for Strengths, Weaknesses, Opportunities, and Threats. Identify current strengths, weaknesses, opportunities for growth, and threats to the community project or program. You can use this analysis as a tool to get you thinking about the program in a broad sense. SWOTs can be used for individual analysis or can be performed by a group of people who then come together to compare and contrast analyses. The SWOT is a tool that is unique to each program and can be used to analyze current infrastructure, strategize future steps, or even simply explore the feasibility of beginning a program.

Strengths	Weaknesses
Opportunities	**Threats**

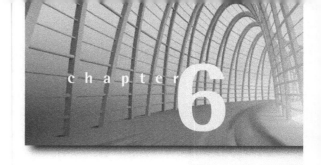

chapter 6

Understanding the Community: A Necessary Step Before Grant Writing

LEARNING OBJECTIVES

By the end of this chapter, the reader will be able to complete the following:

1. Examine the importance of assessing community strengths.
2. Reflect on how to use strengths as a program foundation in practice.
3. Apply the principles of community capacity building through process worksheets.

Key Terms

Capacities
Community assessment
Community capacity building
Community competency
Community mapping
Community stakeholders
Community-based participatory research (CBPR)
Community-centered approach
Needs assessment

Overview

Not only do communities have needs, they also have strengths. In this chapter, the focus is on assessment. But prior to assessment, occupational therapy practitioners need to ascertain their own views of community. In this chapter, the discussion focuses on community needs, strengths, and capacities and provides occupational therapy practitioners with tools for success in community practice.

Introduction

If following a **community-centered approach** to community practice, the occupational therapy practitioner needs to approach the community

---

TABLE 6-1 COMMUNITY CAPACITIES

- Community stakeholders
- Community partnerships
- Physical spaces
- Funding
- Professional expertise
- In-kind donations

---

holistically, exploring all aspects of the community and its members. This process includes identifying challenges and community needs and exploring and discovering community **capacities**. Capacities are strengths or foundations that a program can build upon to meet a need or solve issues (Goodman et al., 1998). Capacities are sometimes identified as strengths or assets (Chaskin, 2001).

Community Capacity Building

Even in poor and underserved communities, strengths exist. Approaches that build upon these strengths have been shown to lead to successful community change. Needs may be easy to identify, but what are community strengths? Strengths and capacities vary among communities, but some examples include **community stakeholders**, community partnerships, physical spaces, and resources such as funding, expertise, and in-kind donations (Goodman et al., 1998).

For example, in a grant project, the community assessment revealed a strong desire in an urban Latino community for access to yoga, but no classes or instructors were available in the community. Through community partnerships, the occupational therapy practitioner was able to find a local church parish that would donate the space, music, and mats for a weekly yoga class. The priest even participated in the yoga classes, which increased parishioner participation. The parish also assisted by advertising the classes in church bulletins and around the community. A small grant was garnered that funded the instructor for multiple sessions. Donations were collected that made the program sustainable beyond the funding period (Voltz, 2003).

In this simple example, it is easy to identify the capacities, including the donation of space and supplies, free community advertising, and stakeholder buy-in, which facilitated increased participation. Without the capacities, the program would not have been nearly as successful because funding would have had to be distributed to space rental, equipment rental, and advertising. If this had been the case, there would have been few funds left to support the instructor, which would have impeded the success of the program. Furthermore, the grant writer was able to demonstrate in the proposal the commitment of the community and the multiple assets the community had to offer.

Occupational therapy practitioners believe in capacity. Collectively, the profession values ability, and occupational therapy practitioners act as facilitators, recognizing and building upon capacity even in traditional practice settings. For example, despite adversities and in the context of problem solving with the patient, practitioners focus on a patient's capacities to attain occupational engagement in a manner that suits the individual's needs. This same concept applies to community practice, and in fact is the theme of community practice because without capacity, there is little opportunity for positive change.

According to Chaskin, Brown, Venkatesh, and Vidal (2001), **community capacity building** is defined as "the interaction of human capital, organizational resources, and social capital existing within a given community that can be leveraged to solve collective problems and improve or maintain the well-being of that community" (p. 7). In other words, community capacity building focuses on the strengths of a community as the starting point for facilitating change. Chaskin and colleagues suggest this occurs through leadership development, organizational development, community organizing, and interorganizational collaboration (Chaskin et al., 2001; Chaskin, 2001). Occupational therapy practitioners in community practice can play a role in each one of these components. As stated by Scaffa (2001), the "community model is dedicated to supporting individuals and communities and empowering them to make their own choices" (p. 7).

Capacity building is simply taking the idea that capacity exists and using it as a foundation for positive change. It is "exemplified by a set of core characteristics and operates through the agency of individuals, organizations, and networks to perform particular functions" (Chaskin, 2001, p. 295). Chaskin (2001) proposes that community capacity building occurs in six interacting dimensions: (1) characteristics of community capacity building; (2) levels of social agency; (3) functions of community capacity; (4) strategies for building community capacity; (5) conditioning influences; and (6) outcomes. According to Chaskin (2001), there are four fundamental characteristics of community capacity building: a sense of community felt by community members, commitment among community members to the community and its well-being, the ability and desire to come together to solve community problems, and the existing capacities and resources in the community. Without these characteristics, a community will struggle to build capacity beyond its current status.

To mobilize a community toward building capacity, capacity must exist on a variety of levels of social agency, including the individual, organizational, and network levels. Capacity building can occur only if commitment exists across all levels. Obviously, individuals need to be committed to the community, and the organizations within the community need to desire to promote and enhance the

TABLE 6-2 DIMENSIONS OF COMMUNITY CAPACITY BUILDING

Dimensions	Description
Dimension 1: Characteristics of community capacity building	• Sense of community • Level of commitment of community members • Ability to solve problems • Access to resources
Dimension 2: Levels of social agency	• Individual • Organization • Network
Dimension 3: Functions of community capacity	• Intent to engage in community capacity
Dimension 4: Strategies for building community capacity	• Unique to each community
Dimension 5: Conditioning influences	• Factors that facilitate or impede capacity building
Dimension 6: Outcomes	• Outcomes for community capacity building

Source: Chaskin, R. J. (2001). Building community capacity: A definitional framework and case studies from a comprehensive community initiative. *Urban Affairs Review, 36*(3), 291–323.

community. The entities must be networked and in a congruent relationship to move toward building capacity.

Similar to community needs, community capacities vary from community to community. Each community has its own strategies for building capacity. Common examples of community capacity include community participation, leadership, access to resources, and a sense of community among members (Chino & DeBruyn, 2006). Many people identify community capacity building as empowerment, but it moves beyond empowerment because it enables community members to take action.

Communities looking to build capacity need to identify the conditioning influences that either facilitate or impede capacity building. Examples of challenges to community capacity building include health disparities, policies, and discrimination (Chaskin, 2001). Last, mentioned as item 6 in the preceding list, communities have to determine their outcomes for community capacity building. Defining the goal and outcome helps mobilize the community toward change.

Kretzmann and McKnight (1993) identify capacity building as "the alternative path," especially in struggling urban neighborhoods (p. 5). They argue that community capacity building is successful for two reasons:

1. History has shown that community change occurs successfully only when community members are committed to investing their own willpower and resources to facilitate change. This means that communities themselves are the change agents, and "experts" from the outside cannot facilitate community change without community buy-in and effort.
2. External assistance may not be an option and neither will it be enough to sustain the change. Community change takes time, and external grants and federal money do not usually last long enough to sustain the transformation (Kretzmann & McKnight, 1993).

According to Kretzmann and McKnight (1993), community assets are of three kinds: individuals, associations, and institutions. This model is similar to the model introduced by Chaskin (2001). In this asset-based approach to community development, McKnight and Kretzmann (1996) acknowledge that each individual in the community has something to offer. Groups of individuals can mobilize to form an association and affect institutions. This is an important approach to take in program development and grant writing in community practice. The issues that these programs propose to solve are usually sizable and require the mobilization of many in the community. Viewing a community for its assets and finding the strengths in all help mobilize the community to change and ensure that the community program utilizes assets from all levels.

In community practice, capacity is a way of looking at a community through a new lens. In health care, providers are trained to look and search for deficits. It can be a true challenge to analyze an individual and group of people for their capacities. However, occupational therapy practitioners are primed to explore capacity and problem solve to facilitate independence among clients in traditional practice settings. The same principles apply to communities, just with a broader perspective (Priest, 2006; Wynn, Stewart, Law, Burke-Gaffney, & Moning, 2006).

As discussed repeatedly in this book, successful community programs are community-driven and follow a community capacity model. In other words, occupational therapy practitioners in community practice should focus on the needs identified by the community and build on existing strengths and infrastructure. It is becoming more relevant to identify needs and focus on resources and capacities in grant proposals as grantors want to ensure funding leads to success as evidence in community capacity building models.

> ### LET'S STOP AND THINK
>
> What challenges do you think occupational therapy practitioners face by using a capacity-building approach?

Types of Community Capacity

In a grant proposal, the grant writer must discuss the resources in a community that provide a foundation for the proposed program. Multiple types of community capacities exist on which to build a program. This approach ensures that the community is viewed as an asset with resources to contribute to the proposed program.

One of the most valuable capacities in a community is its individual community members (McKnight & Kretzmann, 1996). Individual community members have ideas, expertise, and skills to contribute. Community members who choose to engage in community mobilization and program development are often called community stakeholders (Lasker & Weiss, 2003). Community stakeholders are individuals in the community who have demonstrated leadership and who other members of the community trust. These individuals can be a great resource in facilitating community buy-in and also have valuable knowledge about the community. These individuals can provide insight into needs and capacities and even indicate where to find information needed for an assessment or what approaches would work best when developing and implementing programs (Howe, Billingham, & Walters, 2002). In a culturally diverse community, where the occupational therapy practitioner is the minority, community stakeholders can also act as cultural advisors, providing information and consultation related to culture (Jensen & Royeen, 2001). Community stakeholders have unique expertise about the community, so it is wise for practitioners to identify and acknowledge their capacity.

In the next chapter, the importance and process of developing community partners are discussed in detail. Community partners are another form of capacity in communities. According to Walens, Helfrich, Aviles, and Horita (2001), "Partnering with community agencies creates a win-win situation for all parties and when well done expands the context for occupational therapy practice" (p. 73). Relationships across communities with different agencies and individuals can demonstrate to a grant reviewer commitment and community knowledge. These capacities indicate the likelihood that a funded program will be successful. It is crucial to demonstrate in the grant proposal the strength and history of community partnerships as capacity and a basis upon which to build a program.

Community partnerships can supply strong capacity in a community program by sharing resources, staff, and through general collaboration. Academic–community partnerships are one type (Jensen & Royeen, 2001; Suarez-Balcazar, Hammel, & Helfrich, 2005). Another type is community coalitions,

---

LET'S STOP AND THINK

Consider a meaningful community to you. Who are the stakeholders in that community? What roles do they play and why are these roles important to the community?

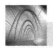

BEST PRACTICE HINT

A stakeholder might not always be the most obvious person or the person with the most education or prestige. Community stakeholders are those who know and love their community. In some communities, stakeholders are evident political leaders, and in others stakeholders are long-standing residents.

where a group of people in the community come together for a specific purpose (Cohen, Baer, & Satterwhite, 2002).

Foster-Fishman and associates (2001) propose that community capacity is collaborative in nature. Members of the collaborative team need to have a shared vision, value diversity, share power, and form positive relationships with those outside the team, including policymakers. Formation of collaborative relationships and partnerships is a strategy that mobilizes community members toward a cause and utilizes the resources of multiple entities.

Cultural traditions and shared culture are capacities that can easily be overlooked. In some cases, Western approaches to health concerns may not be relevant, and traditional cultural practices can be a strong resource to facilitate community change. Culture acts as a community asset by providing a framework for health beliefs and healing (McKnight & Kretzmann, 1996; Penn, Doll, & Grandgenett, 2008). Cultural traditions, rituals, and beliefs can be used as a foundation for community programs and as resources for building community capacity. For example, a community may come together for cultural events, mobilizing members in a unified activity.

An example of the impact of culture as an asset is the Last Buffalo Hunt Program (Ekstrum, 2006). This program uses the cultural traditions of a Plains Indian tribe to promote healthy lifestyles. It focuses on educating Native American community members about the last buffalo hunt and integrates this with a walking program and dietary education. The program is built upon the cultural tradition and value of the buffalo hunt and is successful in engaging many community members because of the meaning this tradition holds and its relevance to the community's culture.

In many communities, physical spaces can be used for programming such as spaces in faith community buildings, public parks, and community centers. These spaces are a form of community capacity. Many organizations can donate or offer space at low cost. These assets can help facilitate program participation by acting as public gathering places that the community trusts and enjoys.

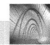

BEST PRACTICE HINT

Remember to ask not only for financial support but also in-kind support and other donations that can facilitate a program.

Other important capacities exist in communities, including funding and in-kind donations. Corporations may be able to offer support for events and activities, and they sometimes can partner on initiatives and be a great resource for a project. Some communities might be rich with in-kind donations including everything from space to a plethora of services. Practitioners must ask and assess what community members can provide to access this wealth of capacities (McKnight & Kretzmann, 1996).

Community Competency

To be successful in both program development and grant writing, occupational therapy practitioners must have knowledge and understanding of the community and the role they can play within the community. To address authentic community needs, their practice must be community-centered and focused on developing programs in partnership with the community. In other words, occupational therapy practitioners must exhibit community competency (Lochner, Kawachi, & Kennedy, 1999).

Community competency is the understanding of the dynamics of a community including its people, resources, and challenges. It requires practitioners to know the community's history, culture, context, geography, language, literacy, views, and diversity (Robinson, 2005, p. 339). With community competency, practitioners can build a structure for occupational therapy that does not damage or destroy the community (Robinson, 2005).

Community competency aligns with capacity building and provides a foundation for program development. Occupational therapy practitioners should follow a community-centered model and focus on the needs and strengths identified with and by the community. Developing community competency is an ongoing process and occurs through experience. Practitioners who wish to develop community competency first acknowledge that community members are the experts about their own problems and that a collaborative solution needs to be developed to address these problems (McKnight & Kretzmann, 1996).

Challenges to Developing Community Competence

Community health problems are large and complex and require an occupational therapy practitioner possess skills for implementing programs and also the desire to grow and to learn about the community. According to McKnight (1995), healthcare professionals sometimes enter a community and explore its problems through the lens of their profession. This view is what McKnight terms "professionalization," and it can break down community relationships and do a community more harm than good.

For example, as described by McKnight (1993), prior to the arrival of a bereavement counselor in a small community, when a loved one passed away neighbors would visit and talk, providing support for each other. Upon the arrival of the counselor, neighbors stopped calling each other, assuming that the bereaved was visiting the bereavement counselor. Because community members perceived the bereavement counselor as the expert in this area, neighbors no longer felt they could provide adequate support for or talk to each other about their grief. Ultimately, the arrival of the bereavement counselor led to a breakdown in relationships and local support in the community.

Healthcare professionals must understand the impact of their role in the community and acknowledge that the impact can be negative. For some practitioners, the concept of professionalization may be difficult to accept because their intentions are not malicious; but healthcare professionals who do not practice in a community-centered way can damage a community consciously or unconsciously (McKnight, 1993).

Another example of the problem of professionalization relates to sustainability. Unfortunately, many times a professional enters a community and sets up a program only to leave when grant funding runs out. This approach is poor and damaging to the community in the following ways:

LET'S STOP AND THINK

Think about a community you belong to. Are there any examples of professionalization? How did it affect the community?

- *A need has been identified.* When a need is identified in the community but no sustainable solution follows, this can leave a community feeling frustrated and overwhelmed. No one in the community may have the ability or expertise to address the problem, leaving the community helpless.
- *The program provided a temporary fix.* The program developed and supported through grant funding may have been a great solution but was not sustainable. This means the program only helped some in the community and was a great solution for a few. Or the program addressed the need only so far and more aspects of the need require intervention. Either way, the community has been left high and dry.
- *A breakdown in trust has occurred.* When an individual or group develops a program for a community and then leaves after grant funding dissolves, the community may develop disdain or mistrust for future groups attempting to address a need in the community. No matter if an entirely new group decides to address a problem, there may be associations, bad feelings, or fear of the same process occurring again. This is why sustainability must be built in from the beginning rather than viewed as an afterthought.

Professionalization can also occur in the identification of needs. As healthcare providers, occupational therapy practitioners are trained to find problems based on occupational engagement. However, the needs identified by the occupational therapy practitioner may not be the same as the needs identified by the community. Implementing a program based on needs identified by the practitioner that do not meld with the community's ideas will lead to the failure of the program. The key to community programs is that they are successful only with community buy-in.

Occupational therapy practitioners working in community settings must work toward community competency and always take a community-centered approach, both for the benefit of the community and for a successful, sustainable practice. Developing community competency requires experience and learning skills in a community practice setting. It also requires that the occupational therapy practitioner face many challenges, build on strengths, and always focus on the identified needs and goals of the community. Understanding the community will lead to successful grant writing as the OT will be able to write effectively describing the community.

TABLE 6-3 PRINCIPLES OF COMMUNITY-BASED PARTICIPATORY RESEARCH (CBPR)

Principle	Description
Community identity	• Community members identify common shared interest, language, values, and possibly geographic location.
Builds on community strengths	• Focus on assets and community resources.
Equitable partnership	• Both researchers and community members collaborate throughout the research process. • This includes identifying the research question, data collection, data analysis, and dissemination.
Co-learning	• Reciprocity in skills and knowledge. • Researchers are not only viewed as experts, but also as community members.
Balance between knowledge and intervention	• Research is to the benefit of the community and not just knowledge for knowledge's sake.
Context	• Focus on context and the multiple determinants of health status.
Systems approach and development	• Integrates all aspects of both the community and the research process.
Dissemination	• All engaged in the project receive the results of the project. • Dissemination is completed in a way that the community understands. • Dissemination may involve community members in scholarly endeavors such as publications and/or presentations.
Commitment	• CBPR takes a long time and researchers must come into relationship with the community.

A Strategy for Building Community Capacity: Community-Based Participatory Research

Community-based participatory research (CBPR) is a collaborative model of research with an aim "to increase knowledge and understanding of a given phenomenon and integrate the knowledge gained with interventions and policy and social change to improve the health and quality of life of community members"

(Israel, Eng, Schulz, & Parker, 2005, p. 5). CBPR is a type of participatory action research that focuses on the inclusion of community members and organization in the development of the research question and research design. By its very nature, participatory action research "involves consumer participation, power, leadership, and knowledge generation in the development, implementation, and evaluation of services" (Taylor, Hammel, & Braveman, 2004, p. 73). This research is community-driven and involves community members in the research process. Those engaged in CBPR may find themselves as a "participant within the community, joining as a partner by assuming various roles, such as community organizer, meeting facilitator, community advocate, activist, or resource person for technical or material aid" (Taylor et al., 2004, p. 74).

According to Israel and associates (2005), CBPR embodies nine principles that establish it as a unique method for exploring community issues. These principles describe the complexity and intensity of the CBPR model. "The knowledge produced from the CBPR experience is intended to be an impetus for increasing critical consciousness among community members, which can lead to the development of sustainable interventions, community-based decisions, and plans for meaningful change" (Foster & Stanek, 2007, p. 43). As stated earlier, this is the role that occupational therapy practitioners want to have in community health and believe can occur if occupations are understood and needs are addressed. CBPR also provides a strategy for attaining community competence and avoiding professionalization.

CBPR is a challenging in-depth research method. It can help practitioners address health disparities and create infrastructure to address actual community needs. This chapter touches only briefly on it as a tool to use in community practice. A strong understanding of research and community is required to engage in successful CBPR. Because CBPR follows a team model, occupational therapy practitioners can be a great asset to a CBPR team in a community practice setting.

Community Capacity Building and Grant Writing

"Many recent grantmaking efforts by foundations and government funding sources have focused on building community capacity," making it relevant to explore the role of community capacity in occupational therapy practice and grant writing (Andrews, Motes, Floyd, Flerx, & Lopez-De Fede, 2005, p. 86; Chaskin et al., 2001). Successful grant proposals outline the resources that will provide support and infrastructure for the proposed project and emphasize community assets as the basis of the program. In every grant proposal, community needs also are fully outlined and discussed.

Identifying Authentic Needs and Capacities

In a grant proposal, the grant writer must identify the community needs. A *need* is simply a gap. For example, a significant number of older adults in a community may lack transportation, so there is a need for a transportation system for seniors. A **needs assessment** is "a systematic set of procedures that serves to identify and describe specific areas of need and available resources in a given population" (Brownson, 2001, p. 101). It is a tool "for identifying local needs, placing needs in order of priority, and targeting resources to help resolve local problems deemed to be of critical importance to the welfare of the community" (Beaulieu, 2002, p. 3). It can assist in establishing which interventions could potentially address community needs. In a grant proposal, the needs assessment drives the goals and objectives and is used to justify the rationale for the program.

A needs assessment paints a picture of the issues a community faces. These challenges can be overwhelming, and only identifying the gaps without also acknowledging community assets does not truly help a community move toward healthy change. Instead of focusing on needs assessment, this chapter focuses on community assessment (Sharpe, Greaney, Lee, & Royce, 2000). A comprehensive **community assessment** focuses on assets and capacities as much as needs.

To understand a community comprehensively, practitioners must follow an approach that explores capacities and needs. Grantors want to know about both so that they can understand the community and the proposed program. Therefore, both should be included in a grant proposal. The job of the grant writer is to describe problems and issues as well as identify strategies to address these problems. A capacity-building approach provides a strong foundation for a program, increasing its likelihood of receiving funding.

A community assessment provides information on current conditions in the community, any issues the community faces, and contributing factors to community issues. The purpose of a community assessment is to identify, support, and mobilize "existing community resources and capacities for the purpose of creating and achieving a shared vision" (Sharpe et al., 2000, p. 206). Assessments can also determine community readiness for change, which is important to know because it can lead to the success or failure of a program (Jumper-Thurman & Plested, 2000).

Communities do not want to be assessed at the drop of a hat, and some communities have faced extensive assessment previously. Some grant RFPs require a new and formalized assessment be performed. But prior to engaging in a new assessment protocol, occupational therapy practitioners should use existing assessment resources and explore what assessment data are already available. Not only does this save time, it ensures that the community does not feel that it is being overassessed or violated by the assessment (Clark et al., 2003). Chapter 9 will discuss data and its use in a grant proposal in more detail.

When a new assessment is not required, it is appropriate to use existing data as part of the assessment. In fact, using existing data is part of the assessment process and a way to come to fully understand the community. Assessment data from only one source is often viewed as weak and does not represent to grant reviewers a comprehensive understanding of the community and its challenges and assets, so practitioners should be sure to gather data from several sources.

In some cases other than when required by the RFP, such as when a community does not have existing assessment data, the existing data are outdated, or data on the issue at hand do not exist, practitioners will need to conduct a new and unique assessment. Practitioners can use multiple approaches to collect community data including surveys, focus groups, interviews, and community forums or town hall meetings (Clark et al., 2003; Timmreck, 2003; Sharpe et al., 2000). Each of these methods asks the community to identify its challenges and assets.

BEST PRACTICE HINT

In the grant proposal, use data from multiple reliable sources to establish the need for funding for the program.

A Community Assessment How-To

Prior to conducting a community assessment, occupational therapy practitioners need to determine the target population being assessed and the approaches to be used in gathering assessment data. The goal of the community assessment is to gain a comprehensive understanding of the community including needs and resources (Timmreck, 2003).

Multiple methods should be used. This means that both quantitative and qualitative approaches should be used. When practitioners choose a method, they should consider the community and the pros and cons of the different approaches. Which approaches have the most likelihood of arriving at a true understanding of the community's needs and resources?

Surveys are a cost-effective and comprehensive way to ascertain community needs and capacities. However, a challenge to using a survey includes developing or finding a reliable questionnaire (Timmreck, 2003). Another consideration is the method of implementation, including how the survey will be distributed, collected, and analyzed. Practitioners should also consider the reading level and primary language of the community to ensure that all community members are assessed accurately. They must determine the sample size and identify the sample population prior to distributing the survey. Last, they must plan for costs including printing and postage. Sometimes incentives increase the response rate, which ensures comprehensive information.

LET'S STOP AND THINK

What strategies for assessment do you think will have the most benefit for gathering data for program development and grant writing?

Focus groups pull together small groups of people to answer a collection of questions (Timmreck, 2003; Sharpe et al., 2000; Clark et al., 2003). These groups are an effective approach to discussing an issue. Strategies to consider when conducting focus group include ensuring that the gathered group represents the community, asking open-ended questions that target information that needs to be gathered, providing for the time it takes to implement and analyze the focus group results, and possibly recording and transcribing the results. To conduct focus groups, a member of the project team should be aware of how to run the group and ask the questions to keep the group on task (Clark et al., 2003). A focus group should be an open forum in which participants feel free to express their opinions openly (Timmreck, 2003). Providing food or another incentive increases participation. Challenges to using a focus group include the time it takes to develop good questions, identify and recruit participants, and interpret the themes from the meeting.

BEST PRACTICE HINT

To avoid bias in responses, the leader of the focus group should be a neutral individual who has no influence on the program or grant.

Interviews gather the opinions of a small group within the larger community (Timmreck, 2003). One strategy is to interview key informants and community stakeholders to gain a representation of the community (Sharpe et al., 2000). Interviews can ask and seek opinions regarding needs and assets. Interviews can be done in person or via phone. A phone interview allows individuals to participate in the interview from any location, which assists in compliance. One benefit to an interview is the opportunity to probe an individual based on the person's unique responses, which can provide valuable data. Interviews are an effective method to use with people who have any kind of sensory disability including vision problems and individuals who may be illiterate or at a low literacy level (Brownson, 2001).

A community forum or town hall meeting gathers individuals from the community to discuss community issues (Sharpe et al., 2000). These meetings can provide a significant amount of information about the community that can be used in a grant proposal or for program planning. If these meetings are formalized and minutes exist, practitioners can pull data directly from the archives to use as assessment data. The challenges to this approach are finding a location, taking the time to educate and invite community members, and taking the risk of low turnout at the meeting. Forums allow for an open space in which community members can provide dialogue and multiple perspectives.

Another effective method for assessing the community is **community mapping**. Community mapping is the process of creating a visual representation of the community's assets (PolicyLink, 2008). Community mapping can be a complex process using geographic information systems (GIS) or it can be done more simply by interviewing stakeholders and identifying capacities in the community (Sharpe et al., 2000). Community mapping does not have to be geographic in nature. Community mapping can be done by simply going out into the community and identifying resources and capacities. Truly, this type of community assessment promotes awareness of what the community has to offer. In the example described earlier in this chapter about the yoga program, community mapping was used to identify potential facilities that would offer space for free or at low cost. Community mapping can also help an organization know which other organizations or

TABLE 6-4 BENEFITS AND CHALLENGES TO COMMUNITY ASSESSMENT METHODS

Method	Benefits	Challenges
Survey	• Collects data from many community members • Time effective • Can provide both quantitative and qualitative data • Can be done using the Internet or via mail	• Response rate might be low • Requires data analysis • Requires understanding of survey design • Community members might not have access to the Internet
Focus groups	• Provides an in-depth perspective • Gains the opinions from a small targeted group	• Time consuming • Recruiting participants
Interviews	• Allows for probing of a problem • Allows participation for individuals with visual disabilities • Low cost	• Time consuming • Requires data analysis • Small representation of community
Community forum	• Allows for dialogue among community members	• Low turnout • Logistical challenges of location and encouraging participation • Requires marketing to community

groups provide similar services or where gaps in services exist in a community (Raise Your Voice, 2005).

One approach to exploring assets and capacities using community mapping is the KEEPRA approach. KEEPRA stands for Kinship, Economic, Education, Political, Religions, and Associations. The purpose of the KEEPRA approach is to ensure that community information is gathered in the main topic areas of interest in a community. The KEEPRA focuses on demographics, epidemiological data, and the beliefs and values of the community.

TABLE 6–5 KEEPRA APPROACH	
Kinship	Includes family structure, housing, food provision, care for children, and so forth
Economic	Includes economic status, earnings, production rates, work quality, job market, unemployment levels, and so forth
Education	Includes beliefs about education, graduation rates, college rates, level of education achieved, and so forth
Political (i.e., government)	Includes policies, regulations, political affiliations, advocacy, and so forth
Religious	Includes religious affiliations, spiritual beliefs, values, norms, morals, customs, and so forth
Associations	Includes community organizations, service provision to community, and so forth

Source: Adapted from Beaulieu, L. J. (2002). *Mapping the assets of your community: A key component for building local capacity*. Retrieved July 12, 2008, from http://srdc.msstate.edu/publications/227/227_asset_mapping.pdf

No one method exists for community assessment. A program or organization may choose to utilize multiple methods. Occupational therapy practitioners ultimately must determine which approaches are most effective in specific communities. In some cases, grant requirements will drive the type of assessment used, but the key is to focus on community capacity and remain community centered.

Conclusion

Multiple approaches for discovering and coming to understand a community comprehensively exist. This chapter focuses on capacity-building approaches to community assessment and program implementation. Community assessment is important for program development and must be included in a grant proposal.

Glossary

Capacities Strengths or foundations that a program can build upon to meet a need or face challenges

Community assessment An assessment performed to identify, support, and mobilize "existing community resources and capacities for the purpose of creating and achieving a shared vision" (Sharpe et al., 2000, p. 206)

Community capacity building "The interaction of human capital, organizational resources, and social capital existing within a given community that can be leveraged to solve collective problems and improve or maintain the well-being of that community" (Chaskin et al., 2001, p. 7)

Community competency The process of understanding the dynamics of a community including its people, its resources, and its challenges and building a structure for occupational therapy within that community that does not damage or destroy the community

Community mapping An assessment method that produces a visual representation of the community's assets

Community stakeholders Individuals in the community who have demonstrated leadership and who other members of the community trust

Community-based participatory research (CBPR) A collaborative model of research that aims "to increase knowledge and understanding of a given phenomenon and integrate the knowledge gained with interventions and policy and social change to improve the health and quality of life of community members" (Israel et al., 2005, p. 5)

Community-centered approach An approach to program development focused on the community's perspective

Needs assessment A tool "for identifying local needs, placing needs in order of priority, and targeting resources to help resolve local problems deemed to be of critical importance to the welfare of the community" (Beaulieu, 2002, p. 3)

References

Andrews, A. B., Motes, P. S., Floyd, A. G., Flerx, V. C., & Lopez-De Fede, A. (2005). Building evaluation capacity in community-based organizations: Reflections of an empowerment evaluation team. *Journal of Community Practice, 13*(4), 85–104.

Beaulieu, L. J. (2002). *Mapping the assets of your community: A key component for building local capacity.* Retrieved July 12, 2008, from http://srdc.msstate.edu/publications/227/227_asset_mapping.pdf

Brownson, C. A. (2001) Program development: Planning, implementation, and evaluation strategies. In M. Scaffa (Ed.), *Occupational therapy in community-based practice settings.* Philadelphia: F. A. Davis.

Chaskin, R. J. (2001). Building community capacity: A definitional framework and case studies from a comprehensive community initiative. *Urban Affairs Review, 36*(3), 291–323.

Chaskin, R. J., Brown, P., Ventakesh, S., & Vidal, A. (2001). *Building community capacity.* New York: Walter de Gruyer.

Chino, M., & DeBruyn, L. (2006). Building true capacity: Indigenous models for indigenous communities. *American Journal of Public Health, 96*(4), 596–599.

Clark, M. J., Cary, S., Diemert, G., Ceballos, R., Sifuentes, M., Atteberry, M., et al. (2003). Involving communities in community assessment. *Public Health Nursing, 20*(6), 456–463.

Cohen, L., Baer, N., & Satterwhite, P. (2002). Developing effective coalitions: An eight step guide. In M. E. Wurzbach (Ed.), *Community health education and promotion: A guide to program design and evaluation* (2nd ed., pp. 144–161). Gaithersburg, MD: Aspen Publishers.

Ekstrum, J. (2006). *The Last Buffalo Hunt Program.* Unpublished program.

Foster, J., & Stanek, K. (2007). Cross-cultural considerations in the conduct of community-based participatory research. *Family and Community Health, 30*(1), 42–49.

Foster-Fishman, P. G., Berkowitz, S. L., Lounsbury, D. W., Jacobsen, S., & Allen, N. A. (2001). Building collaborative capacity in community coalitions: A review and integrative framework. *American Journal of Community Psychology, 29*(2), 241–261.

Goodman, R. M., Speers, M. A., McLeory, K., Fawcett, S., Kegler, M., Parker, E., et al. (1998). Identifying and defining the dimensions of community capacity to provide a basis for measurement. *Health Education Behaviors, 25*(3), 258–278.

Howe, A., Billingham, K., & Walters, C. (2002). Helping tomorrow's doctors to gain a population health perspective—good news for community stakeholders. *Medical Education, 36*(4), 325–333.

Israel, B. A., Eng, E., Schulz, A. J., & Parker, E. A. (2005). Introduction to method in community-based participatory research for health. In B. A. Israel, E. Eng, A. J. Schulz, & E. A. Parker (Eds.), *Methods in community-based participatory research for health.* San Francisco: Jossey-Bass.

Jensen, G. M., & Royeen, C .B. (2001). Analysis of academic–community partnerships using the integration matrix. *Journal of Allied Health, 30,* 168–175.

Jumper-Thurman, P., & Plested, B. A. (2000). Community readiness: A model for healing in a rural Alaskan community. *Family Psychologist,* Summer, 8–9.

Kretzmann, J. P., & McKnight, J. L. (1993). *Building communities from the inside out: A path toward finding and mobilizing a community's assets.* Skokie, IL: ACTA Publications.

Lasker, R. D., & Weiss, E. S. (2003). Creating partnership synergy: The critical role of community stakeholders. *Journal of Health and Human Services Administration, 26*(1), 119–139.

Lochner, K., Kawachi, I., & Kennedy, B. P. (1999). Social capital: A guide to its measurement. *Health and Place, 5*(4), 259–270.

McKnight, J. (1995). *Careless society: Community and its counterfeits.* New York: Basic Books.

McKnight, J. L., & Kretzmann, J. P. (1996). *Mapping community capacity.* Evanston, IL: Institute for Policy Research.

Penn, J., Doll, J. D., & Grandgenett, N. (2008). Culture as prevention: Assisting high-risk youth in the Omaha Nation. *Wicazo Sa Review, 23*(2), 43–61.

PolicyLink. (2008). *Community mapping.* Retrieved July 18, 2008, from http://www. policylink.org/EDTK/Mapping/

Priest, N. (2006). "Motor Magic": Evaluation of a community capacity building approach to supporting the development of preschool children. *Australian Occupational Therapy Journal, 53,* 220–232.

Raise Your Voice. (2005). *Community mapping guide compass.* Retrieved July 18, 2008, from http://www.actionforchange.org/mapping/

Robinson, R. (2005). Community development model for public health applications: Overview of a model to eliminate population disparities. *Health Promotion Practice, 6*(3), 338–346.

Scaffa, M. (Ed.). (2001). *Occupational therapy in community-based practice settings.* Philadelphia: F. A. Davis.

Sharpe, P. A., Greaney, M. L., Lee, P. R., & Royce, S. W. (2000). Assets-oriented community assessment. *Public Health Reports, 115,* 205–211.

Suarez-Balcazar, Y., Hammel, J., & Helfrich, C. (2005). A model of university-community partnerships for occupational therapy scholarship and practice. *Occupational Therapy in Health Care, 19,* 47–70.

Taylor, R., Hammel, J., & Braveman, B. (2004). Developing and evaluating community-based services through participatory action research: Three case examples. *American Journal of Occupational Therapy, 58*(1), 73–82.

Timmreck, T. C. (2003). *Planning, program development and evaluation* (2nd ed.). Sudbury, MA: Jones and Bartlett.

Voltz, J. D. (2003). Nebraska Health Ministry Network through Interchurch Ministries of Nebraska request for health ministry program support, yoga programming for Iglesia de Cristo Rey Omaha, Nebraska. Coordinated with Interfaith of South Omaha.

Walens, D., Helfrich, C. A., Aviles, A., & Horita, L. (2001). Assessing needs and developing interventions with new populations: A community process of collaboration. *Occupational Therapy in Mental Health, 16*(3-4), 71–95.

Wynn, K., Stewart, D., Law, M., Burke-Gaffney, J., & Moning, T. (2006). Creating connections: A community capacity-building project with parents and youth with disabilities in transition to adulthood. *Physical and Occupational Therapy in Pediatrics, 26*(4), 89–103.

Instructions: Identify community capacities of a chosen community using the following table.

Category	Community Capacity
Community stakeholders	
Community members	
Community partnerships	
Physical spaces	
Funding resources	
Community experts	
In-kind donations	
Other	

PROCESS WORKSHEET 6-2 **IDENTIFYING THE DIMENSIONS OF COMMUNITY CAPACITY**

Instructions: To assess community capacities, describe your community according to the six dimensions proposed by Chaskin (2001).

Dimensions	Community Description
Dimension 1: Characteristics of community capacity building	
Dimension 2: Levels of social agency	
Dimension 3: Functions of community capacity	
Dimension 4: Strategies for building community capacity	
Dimension 5: Conditioning influences	
Dimension 6: Outcomes	

PROCESS WORKSHEET 6-3 CRITIQUING COMMUNITY ASSESSMENT TECHNIQUES

Instructions: Identify the benefits and challenges of each assessment technique related to your community.

Method	Benefits	Challenges
Survey		
Focus groups		
Interviews		
Community forum		
Asset mapping		
Other: _____		

PROCESS WORKSHEET 6-4   COMMUNITY MAPPING

Instructions: Complete the community map following the KEEPRA approach. Identify assets of the community in each category in the following circles.

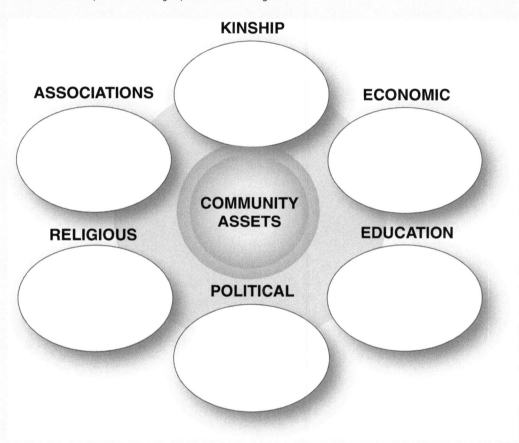

KINSHIP

ASSOCIATIONS

ECONOMIC

COMMUNITY ASSETS

RELIGIOUS

EDUCATION

POLITICAL

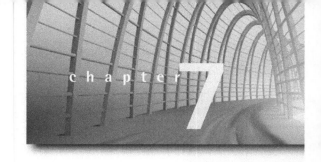

chapter 7

Community Partnerships: A Key to Success

LEARNING OBJECTIVES

By the end of this chapter, the reader will be able to complete the following:

1. Discuss how to develop community partnerships.
2. Analyze the role of the community as an expert in its own health care.
3. Reflect on the challenges and strategies of developing community partnerships.

Key Terms

Academic–community partnership
Advisory board
Board of directors
Communication plan
Community coalition
Community engagement
Community partnerships
Community stakeholders
Memorandum of understanding (MOU)

Overview

This chapter discusses the importance of community partnerships, how they develop, and pitfalls to avoid. Community partnerships are a strategy for developing successful community programs and writing grants to support these programs. This chapter assumes that occupational therapy practitioners are community-centered and focus on community-identified needs and capacities.

Introduction

As discussed in the previous chapter, successful grant programs match the needs and capacities of a community with the grant funding requirements.

171

Making this match is a challenge because it calls on those implementing the community program to understand the community fully on a deep and profound level. To do so, healthcare professionals and others have to step back and focus on needs identified by outsiders as well as community-identified needs. Many times the needs identified by outsiders differ from those identified by community members. When practitioners try to implement a program that does not match community desires, the results can be destructive and even oppressive (Lasker & Weiss, 2003; Israel, Eng, Schultz, & Parker, 2005). Furthermore, communities have to be ready to engage in behavior change, and occupational therapy practitioners must be aware of the community's readiness to engage in change (Edberg, 2007; Jumper-Thurman & Plested, 2000).

Occupational therapy practitioners who want to explore and understand community needs so that they can develop a meaningful and relevant program should focus on developing viable **community partnerships**. Challenges to community health cannot be addressed alone, and occupational therapy practitioners need to engage in collaboration to be successful in community work (Fazio, 2008; Becker, Israel, & Allen, 2005). Despite the benefits, collaborating and developing community partnerships can be time consuming and challenging.

Community Partnerships: Why They Matter

To work in community practice, occupational therapy practitioners must come to know and understand communities (Elliott, O'Neal, & Velde, 2001). Ultimately, to be successful in a community, practitioners have to engage and deeply understand the community to develop programs that address occupational needs. By developing and maintaining community relationships through partnerships, practitioners can come to fully understand the community and develop meaningful and relevant programming (Fazio, 2008).

Partnerships are entities "formed between two or more sectors to achieve a common goal that could not otherwise be accomplished separately" (Meade & Calvo, 2001,

p. 1578). Community partnerships have been demonstrated to be a successful approach to addressing health concerns (Becker et al., 2005; Roussos & Fawcett, 2000). Furthermore, partnerships pull together the expertise of a diverse group to address a problem (Becker et al., 2005). Although no definitive structure for community partnerships exists, community partnerships commonly include community coalitions, academic–community partnerships, healthcare consortiums, advocacy groups, and other grassroots organizations (Roussos & Fawcett, 2000). Partnerships can be formal or informal depending on the community and its needs.

TABLE 7-1 THE ROLE OF OCCUPATIONAL THERAPY PRACTITIONERS IN COMMUNITY PARTNERSHIPS
• Faculty member as part of an academic–community partnership • Community coalition member • Advisory board member • Nonprofit board of directors member • Member of the community

Participants in community partnerships also vary, including private, public, for-profit, and not-for-profit organizations (Shortell et al., 2002).

Collaboration is the foundation of partnerships, and successful collaboration is fundamental to a partnership's success (Fazio, 2008; Ansari, Phillips, & Hammick, 2001). In traditional practice, occupational therapy practitioners are called to collaboration and partnerships to work as part of the healthcare team (Baum, 2002), so they understand the concept of partnership in the traditional practice setting as discussed in the literature on client-centered practice and interprofessional practice (Law, 1998). In these discussions on client-centered practice, the practitioner is in partnership with the client to ensure that the client's therapeutic goals are addressed (Law, 1998; Sumsion, 1999).

Partnerships form between groups or organizations. Occupational therapy practitioners can play many roles in community partnerships through academic–community partnerships, community coalition membership, advisory board membership, nonprofit board membership, or simply as members of the community. Each different type of partnership is described later in this chapter. Partnerships have many benefits because they utilize the capacities of at least two different organizations to address needs. Collaboration of this nature maximizes resources by using the strengths of a mobilized group of people. In many cases, one agency alone cannot address a need, but in collaboration, community needs can be addressed efficiently. Furthermore, partnerships created to address health-related issues can "aim to create a seamless system of relevant healthcare services for the community" (Meade & Calvo, 2001, p. 1578).

Community partnerships, in themselves, can be complicated to develop and maintain (Becker et al., 2005). As with any team, a significant investment is required to develop trust and relationships and to face the challenges of effective collaboration (Becker et al., 2005). Research shows that developing and maintaining partnerships take time, commitment, and open communication to foster

> **LET'S STOP AND THINK**
>
> What challenges exist in client-centered practice in traditional occupational therapy practice settings? Evaluate whether these same challenges apply to community partnerships.

LET'S STOP AND THINK

Which parts of the Occupational Therapy Practice Framework are important when developing and maintaining community partnerships?

mutual trust required for true exchange (Burhansstipanov, Dignan, Bad Wound, Tenney, & Vigil, 2000; Kagawa-Singer, 1997; LaMarca, Wiese, Pete, & Carbone, 1996; Poole & Van Hook, 1997). Occupational therapy practitioners included in collaborations need to commit the time and their problem-solving abilities to be effective community partners.

Establishing Partnerships

Community partnerships are an effective method for addressing community health issues. Successful community partnerships exist because of successful management of group dynamics (Becker et al., 2005). Community partnerships consist of relationships among a diverse group of people (Bringle & Hatcher, 2002). These individuals and groups come together with a goal to address community needs. Throughout this book, the concept of maintaining a community-centered approach dominates. This concept applies to developing and maintaining community partnerships as well. Community partnerships need to be equitable, allowing each party to engage equally and have a say in the direction and activities of the partnership (Becker et al., 2005).

In developing community partnerships, the members of the partnership need to be clearly identified. The partnership model determines who is involved in the partnership, and members of the partnership must be identified clearly. After identifying the partners, the group must identify a collective mission (Bringle & Hatcher, 2002). The mission of the partnership depends on the community need being addressed by the group. In some cases, the group may address multiple needs or may be very focused on one specific community need. All of these aspects are driven by the community and the partners.

Once a mission is finalized, the group must develop and agree on the infrastructure for working together. The infrastructure must be collectively agreed upon and includes a structure for how the group will meet and follow its mission, decision-making protocols, and a plan for how conflicts will be resolved (Becker et al., 2005). The group may want to engage in some brief assessment to identify the strengths each team member brings to the partnership to aid in delineating tasks and activities. Trust building is also an essential activity at this stage and should include respecting differences, confidentiality, addressing the needs of the group, and completing assigned tasks in an effective and timely manner (Becker et al., 2005).

Partners should develop a system to communicate the progress of the program and grant and to address issues that may arise. Sometimes a written **communication plan** must be included in a grant proposal. The communication plan should include simple information such as who to contact in an emergency, a schedule of meetings, and deciding who will call and run meetings. In communications, practitioners should avoid using occupational therapy terminology or other health-related terminology that community members do not understand. The group must consider community member health literacy level, or the level of understanding of written and verbal health terminology, when conducting meetings and creating the content of the meeting agenda. Occupational therapy practitioners must be especially cognizant of this because many people are unfamiliar with the profession of occupational therapy and its language (Suarez-Balcazar, 2005).

As mentioned, partnerships can be very formal or very informal depending on the partners involved, the community need, and the program. If partnerships are formal, then the partners may develop a strategic plan that identifies goals and objectives for the partners based on the group's mission (Becker et al., 2005). They should maintain formal agendas and meeting minutes to track their efforts. In some cases, this documentation may be part of a program's evaluation plan and may provide valuable information for a grant report. Granting agencies that require partnerships will want documentation of the success of the partners in reaching their goals.

Developing community partnerships requires commitment and care for the community. Occupational therapy practitioners can play a critical role with their expertise in occupation (Fazio, 2008). Practitioners must remember that there are many aspects of developing a community partnership. Partnerships should be thoughtfully developed, especially if a community is underserved. And, once a partnership is developed, it needs to be maintained.

Community Involvement: Becoming a Part of the Partnership

Practitioners or community members can initiate community partner relationships (Bringle & Hatcher, 2002). These relationships can begin related to an immediate need, by desire of the community members, or as a requirement of a grant. Relationships may emerge slowly or come together quickly depending on the group dynamics and the community. Practitioners can develop community relationships by accident, by being sought by the community, through community engagement, or by simply being a member of the community.

Occupational therapy practitioners may become involved in a community partnership by accident or personal interest. A practitioner may identify community needs by recognizing patterns with patients in traditional practice settings. For example, a practitioner who finds multiple admissions for hip fractures secondary to a fall among older adults may want to address the larger problem. As a result of this interest, he or she may become involved in a local fall prevention coalition. In this example, the practitioner becomes involved in a community partnership and collaborates with other experts to address a community need.

In communities, healthcare providers are often viewed as experts, and communities, especially underserved communities, may seek out experts for assistance in addressing needs (Baum, 2002). In such cases, occupational therapy practitioners can serve the community using their expertise in an almost endless array of possibilities (Voltz-Doll, 2008).

BEST PRACTICE HINT

Want to get involved in the community? Volunteer to be part of a local speakers' bureau where you can go present on health topics related to occupational therapy practice. Through these speaking engagements, you can get to know community members and educate them about the possibilities of occupational therapy in community settings.

Another effective approach for becoming involved in community partnerships is through community engagement in which practitioners identify where they best fit in community collaborative efforts. **Community engagement** is "the process of working collaboratively with and through groups of people affiliated by geographic proximity, special interest, or similar situations to address issues affecting the well-being of those people" (Centers for Disease Control and Prevention, 1997). Community engagement implies that the practitioner is engaged in the community instead of serving it or applying treatment strategies to it. As in traditional practice, where occupational therapy practitioners define themselves as facilitators of occupation, the same is true in community (Wittman & Velde, 2001). Practitioners can engage with the community to come to know and understand the community through volunteerism, provision of pro bono services, community organization participation, and many other activities.

Communities can be viewed through a variety of lenses including the community member and occupational therapy practitioner. Most simply, understanding community needs can come from being a part of a community. Occupational therapy practitioners may be community members before they are professionals in the community. Being a member of a community provides a deep experience of the community's strengths and challenges. Occupational therapy practitioners can view the community through their professional lens to explore occupational needs or issues that can be addressed (Fazio, 2008). As a member of the community, the occupational therapy practitioner may be able to understand the community from the inside and as an expert in occupation.

BEST PRACTICE HINT

Provide pro bono or volunteer services to a local free health clinic as a way to get to know the community as well as its needs and capacities.

Partnering with Community Stakeholders

To work with a community toward success in addressing needs, collaboration is necessary (Fazio, 2008). But who in the community should the occupational therapy practitioner seek as collaborators? Practitioners can work with **community stakeholders**, individuals in the community who are respected by others and who hold significant knowledge about community needs and assets. A key strategy for success in community practice is working with these community stakeholders (Lasker & Weiss, 2003).

Stakeholders depend on the community and the culture of the community. Stakeholders in one community might not be viewed as stakeholders in another community. In some communities, elders are viewed as stakeholders because of their knowledge and experience. In others, stakeholders are those who work directly with community members to provide services. In the case of health-related services, stakeholders may include community members and healthcare providers. Other examples of stakeholders include long-time community residents, religious leaders, neighborhood association leaders, and political leaders.

Getting to know the community stakeholders is part of the process of coming to know the community (Murry & Brody, 2004). In some communities, stakeholders may self-identify or others may identify these individuals. Usually, spending some time in the community can quickly reveal stakeholders. In other situations, occupational therapy practitioners may not be able to simply ask community members to identify stakeholders and stakeholders may not be self-evident. Also, individuals may identify themselves as stakeholders, but others in the community may not view them as so. Occupational therapy practitioners must be careful and be sure to work with individuals who have the community's best interest in mind (Foster-Fishman, Berkowitz, Lounsbury, Jacobsen, & Allen, 2001). Although it may be difficult to identify stakeholders, leaders in the community usually emerge in time.

Stakeholders are key resources for occupational therapy practitioners in all stages of program development and the grant writing process. Practitioners should view these individuals as "community experts" who can provide invaluable insight into the community and assist in facilitating buy-in from other members of the community. The number of stakeholders should not be limited and the occupational therapy practitioner should get to know many individuals to get to know the community (Suarez-Balcazar, Harper, & Lewis, 2005). By including multiple stakeholders, practitioners can ensure that the program captures multiple points of view and is sustainable even if a stakeholder moves, retires, or changes positions (Wells, Miranda, Bruce, Alegria, & Wallerstein, 2004). Practitioners should always keep in mind that everyone has capacity and assets to offer, so exploring these for the benefit of the program and the greater community is a necessary step in building an effective partnership (Kretzmann & McKnight, 1993).

When the practitioner partners with an established nonprofit agency, the practitioner should become familiar with the agency and should learn its mission and goals and the services it provides. Practitioners can explore these details during the community assessment stage of program development and grant writing. One method for learning about a nonprofit agency is to volunteer to provide services or to join the board of directors. A **board of directors** is a group of individuals who guide the organization in its mission, finances, and programming. Nonprofit agencies use boards of directors to aid them in planning and ensuring financial viability of the organization. Members of a board of directors are volunteers who have

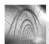

BEST PRACTICE HINT

To join a board of directors, contact the local United Way, which can identify organizations that need board members.

expertise and can help the organization. By serving on a board, the occupational therapy practitioner can come to fully understand the agency, meet community stakeholders, and engage in community activities. All of these activities assist the practitioner in learning about the community and building the groundwork for future partnerships.

Another strategy is to make sure partners are "involved in every step of the research, educational and practice process" in community practice (Suarez-Balcazar, Hammel, & Helfrich, 2005, p. 49; Becker et al., 2005). Community stakeholders must be involved early in the program development process. By involving stakeholders, practitioners can ensure that the program addresses community needs and facilitates social change (Suarez-Balcazar, Harper, & Lewis, 2005). As discussed in other chapters, stakeholders should be included even as early as brainstorming and beginning program development. Involving stakeholders is necessary and a smart strategy in developing a community partnership that will help sustain community programming.

Academic–Community Partnerships

Academic–community partnerships, also called community–campus partnerships, are a common community partnership model (Bringle & Hatcher, 2002; Suarez-Balcazar, Hammel, & Helfrich, 2005; Suarez-Balcazar, Harper, & Lewis, 2005; Suarez-Balcazar & Orellana, 1999). Academic–community partnerships exist when an academic institution and a community or community agency work together to address a community need (Erwin, Blumenthal, Chapel, & Allwood, 2004; Benoit, Jansson, Millar, & Phillips, 2005). A variety of models of academic–community partnerships exists, and occupational therapy practitioners in academic settings may find these models the most viable for community practice.

The mission of many academic institutions is to serve the community. In most cases, academic institutions aid communities by conducting research or implementing important programs, and communities aid academic institutions by providing real-world learning experiences for students. Some academic–community partnerships focus on research. In such cases, the academic institution may use a community-based participatory research (CBPR) model to engage in collaborative research with a community. In fact, most of the values of academic–community partnerships are similar to the values of CBPR discussed in earlier chapters, including equitable work and a focus on the community's needs and capacities rather than the institution's. Other partnerships follow a service learning model. In such cases, students provide services to the community and address learning objectives through community immersion. Examples include health screenings in which students learn to administer the screening and community members receive the needed screening free of charge or for a reduced fee. The service–learning partnership model can work well for community practice and education of occupational therapy students.

Research has shown that academic–community partnerships can improve student education, address health disparities, and increase healthcare access for communities
(Commission on Community-Engaged Scholarship in the
Health Professions, 2005). The strategies for building an
academic–community partnership are similar to those of
other models. However, the academic institution has significant resources both in the expertise of faculty and students
who can provide necessary services while meeting learning
objectives.

BEST PRACTICE HINT

To learn more about
academic–community partnerships,
explore Community-Campus
Partnerships for Health, available
online at http://www.ccph.info/.

Engaging the Community

Once a community partnership has been developed and each partner fully under-
stands their roles and responsibilities, activities need to take place to engage the
community to maintain the partnership. All parties involved should monitor the
partnership to assess its success and ability to reach its goals and objectives (Bringle
& Hatcher, 2002). Individuals remain in a partnership when they feel engaged and
like they contribute to the mission of the group. The project team can engage community members in the partnership and program by developing an advisory board
and/or a community coalition.

An **advisory board** is a collection of community members who provide feedback on a program (MacQueen et al., 2001). These individuals may be community
stakeholders or community members. The advisory board is a resource to the program team and connects the team with community members. Advisory boards are
not the same thing as a board of directors in a nonprofit organization and do not
require necessarily the same formality. In some cases, a program may have a board
of directors and an advisory board, depending on its needs.

Prior to convening an advisory board, the project team should take time to
establish the role of the advisory board, goals of the advisory board, and a description of the roles of members on the advisory board. Advisory boards usually consist of experts who know the community and the organization so that these
individuals can make recommendations and guide the organization or program.
An advisory board demonstrates quality assurance and that the organization is listening to the voice of the community. When inviting individuals to participate on
an advisory board, the leader of the advisory board needs to ensure that the participants are individuals who will provide constructive and critical feedback and
also have the time to devote to advisory board activities. Advisory boards typically
do not meet often and do not require a significant amount of time, which is a benefit when recruiting members. (This is in contrast to a board of directors, who
meet more regularly, usually on a monthly or bimonthly basis.) It is important to
note that some grantors may require an advisory board as part of a grant funded
program.

A **community coalition** is an organized group with strong leadership and multiple partners that has a planning process that is usually revised annually (Wolff, 2001). According to Cohen, Baer, and Satterwhite (2002), a coalition "is a union of people and organizations working to influence outcomes on a specific problem" (p. 144). Coalitions usually have a mission statement and an action plan with goals, objectives, and outcomes related to a community need. Coalitions harness the power of multiple partners in an organized fashion. Sometimes coalitions emerge out of community partnerships or advisory boards. Sometimes a community coalition is part of an academic–community partnership.

Community coalitions are unique because they include community members, focus on community issues, and focus on a community-wide effort (Wolff, 2001). Community coalitions exist for a variety of reasons. The collaboration of a community coalition allows for more to be done with fewer resources. Interventions addressing needs derive from and address the entire community, allowing for community members to engage in addressing their own community challenges. This, in turn, promotes empowerment of community members (Wolff, 2001).

Occupational therapy practitioners can be part of a community coalition or help organize the coalition. There are some strategies for forming a coalition. First, as with partnership development, is to identify a collective mission for the coalition. A coalition might also include written memoranda of understanding or draft by-laws that outline how the coalition will run. Some coalitions go as far as to attain nonprofit status.

Cohen, Baer, and Satterwhite (2002) developed definitive steps for forming a community coalition: analyze the program's objectives and determine whether to form a coalition; recruit the right people; devise a set of preliminary objectives and activities; convene the coalition; anticipate necessary resources; define a successful coalition structure; maintain the coalition; and evaluate the coalition.

In coalitions, every member should know their role. In some cases, defining specific leadership roles with identified responsibilities may be effective. Some coalitions elect officers and follow formal guidelines of running meetings, recording minutes, and voting formally on decisions (National Cancer Institute, 2008). These procedures should be defined as the coalition forms (Granner & Sharpe, 2004). The process of decision making should be determined to make sure the coalition communicates well and makes decisions with the community's best interest in mind. Members of the coalition should determine communication methods. Coalitions should act as a forum for information sharing about what is going on in the community. Some suggestions for facilitating communication include using a wiki or establishing a website.

Community coalitions are an appropriate way to address some community needs. However, community coalitions require significant human resources and time to develop. If a grant requires a community coalition, the justification and

TABLE 7-2 STEPS TO FORMING A COALITION

Step	Description
Analyze the program's objectives and determine whether to form a coalition.	• Determine reason for forming coalition. • Determine if a coalition is appropriate for the community. • Determine the cost and resources needed for the coalition.
Recruit the right people.	• Determine potential members. • The right people determine the success of the group. • Determine size of coalition (i.e., number of members).
Devise a set of preliminary objectives and activities.	• Develop collective goals and objectives among members. • Determine coalition activities (action items).
Convene the coalition.	• At the first meeting, review the coalition's purpose and objectives. • After this meeting, finalize members.
Anticipate the necessary resources.	• The most valuable resource is time. • Determine monetary resources needed.
Define elements of a successful coalition structure.	• Determine how long the coalition will exist (for example, it may only be necessary during a grant period to meet requirements). • Specify meeting location and frequency. • Determine decision-making processes. • Specify actions between meetings.
Maintain coalition vitality.	• Address challenges. • Celebrate successes.
Make improvements through evaluation.	• Determine evaluation methods. • Evaluation should be ongoing.

Source: Adapted from Cohen, L., Baer, N., & Satterwhite, P. (2002). Developing effective coalitions: An eight step guide. In M. E. Wurzbach (Ed.), *Community health education and promotion: A guide to program design and evaluation* (2nd ed., pp. 144–161). Gaithersburg, MD: Aspen.

funding required to run the coalition should be described in the grant proposal. If the project team determines that a community coalition is an effective partnership model, the project team must recruit coalition members. The coalition leaders need to identify how many members should be a part of the coalition to be effective. Then, potential members need to be identified and invited.

At the initial meetings, coalition membership should be finalized. Coalitions need to be somewhat flexible but should have requirements for membership (Wolff, 2001). There may be times when members need to leave the coalition or when they find their objectives do not match with the objectives and activities of the coalition. Although coalitions should be stable entities, successful coalitions allow members to come and go if a match does not work (Wolff, 2001). However, members cannot constantly join and exit if the coalition is to be effective. Coalitions are action oriented, focus on tasks, and do not meet simply to meet.

Once individuals are called to the table, objectives and activities for the coalition should be developed. These objectives and activities should be collective and are usually in the form of a written action plan. If a coalition is a requirement of a grant, the objectives and activities may be included in the grant proposal. All members should be educated on the mission and objectives of the partnership. Members of the coalition need to determine resources required based on the actions desired, including time and money. In most cases, members of coalitions volunteer to participate or participate as part of their existing job responsibilities. Coalition members should identify the time commitment required to complete the coalition's activities and clearly communicate this to members to ensure that everyone can participate appropriately. The group may also devise a budget and seek external funding resources either through donations or grant funding.

The group must clearly identify the logistics of the coalition, including meeting times and locations, reporting requirements, communication structure, and decision-making processes. As the coalition moves along accomplishing activities related to its objectives, the partners should take time to celebrate successes and address problems that impede outcomes. To measure successes and challenges, the community coalition needs an evaluation plan that can describe its impact. All of these steps and actions can ensure a community coalition is formed that has a sound infrastructure to address community needs (Cohen et al., 2002).

In some cases, coalitions can access more opportunities for funding than community organizations can alone. Grantors may feel that a coalition is more likely to get things done than a single organization is. Not only is this relevant to grant funding but also to advertising a program to the community. Community members may be willing to collaborate and work with a coalition rather than a single organization. Coalitions have implications for policymakers as well, and coalitions may find their voice heard more readily than that of a single community organization (Wolff, 2001).

TABLE 7-3 TYPICAL COMPONENTS OF AN MOU

- Name of partners
- Brief history of partnership
- Brief description of how the partners work together
- The proposed or existing activities of the partnership
- Official signatures with dates from representatives of both partners

---

Memorandums of Understanding

Documentation of partnerships demonstrates a commitment and can be included in a grant to demonstrate community collaboration. There are several ways to document a partnership. A common method for documenting evidence of a partnership is the use of a memorandum of understanding (Adams, Miller-Korth, & Brown, 2004). A **memorandum of understanding (MOU)** is not a contract but simply a written agreement between two agencies outlining how each will work together in a community partnership. Memorandums of understanding (MOUs) are common in the community setting where contracts for services may not be necessary or applicable (Holkup, Tripp-Reimer, Salois, & Weinert, 2004).

MOUs provide formal documentation of each community partner's responsibilities and the structure of the collaboration. MOUs can be completed among agencies that want to document a partnership. In some grant proposals, a formal MOU is required. In most cases, the MOU is included in the grant proposal appendices. Some granting agencies require that partners use a specific MOU document as outlined in the submission guidelines or request for proposals (RFP); however, others allow community agencies to develop their own.

Although community partners may have general MOUs for their partnership, they may choose to draft an MOU specific to grant activities to document how they will work together with the grant funding.

An MOU usually includes the following components: names of the partners involved, a brief history of the partnership, a brief description of how the partners work together, the proposed activities of the partnership, and signatures of representatives from both partners. See Table 7-4 for a sample form of an MOU.

Challenges to Community Partnerships

Developing and maintaining viable community partnerships can be challenging. Bringing multiple individuals together to address a problem presents issues in meeting every participant's needs while addressing the community-wide objective. Some difficulties may include lack of trust, power struggles among group members, lack of respect for differences, and poor management of partnership activities (Erwin et al., 2004). Other challenges include a lack of financial support and a poorly designed partnership (Butterfoss & Francisco, 2004). However, some of these challenges are also what lead to successful partnerships. For example, research shows that diverse partnerships can be successful because they accurately represent the community (Shortell et al., 2002).

Partnerships may be unsuccessful because of poor management; however, the partners can remedy this situation by appointing leaders to be responsible for managing the partnership. In some cases, the leader is an executive director or other specially appointed individual (Shortell et al., 2002). The group must define the responsibilities of the leadership role clearly and discuss them with all members of the partnership. A focused partnership promotes success because all members know the direction of the group. A partnership without a definitive focus is likely to make group members feel like their contributions are fruitless.

Conflict occurs in all groups and is often related to power struggles among group members. Power conflicts lead to a lack of trust, which breaks down the relationships crucial to a partnership's success. Successful partnerships anticipate challenges and develop procedures for addressing them before they become major problems (Shortell et al., 2002). Distrust can also be alleviated by ensuring that all partners are aware of the activities of the partnership (Adams et al., 2004). Effective communication helps avoid the development of distrust.

Distrust among community partnerships can also be caused by lack of cultural awareness and cultural sensitivity that result from cultural differences (Bringle & Hatcher, 2002). In some cases, practitioners and other professional team partners may come from a different cultural background than the community being served. It can be difficult for outsiders to learn the culture and deal with cross-cultural relationships because of the differences in communication and health beliefs among cultural groups (Bringle & Hatcher, 2002). Furthermore, practitioners must recognize their cultural biases and not let them influence the program or grant. Practitioners must also recognize their own values and how these interplay with values of the community. They must respect diversity to work in diverse communities and must be able to embrace different ways of doing things (Black & Wells, 2007). Practitioners can perform a self-assessment to reflect on their values (Black & Wells, 2007).

Many community development models argue that cultural competence is essential to success among partnerships (Wittman, O'Neal, & Velde, 2001). The word *competence* may be a bit of a misnomer; however, the occupational therapy practitioner should

TABLE 7-4 SAMPLE MEMORANDUM OF UNDERSTANDING

This document constitutes a Memorandum of Understanding (MOU) between the University and the Community Response Team regarding the Suicide Prevention Plan.

The University has an established partnership with the Community Response Team and a historical partnership with the community of more than 14 years. For the purpose of the Prevention Plan, the University indicates a willingness to work with the Community Response Team to address the critical issue of suicide prevention in the community.

Roles and Responsibilities:

University agrees to implement the following:

- Develop and implement an evidence-based and culturally relevant stress management program for the prevention of suicide.
- Develop sensory rooms and a traveling sensory workshop for the purpose of stress management as a tool for suicide prevention in the local schools.
- Conduct stress management workshops four times per year in the community.
- Engage in planning and development as needed in partnership with the Community Response Team.
- Provide training to Community Response Team staff and school staff in the stress management program for sustainability.

Planning and Development Contact Person:

- Joy D. Doll, OTD, OTR/L, Assistant Professor, Clinical Education, Department of Occupational Therapy, University
- Staff/Faculty as needed

Resources Provided by University:

- Expertise of Dr. Joy Doll, who has an established relationship in the community and experience with program development and implementation in several underserved communities
- Doctor of Occupational Therapy students, who have received cultural awareness training to assist in program implementation
- Transportation of students and faculty to the community

I hereby agree to fulfill my sections of this project, and I agree to abide by the terms and conditions contained in this Memorandum of Understanding between the University and the Community Response Team.

Signature: _____

Signature: _____

TABLE 7-5 SUGGESTED MEMBERS OF SUCCESSFUL PARTNERSHIPS

- Representatives from health care including hospitals, insurers, health systems, and clinicians
- Representatives of social services including government and not-for-profit agencies
- Representatives of the business community including local corporations and small businesses
- Local and state government leaders including the mayor, city council members, the board of supervisors, and state representatives

Source: Shortell, S. M., Zukoski, A. P., Alexander, J. A., Bazzoli, G. J., Conrad, D. A., Hasnain-Wynia, R., et al. (2002). Evaluating partnerships for community health improvement: Tracking the footprints. *Journal of Health Politics, Policy and Law, 27*(1), 49–91.

TABLE 7-6 STRATEGIES FOR WORKING IN A DIVERSE COMMUNITY

- Seek out experiences with diverse communities.
- Reflect on cross-cultural experiences.
- Speak to cultural experts.
- Read reliable cultural resources.
- Engage in cultural immersions.
- Be observant of cultural practices.
- Ask questions or seek clarification if ever confused.
- Use reliable cultural theoretical approaches.

---

at least become knowledgeable in the cultural nuances and cultural practices of a community. Many models regarding health and cultural competency exist, but nothing replaces experience with diverse individuals. Experience teaches the nuances and ways in which a community functions (Masin, 2006). Practitioners should recognize that cultural differences can present communication issues and very different views of community needs and assets. As stated by Padilla and Brown (1999), gaining "cultural sensitivity is a lifelong process that involves both learning how to gain information from clients and unlearning personal assumptions and stereotypes that interfere with the professional's ability to see clients for who they are" (p. 29).

BEST PRACTICE HINT

Do not be afraid to ask questions about the culture and its impact on the community to gain knowledge and become culturally aware and sensitive.

TABLE 7-7 KLEINMAN'S QUESTIONS

- What do you call your problem? What name does it have?
- What do you think caused your problem?
- Why do you think it started when it did?
- What does your sickness do to you? How does it work?
- How severe is it? Will it have a short or long course?
- What do you fear most about your disorder?
- What are the chief problems that your sickness has caused for you?
- What kind of treatment do you think you should receive?
- What are the most important results you hope to receive from the treatment?

Source: Kleinman, A., Eisenberg, L., & Good, B. (1978). Culture, illness and care: Clinical lessons from anthropologic and cross-cultural research. *Annals of Internal Medicine, 88,* 251–258.

Occupational therapy practitioners can facilitate cross-cultural communication by using existing cultural models. The explanatory model, developed by physician and medical anthropologist Arthur Kleinman and colleagues (1978), provides a model for enhancing cross-cultural communication in community partnerships. The questions used in this model (as shown in **Table 7-7**) provide a format for exploring needs based on the cultural perspective of the community members being asked. Many other cultural models exist to aid occupational therapy practitioners in gaining cultural awareness, including the Sunrise Model, the Purnell Model of Cultural Competence, and the Cultural Competency Continuum (Craig, 2001; Purnell, 2002; Cross, Bazron, Dennis, & Isaacs, 1989). Practitioners should choose the approach that best suits their community and cultural knowledge.

Healthcare providers, including occupational therapy practitioners, may discover unique challenges to involvement in a community partnership. Healthcare providers are taught to think in a reductionistic manner that can conflict with community health models (Lasker & Weiss, 2003). In the traditional medical model, healthcare providers look for disease and disability along with the dysfunction causing the problems. For healthcare providers, it may be difficult to view a community's capacities when their education has focused on finding problems and seeking answers to the problems. The medical model approach is linear and reductionistic, sometimes limiting the ability to view the complexity of the system.

LET'S STOP AND THINK

Reflect on your own cultural values. How would you answer Kleinman's questions? Interview a partner using Kleinman's questions.

In communities, practitioners are called to take in the big picture and try to understand the community as a whole. Communities are open, complex systems that function in a nonlinear fashion. According to Elliott, O'Neal, and Velde (2001), community programs are "open systems in constant interaction with their physical, natural, temporal, social and political environment" (p. 106). This makes it hard to propose cause-and-effect answers to problems, as the medical model does. Therefore, occupational therapy practitioners must not dissect the community to find the parts that equal a predictable sum. Reducing the community does not do it justice and prevents understanding. Furthermore, a reductionist view conflicts with the community view, causing distrust and problems within community partnerships.

Practitioners in the community setting sometimes find it difficult to acknowledge that their expertise is not as crucial as that of the community members' (Lasker & Weiss, 2003; Wells et al., 2004). A community-centered approach maintains the community's values at the forefront, as discussed in detail in Chapter 1. Healthcare providers can find it very challenging and humbling to realize that, although some ideas might be useful, the community truly knows its issues and practitioners are only vehicles for programs that address these issues. Although this sounds harsh and may be hard to digest, healthcare practitioners must understand the relationship and the reality of communities. Occupational therapy practitioners are familiar with educating patients, but in community settings to succeed practitioners have to be open to learning. They must go beyond being client-centered and must focus on the needs and wants of the community and allow the community to drive the focus of the program and its outcomes (Fazio, 2008).

A relationship should exist in a community partnership where the exchange is mutual (Becker et al., 2005). Occupational therapy practitioners should never assume that they are the only experts who can provide solutions to problems. Community members' ideas should be valued even though the practitioner is the one with the degree and experience. Nothing replaces experience in the community as the strongest source of expertise. Practitioners that have spent time in a community recognize that they have grown professionally and learned much from the community. In these lessons, they recognize the constant exchange between partners. By maintaining an openness to learning, practitioners can discover community-driven solutions to community issues and ensure that the developing program aligns with the community.

Grants and Partnerships

In a grant proposal, the grant writer should discuss and demonstrate how partnerships have evolved, their history, and how the partners work together. As grant funding becomes increasingly competitive, partnerships prove to be a method for approaching funding agencies to maximize both resources and positive outcomes for the community (Roussos & Fawcett, 2000). A description of these aspects of the partnership can be included in the grant narrative or may be made more evident though a subcontract or memorandum of understanding. It is important to read the grant request for proposals (RFP) carefully to ensure that a partnership is supported. Progress and outcomes of partnerships need to be outlined in grant reports.

Sometimes the RFP may specifically request that information about community partnerships be provided. In this case, the RFP will outline what needs to be included in the proposal to document evidence of the community collaboration. However, even when not specifically required, documenting partnerships can enhance a grant proposal and can be a crucial aspect in securing funding. Partnerships make programs worth funding and many funders seek out community collaborations.

Conclusion

Community practice is successful when strong partnerships form between individuals and agencies within a community. This chapter discusses the role of occupational therapy practitioners in community partnerships where they remain community-centered and utilize an asset-based approach to address community needs.

Glossary

Academic–community partnership A partnership between an academic institution and a community or community agency that works to address a community need

Advisory board A collection of community members who provide feedback on a program

Board of directors A group of individuals who guide a nonprofit organization in its mission, finances, and programming

Communication plan A comprehensive plan describing how members of a partnership will communicate. The plan includes who to contact in an emergency, a schedule of meetings to update and discuss the program and/or grant, and deciding who will call and run meetings

Community coalition An organized group of people who address a community problem

Community engagement "The process of working collaboratively with and through groups of people affiliated by geographic proximity, special interest, or similar situations to address issues affecting the well-being of those people" (Centers for Disease Control and Prevention, 1997)

Community partnerships Entities "formed between two or more sectors to achieve a common goal that could not otherwise be accomplished separately" (Meade & Calvo, 2001, p. 1578)

Community stakeholders Individuals in the community who are respected by others and hold significant knowledge about community needs and assets

Memorandum of understanding (MOU) An agreement between two agencies outlining how each will work together

References

Adams, A., Miller-Korth, N., & Brown, D. (2004). Learning to work together: Developing academic and community research partnerships. *Wisconsin Medical Journal, 103*(2), 15–19.

Ansari, W. E., Phillips, C. J., & Hammick, M. (2001). Collaborating and partnerships: Developing the evidence base. *Health and Social Care in the Community, 9*(4), 215–227.

Baum, C. (2002). Creating partnerships: Constructing our future. *Australian Occupational Therapy Journal, 49*, 58–62.

Becker, A. B., Israel, B. A., & Allen, A. J. (2005). Strategies and techniques for effective group process in CBPR partnerships. In B. A. Israel, E. Eng, A. J. Schulz, & E. A. Parker (Eds.), *Methods in community-based participatory research for health* (pp. 52–72). San Francisco: Jossey-Bass.

Benoit, C., Jansson, M., Millar, A., & Phillips, R. (2005). Community–academic research on hard-to-reach populations: Benefits and challenges. *Qualitative Health Research, 15*(2), 262–282.

Black, R. M., & Wells, S. A. (2007). *Culture and occupation.* Bethesda, MD: AOTA Press.

Bringle, R. G., & Hatcher, J. A. (2002). Campus–community partnerships: The terms of engagement. *Journal of Social Issues, 58*(3), 503–516.

Burhansstipanov, L., Dignan, M. B., Bad Wound, D., Tenney, M., & Vigil, G. (2000). Native American recruitment into breast cancer screening: The NAWWA project. *Cancer Education, 15*, 28–52.

Butterfoss, F. D., & Francisco, F. T. (2004). Evaluating community partnerships and coalitions with practitioners in mind. *Health Promotion Practice, 5*(2), 108–114.

Centers for Disease Control and Prevention. (1997). Principles of community engagement. Retrieved July 12, 2008, from http://www.cdc.gov/phppo/pce/

Cohen, L., Baer, N., & Satterwhite, P. (2002). Developing effective coalitions: An eight step guide. In M. E. Wurzbach (Ed.), *Community health education and promotion: A guide to program design and evaluation* (2nd ed., pp. 144–161). Gaithersburg, MD: Aspen.

Commission on Community-Engaged Scholarship in the Health Professions. (2005). *Linking scholarship and communities: Report of the Commission on Community-Engaged Scholarship in the Health Professions.* Seattle: Community-Campus Partnerships for Health.

Craig, G. (2001). Sunrise model. Retrieved September 24, 2008, from http://learn.sdstate.edu/share/Sunrise.html

Cross, T., Bazron, B., Dennis, K., & Isaacs, M. (1989). *Toward a culturally competent system of care.* Washington, DC: CAASP Technical Assistance Center, Georgetown University Child Development Center.

Edberg, M. (2007). *Essentials of health behavior: Social and behavior health in public health.* Sudbury, MA: Jones and Bartlett.

Elliott, S., O'Neal, S., & Velde, B. P. (2001). Using chaos theory to understand a community-built occupational therapy practice. *Occupational Therapy in Health Care, 13*(3/4), 101–112.

Erwin, K., Blumenthal, D. S., Chapel, T., & Allwood, L. V. (2004). Building an academic–community partnership for increasing the representation of minorities in the health professions. *Journal of Health Care for the Poor and Underserved, 15*, 589–602.

Fazio, L. (2008). *Developing occupation-centered programs for the community* (2nd ed.). Upper Saddle River, NJ: Prentice Hall.

Foster-Fishman, P. G., Berkowitz, S. L., Lounsbury, D. W., Jacobsen, S., & Allen, N. A. (2001). Building collaborative capacity: A review and integrative framework. *American Journal of Community Psychology, 29*(2), 241–261.

Granner, M. L., & Sharpe, P. A. (2004). Evaluating community coalition characteristics and functioning: A summary of measurement tools. *Health Education Research, 19*(5), 514–532.

Holkup, P. A., Tripp-Reimer, T., Matt Solois, E., & Weinert, C. (2004). Community-based participatory research: An approach to intervention research with a Native American community. *Advances in Nursing Science, 27*(3), 162–175.

Israel, B. A., Eng, E., Schulz, A. J., & Parker, E. A. (2005). *Methods in community-based participatory research for health.* San Francisco: Jossey-Bass.

Jumper-Thurman, P., & Plested, B. (2000). Community readiness: A model for healing in a rural Alaskan community. *Family Psychologist,* Summer, 8–9.

Kagawa-Singer, M. (1997). Addressing issues for early detection and screening in ethnic populations. *Oncology Nursing Forum, 24*(10), 1705–1711.

Kleinman, A., Eisenberg, L., & Good, B. (1978). Culture, illness and care: Clinical lessons from anthropologic and cross-cultural research. *Annals of Internal Medicine, 88,* 251–258.

Kretzmann, J. P., & McKnight, J. L. (1993). *Building communities from the inside out: A path toward finding and mobilizing a community's assets.* Skokie, IL: ACTA Publications.

LaMarca, K., Wiese, K. R., Pete, J. E., & Carbone, P. P. (1996). A progress report of cancer centers and tribal communities: Building a partnership based on trust. *Cancer, 78*(Suppl. 7), 1633–1637.

Lasker, R. D., & Weiss, E. S. (2003). Broadening participation in community problem solving: A multidisciplinary model to support collaborative practice and research. *Journal of Urban Health, 80*(1), 14–47.

Law, M. (1998). *Client-centered occupational therapy.* Thorofare, NJ: Slack.

MacQueen, K. M., McLellan, E., Metzger, D. S., Kegeles, S., Strauss, R. P., Scotti, R., et al. (2001). What is community? An evidence-based definition for participatory public health. *American Journal of Public Health, 91*(12), 1929–1938.

Masin, H. L. (2006). Communicating with cultural sensitivity. In C. M. Davis (Ed.), *Patient practitioner interaction: An experiential manual for developing the art of health care.* Thorofare, NJ: Slack.

McKnight, J. (1995). *Careless society: Community and its counterfeits.* New York: Basic Books.

Meade, C. D. & Calvo, A. (2001). Developing community–academic partnerships to enhance breast health among rural and Hispanic migrant and seasonal farmworker women. *Oncology Nursing Forum, 28*(10), 1577–1584.

Minkler, M., & Wallerstein, N. (1997). Improving health through community organization and community building. In M. Minkler (Ed.), *Community organizing and community building for health* (pp. 30–52). New Brunswick, NJ: Rutgers University Press.

Murry, V. M., & Brody, G. H. (2004). Partnering with community stakeholders: Engaging rural African American families in basic research and the Strong African Families Preventive Intervention Program. *Journal of Marital and Family Therapy, 30*(3), 271–283.

National Cancer Institute. (2008). Making health communication programs work. Retrieved July 21, 2008, from http://www.cancer.gov/PDF/41f04dd8-495a-4444-a258-1334b1d8 64f7/Pink_Book.pdf

Padilla, R., & Brown, K. (1999). Culture and patient education: Challenges and opportunities. *Journal of Physical Therapy Education, 13*(3), 23–30.

Poole, D., & Van Hook, M. (1997). Retooling for community health partnerships in primary care and prevention. *Health and Social Work, 22*(1), 2–4.

Purnell, L. (2002). The Purnell model for cultural competence. *Journal of Transcultural Nursing, 13*(3), 193–196.

Roussos, S. T., & Fawcett, S. B. (2000). A review of collaborative partnerships as a strategy for improving community health. *Annual Reviews of Public Health, 21,* 369–402.

Shortell, S. M., Zukoski, A. P., Alexander, J. A., Bazzoli, G. J., Conrad, D. A., Hasnain-Wynia, R., et al. (2002). Evaluating partnerships for community health improvement: Tracking the footprints. *Journal of Health Politics, Policy and Law, 27*(1), 49–91.

Suarez-Balcazar, Y. (2005). Empowerment and participatory evaluation of a community health intervention: Implications for occupational therapy. *Occupational Therapy Journal of Research, 25*(4), 1–10.

Suarez-Balcazar, Y., Hammel, J., & Helfrich, C. (2005). A model of university–community partnerships for occupational therapy scholarship and practice. *Occupational Therapy in Health Care, 19,* 47–70.

Suarez-Balcazar, Y., Harper, G., & Lewis, R. (2005). An interactive and conceptual model of community–university collaborations for research and action. *Health Education and Behavior, 32,* 84–101.

Suarez-Balcazar, Y., & Orellana, L. (1999). A university–community partnership for empowerment evaluation with a community housing organization. *Sociological Practice. A Journal of Clinical and Applied Sociology, (1),*115–132.

Sumsion, T. (1999). *Client-centered practice in occupational therapy.* Edinburgh: Churchill Livingstone.

Voltz-Doll, J. D. (2008). Professional development: Growing as an occupational therapist. *Advance for Occupational Therapy Practitioners, 24*(5), 41–42.

Wells, K., Miranda, J., Bruce, M. L., Alegria, M., & Wallerstein. N. (2004). Bridging community intervention and mental health services research. *American Journal of Psychiatry, 161,* 955–963.

Wittman, P. P., & Velde, B. P. (2001). Occupational therapy in the community: What, why, and how. *Occupational Therapy in Health Care, 13*(3/4), 1–5.

Wolff, T. (2001). Community coalition building: Contemporary practice and research: Introduction. *American Journal of Community Psychology, 29*(2), 165–172.

PROCESS WORKSHEET 7-1 **DEVELOPING A COMMUNICATION PLAN**

Instructions: Complete this worksheet as a way to think about and develop a communication plan for a partnership.

1. Identify types communication (for example, e-mail, text messaging, meetings) to be used by staff and community members.

   _____

   _____

2. Identify how often meetings will be conducted.
   Meeting Schedule (circle one)

   Daily   Weekly   Monthly   Quarterly   Yearly

3. Identify who will need to attend these meetings.

   _____

   _____

4. Identify the type of meetings you will conduct.

Type of Meeting	When
Brainstorming	
Strategic planning	
Logistical	
Planning	
Informational	
Other	
Other	
Other	

5. Identify anything else you want to include in your communication plan.

   _____

   _____

PROCESS WORKSHEET 7-2 **EMERGENCY PHONE TREE**

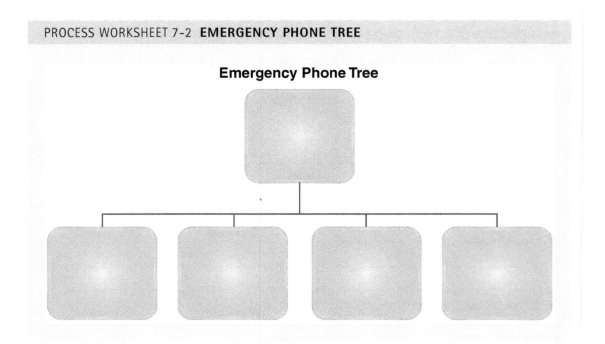

PROCESS WORKSHEET 7-3 **MEMORANDUM OF UNDERSTANDING WORKSHEET**

Instructions: Complete the following memorandum of understanding (MOU), which can be used in general or as part of a grant application. Fill in the document with the names of the community partners that you work with. This document can be modified to meet the needs of your partnership. Typically, MOUs are completed on letterhead. Please note: A memorandum of understanding is not a contract.

Memorandum of Understanding

This is a memorandum of understanding between _____ and

_____ (identify partners in blanks).

As an active community partner, the _____ in _____ (city,

state) fully supports the _____ application to the

_____ (name of funding agency).

Since _____ (length of partnership), the _____ has played an active

role in developing community efforts for the _____ (describe program efforts).

_____ (name of partner) agrees to contribute to the

_____ (name of program) by providing:

_____ (identify what will be provided by your agency in

support of the partnership).

_____   _____

Signature   Signature

Date: _____

PROCESS WORKSHEET 7-4 **CONVENING AN ADVISORY BOARD**

Instructions: Complete this worksheet to assist in development of an advisory board.

Goals of Advisory Board

Potential Activities of Advisory Board

Potential Members of Advisory Board

PROCESS WORKSHEET 7-5   **POSTMEETING REFLECTION**

Instructions: This worksheet can be used to conduct a reflection after advisory board or coalition meetings. This document can be used for either individual or group reflection.

1. What went well in today's meeting?

   _____

   _____

   _____

   _____

2. Describe any outcomes or completed activities from today's meeting.

   _____

   _____

   _____

   _____

3. What challenges can be identified from today's meeting?

   _____

   _____

   _____

   _____

4. How does the group think these challenges can be resolved?

   _____

   _____

   _____

   _____

5. If anything, what will we do differently in the next meeting?

   _____

   _____

   _____

   _____

   _____

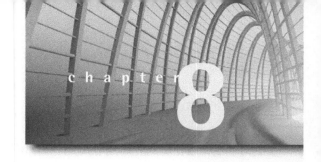

chapter 8

Piecing Together the Grant Proposal

LEARNING OBJECTIVES

By the end of this chapter, the reader will be able to complete the following:

1. Identify all the components of a strong grant proposal.
2. Develop a problem statement or statement of need.
3. Draft a sample grant proposal.

Key Terms

Abstract
Activity
Budget justification
Cover letter
Direct cost
Goal
Grant narrative
Grant proposal
Implementation plan
Indirect cost
Letter of intent
Logic model
Objective
Outcome
Problem statement or
    needs statement

Overview

This chapter covers the components involved in a typical grant proposal. The chapter discusses suggestions and tips on how to draft each component and integrate program development components for the occupational therapy practitioner.

Introduction

Grant proposals appear in all shapes and sizes with a vast variation in requirements and guidelines. Despite the differences, many grant proposals follow similar formats and include common components. Most grant proposals require the grant writer to draft sections on goals, objectives, activities, implementation plans, budgeting, and timelines. This chapter describes each component and how to maximize its potential for impressing grant reviewers.

The Grant Writing Process

Every grant writer develops their own process for drafting a grant proposal. Similar to how writers have their own creative process, each grant writer needs to identify what maximizes the grant writing process (Mosey, 1998; Hocking & Wright St. Clair, 2007). For some grant writers, shutting the office door and having uninterrupted time to write are key. For others, the grant writing process is a collaborative effort, where team members spur ideas in each other and one person formats and pulls the thoughts together (Beitz & Bliss, 2005; Holtzclaw, Kenner, & Walden, 2009). Still other grant writers may divvy portions of the grant proposal among team members, targeting each team member's expertise with one person charged with collating and collecting all the pieces into one document.

> **LET'S STOP AND THINK**
>
> What approaches and strategies will you employ in your grant writing process? Brainstorm a few options.

Whatever the approach, the grant writer or writers need to find the process that leads to success. In most cases, requests for proposals (RFPs) are released with a short turnaround time in which to draft a hefty grant proposal. Practitioners working on a team must ensure that all the team members have read the RFP, specific tasks have been distributed appropriately, and one person oversees the operation (Holtzclaw et al., 2009). Remember, a grant proposal "constitutes a bond of agreement between the proposal developers and the funding agency and serves as the blueprint for the project" (Ingersoll & Eberhard, 1999).

Components of a Grant Proposal

Most grant proposals have a standard format, yet no standards exist across all grant guidelines, and even federal grants vary in their requirements. Typically, a grant proposal includes the following components: title, abstract, introduction, goals/objectives, background, literature review, theoretical foundation, methodology or implementation plan, timeline, dissemination plan, project team bios, institutional information and paperwork, budget, budget justification, references, and appendices.

> **BEST PRACTICE HINT**
>
> Develop a checklist of all the items required by the RFP to ensure that you include all components in the final proposal.

Grant proposals are usually divided into several main sections. The **grant narrative** is the section that includes the goals, objectives, activities, proposed outcomes, background, needs statement or problem statement depending on the RFP, literature review, theoretical foundation, methodology or implementation plan, timeline, and dissemination plan. The budget is usually contained in a separate section with spe-

TABLE 8-1 TYPICAL COMPONENTS OF A GRANT PROPOSAL

Common Components of a Typical Grant Proposal

- Title
- Abstract
- Introduction
- Goals/objectives/activities
- Outcomes
- Background/needs statement/problem statement
- Literature review/theoretical foundation
- Methodology or Implementation plan
- Evaluation plan
- Timeline
- Dissemination plan
- Project team bios
- Institutional information and paperwork
- Budget
- Budget justification
- References
- Appendices

Less Common Components of a Grant Proposal

- Logic model
- Image or visual of project
- Detailed budget with specific items being purchased

Source: Gitlin, L. N., & Lyons, K. J. (2004). *Successful grant writing: Strategies for health and human service professionals* (2nd ed). New York: Springer; and Holtzclaw, B. J., Kenner, C., & Walden, M. (2009). *Grant writing handbook for nurses* (2nd ed.). Sudbury, MA: Jones and Bartlett.

cific forms or following a specific format. The program team's biographies and qualifications are usually in a separate section and are sometimes included in the appendices. The appendices are the last section and vary with grant requirements. There is no standard formatting for a grant proposal, so grant writers should review the RFP and follow the appropriate guidelines (Inouye & Fiellin, 2005; Dahlen, 2001; Lusk, 2004).

TABLE 8-2 GRANT PROPOSAL FORMATTING	
Section	**Components of Section**
Grant proposal narrative	• Goals
	• Objectives
	• Grant activities
	• Outcomes
	• Background/literature review
	• Needs statement/problem statement
	• Theoretical foundation
	• Methodology
	• Implementation plan
	• Timeline
	• Dissemination plan

Title

To the novice grant writer, it might sound outlandish to put a lot of thought into the title of the grant proposal, but it is very important. The title of the grant proposal should provide a short, concise glimpse of the purpose and outcome of the program (Gitlin & Lyons, 2004). Some grant funders limit the length of the title, but others allow any number of characters. The key to garnering funding is to capture the grant reviewers' attention (Barnard, 2002). A catchy and thoughtful title shows creativity and a passion for the proposed program. However, the grant writer needs to ensure that the title accurately describes the program and does not detract from the overall proposal.

BEST PRACTICE HINT

Ask community members to identify a title for the project that is meaningful and represents both the community and the proposal.

Letter of Intent

Some funding agencies require applying agencies to submit a **letter of intent**, which is simply a letter to the funding agency informing it of the organization's intent to apply for the grant (Holtzclaw et al., 2009; Coley & Scheinberg, 2008). In a sense, a letter of intent is a shortened grant proposal that typically includes a description of the applying agency and a brief description of the proposed program. Letters of intent ask whether the funding agency is interested in funding the project. They

> ### TABLE 8-3 EXAMPLES OF FUNDED GRANT TITLES
>
> - *Engaging Students: The Community as Classroom* (Flecky & Doll, 2008)
> - *A Heart for Health: The Health Report Card Project* (Voltz, Ryan Haddad, Hohnstein, & Martens Stricklett, 2007)
> - *Caring for the Caregiver: An Outreach Program for Caregivers* (Ryan Haddad, Koenig, & Voltz, 2007).
> - *Brain Bash—An Interactive Interprofessional Educational Outreach for the Prevention of Youth Substance Abuse and the Promotion of Healthy Living* (Cochran, Goulet, Voltz, Jensen, Ryan Haddad, & Wilken, 2006)

may also describe additional information required by the funding agency, including the agency budget and tax identification number (Non-Profit Guides, 2008). The funding agency outlines the requirements of the letter of intent.

In many cases, agencies that require a letter of intent filter through these letters, and then invite only certain projects to apply. A letter of intent is much shorter to draft than a full proposal and can save the project team time when choosing agencies from which to seek funding. Letters can range in length from one page to several pages. The challenge is fitting a description of a program into a short letter!

Abstract

The **abstract** is a "brief description of the proposal" (Gitlin & Lyons, 1996, p. 66; Gitlin & Lyons, 2004; Holtzclaw et al., 2009). The purpose of the abstract is to provide an abbreviated description of the proposed program. In other words, the abstract is the executive summary of the proposal. An abstract summarizes the key points such as the program purpose and outcome along with a brief description of the need for the program. Even though the abstract appears at the beginning of the grant proposal, it is best for the project team to write the abstract last when all other components of the grant are complete to make sure it accurately summarizes the proposed program (Holtzclaw et al., 2009). Most RFPs set a word limit on abstracts (Gitlin & Lyons, 2004).

Abstracts are an extremely important component of the grant proposal and the grant writing team should never overlook them. The abstract may very well be the first part of the proposal that the reviewer sees, so it must be nicely organized, provide a succinct but powerful description, and flow with the rest of the proposal. A poorly written abstract insinuates a poorly written grant proposal (Holtzclaw et al., 2009). Furthermore, if the program is funded, the funder may publish the abstract, so the abstract may travel beyond the reviewer's desk. In this case, the abstract represents the program to the scholarly community and other grantees.

TABLE 8-4 SAMPLE GRANT ABSTRACTS

Sample Abstract #1

The Community Response Team (CRT) is proposing to enhance their ongoing Community Mobilization Initiative by assisting Native American youth ages 12–18 in the substance abuse recovery process by initiating the "Sacred Child" program. The program will utilize an evidence-based approach in providing outpatient treatment, community outreach, and peer-to-peer recovery services for youth and their families. Program activities will assist the community in developing a recovery support infrastructure on the reservation. This recovery support system will directly assist youth in developing their cultural knowledge and skills to make better decisions regarding substance abuse and will provide a framework to change community norms regarding substance abuse and recovery.

The CRT vision is to provide a culturally appropriate system of care that connects successful evidence-based approaches with core values and teachings of culture to provide a framework to change community norms regarding substance abuse and recovery. Through partnerships with the Tribal Court, Public Schools, and the Tribe, the CRT will incorporate the program into outpatient treatment, outreach, and peer-to-peer services while engaging tribal leaders and community stakeholders, focusing on a community change process regarding attitudes toward substance abuse.

One specific goal and three objectives will be pursued through this effort: **Project Goal:** To provide an effective and comprehensive recovery support infrastructure on the reservation. **Objective 1:** To undertake the culturally relevant, evidence-based substance abuse program for youth ages 12–18 on the Omaha reservation; **Objective 2:** To integrate the program into new and existing youth outreach programs to provide a comprehensive approach to building youth awareness, recruitment, and referral into this substance abuse program; and **Objective 3:** To establish Child Center, to coordinate the program, and to facilitate youth involvement, mentoring, and recovery support services.

The evaluation for this project will be ongoing and consist of two parts: (1) a process evaluation that examines whether the implementation of the project is successful in matching the plans with the actual services and activities as well as tracking progress on project goals over time, and (2) an outcome evaluation that features a core data collection effort using the Discretionary Services Client Level GPRA Tool. This instrument will be administered to participants according to the baseline, 6-month, and 12-month intervals of participant involvement. It is expected that at least 100 youth will participate in treatment yearly over the 3 years of the grant. In addition, it is expected that 400 community members will participate in community-based outreach and peer-to-peer recovery activities.

TABLE 8-4 SAMPLE GRANT ABSTRACTS (CONTINUED)

Sample Abstract #2

The purpose of this project is to explore the role of the "community as classroom" as a curricular process in the Department of Occupational Therapy. The research team proposes to explore and define a model for faculty in occupational therapy, and intended for replication by faculty across the health sciences, to engage in community-based learning with health professions students. The proposed model will explore how to develop partnerships, explore the role of students in meeting community needs, and provide tips and techniques for bridging community service to scholarship. This model is needed to support faculty desiring to employ the Scholarship of Engagement as an approach to the Scholarship of Teaching and Learning. Outcomes of the project will include the development of sustainable community partners that support community needs and the occupational therapy curriculum, and an assessment plan for assessing the impact of community-based learning for students, community members, and faculty.

Occupational therapy is a profession that uses "human 'doing' as both the means and ends of intervention" (Pierce, 2003, p. 4). Based on this basic tenet of the profession, occupational therapy education needs to be active, experiential, hands-on, and reflective. The grant team proposes that service learning acts as a strong pedagogical approach for teaching important aspects of the occupational therapy profession. Our proposed project involves implementing a developed model entitled Community as Classroom that integrates best practices for occupational therapy education in planning and implementation of community engagement/service learning as a valuable pedagogical approach. The grant team wants to take the results of a pilot project to implement this model fully throughout the occupational therapy curriculum.

Cover Letter

In some cases, grant RFPs require a **cover letter** included at the front of the proposal that simply describes to reviewers the intent to apply for the grant funding, the organization applying for funding, and the proposed program (Berg et al., 2007; Barnard, 2002; Coley & Scheinberg, 2008). A cover letter can go into more detail than an abstract can, but the cover letter does not replace the abstract. The requirements for the cover letter are usually outlined in the grant guidelines.

BEST PRACTICE HINT

Even if not required, include a cover letter with a grant proposal to introduce the grant proposal and let the reviewers know more about the organization applying for funding.

TABLE 8-5 SAMPLE COVER LETTER
Dear Sir or Madam, Please accept this proposal entitled *A Heart for Health: The Health Report Card Project* to the Minority Public Health Association. This proposal is to support healthcare services to the underserved African American population located in North Omaha, Nebraska, focusing on cardiovascular disease, diabetes, and fostering community collaboration to meet community needs. We propose to complete this project in partnership with the Ministry Center, a local nonprofit, located in the heart of the North Omaha community. Our approach utilizes the strengths of all the entities involved to make this project a success, including the needs expressed by community members, the staff and facilities at the Ministry Center, faculty within the school, and health professions students in pharmacy, physical therapy, and occupational therapy. The Health Report Card is an innovative method to ensure that beyond receiving health screenings, community members can begin to become more knowledgeable about their health status and begin to command their health. The project team believes the Health Report Card will make a sustainable impact on both individuals and the community as a whole, increasing awareness and control of one's own health. We have enclosed a sample of the Health Report Card for your review as a health education tool. Thank you for your consideration of *A Heart for Health: The Health Report Card Project.* We look forward to working together to address health disparities and improve the health of minorities in our own community. Sincerely,

Optional Components of Research and Program-Based Grants

Because no standardized requirements for grants exist, some components may vary based on the type of grant proposal. In a research grant, the first section includes a background and literature review. In a program-based or demonstration grant, the grant proposal includes a problem statement or statement of need that describes the community need with data. Each section has its own unique purpose, and the grant writer must review the RFP to determine which sections and what information in each section is required.

Background

All grant proposals require the grant writer to describe the community, the program, and the needs the program will address in a section often referred to as the background. The background describes the community and its needs with supportive data and then identifies how the needs should be addressed. The background should do the following: demonstrate the need, identify community capacity, demonstrate the organization's understanding of the need, inform grant reviewers about the need in a clear and straightforward manner, and make a case to the reviewers as to why these challenges should be met (Environmental Protection Agency, 2007).

BEST PRACTICE HINT

Although the background, literature, and needs statements may require similar information, the requirements of each will vary based on the grant requirements. Thoroughly review the RFP to determine which components are required for each grant and what is required in each grant proposal section.

Depending on the granting agency, the background section may be called different names. In some cases, it is simply called the background. In others, it is called the literature review. Still other granting agencies title this section the **needs statement** or **problem statement**. In the case of a research-based grant, this section may be called the rationale. The RFP guidelines will reveal the title of this section and describe what should be included in the proposal.

The background should include facts from reliable sources about the community that establish the challenges the community faces. The grant writer must determine which sources provide the most reliable support for the proposal (Gitlin & Lyons, 2004). Data in the background should represent the needs both nationally and related to the community. The grant writer needs to describe the community, including demographics and other facts. The RFP will outline specific requirements for data, if any, and what should be included in this section. Grant writers must follow all guidelines including the page number limit for this section.

In addition to supportive data, the background also should include a literature review that summarizes the literature that supports the proposal. A separate literature review section might sometimes be required, or this section can meld with the section outlining the theoretical foundations. The purpose of the literature review is to describe programs that are similar to the proposed program and to provide evidence of successful models that have been documented in the literature (Gitlin & Lyons, 2004; Barnard, 2002). The grant writer needs to reference sources according to the RFP guidelines and use literature that fully supports the proposed program. Literature reviews can assist a grant proposal in several ways: by identifying how much the topic has been discussed in the literature, assisting with pro-

BEST PRACTICE HINT

Never exceed RFP page number requirements. If a proposal exceeds these requirements, often it will be discarded and will not be reviewed.

viding a rationale for the proposed project, identifying strategies for implementation, and demonstrating a widespread knowledge of the topic (Gitlin & Lyons, 2004). If the proposed program does not have a lot of literature available, it is best

TABLE 8-6 RELIABLE SOURCES OF DATA

National data sources	• National reliable health organizations such as the Centers for Disease Control and Prevention or Healthy People 2020
	• Census Bureau
Local data sources	• Health departments
	• Hospital reports
	• University research
	• Community assessments

TABLE 8-7 EXAMPLE OF A PORTION OF A GRANT BACKGROUND

Approximately 19.2 million Asian Americans live in the United States, with individuals from China making up the largest subset of all Asian Americans (24%). Of the Chinese living in the United States, 38% are foreign-born with citizenship and 33% are foreign-born without citizenship. According to the U.S. Census Bureau, 43% of Asian Americans arrived in the United States between 1990 and 2000, with 43% of Chinese Americans arriving during these years. Fifty percent of Chinese Americans are not considered to be "good" English speakers and still speak their native Chinese at home. Of Chinese Americans 25 and older, 23% have less than a high school education, and of all Asian American groups, Chinese fall third for collegiate education with 48% having completed bachelor's degrees. Many Chinese who choose to get an education in the United States decide to stay when their education is complete. Among Chinese Americans 16 and older, 69% of men and 57% of women are employed. Over half of Chinese Americans work in a professional environment, but only 14% are employed in service-related jobs, like health care. Despite having a higher earning ratio than other groups in the United States, poverty levels compare to the national average with 14% of Chinese Americans living in poverty. Although the population of Chinese in the state of Nebraska is small (in 2005, 1.5% of Nebraskans identified themselves as Asian), the number of Chinese in the Midwest is growing with Chicago, Illinois, ranking seventh nationally in the amount of Chinese now residing in an urban area.

Source: Reeves, T. J., & Bennett, C. E. (2004). We the People: Asians in the United States: Census 2000 Special Reports. Retrieved March 24, 2009, from http://www.census.gov/prod/2004pubs/censr-17.pdf; and Mu, K., Bracciano, A., Goulet, C., & Voltz, J. D. (2007). *Chinese Study in Health Care: An Innovative Approach for Teaching Health Care Professionals.* Submitted to the United States Department of Education.

to state this in the proposal. Grant writers can also identify in this section how they plan to contribute to the literature by disseminating the information.

Problem Statement/Needs Statement

The problem statement or needs statement describes the community and the problem or need that affects the community (Coley & Scheinberg, 2008). The needs or problem statement is the call for assistance for funding to help meet community need (Notario-Risk & Ottenwess, 2000). Problem statements in grants focused on program development differ from those in research grants, where this section focuses on establishing a need for the proposed research (Writing Center—University of North Carolina at Chapel Hill, 2007). In a community program development grant proposal, the problem statement describes "the critical conditions that are affecting certain people or things in a specific place at a specific time" (Notario-Risk & Ottenwess, 2000, p. 4).

The needs or problem statement is the true meat of the grant proposal because the applying agency is seeking funding from the granting agency to address this community problem or need. In many cases, this statement is a component of the grant narrative, as described in the RFP. If a problem or need is not well defined, then the rest of the proposal holds little purpose. Likewise, a well-designed program with a clear problem statement that addresses an unimportant need or trivial problem will not be funded.

The terms *problem statement* and *needs statement* might be used interchangeably among granting agencies. Problem statements need to cover the issue at hand but not be too broad (Bordage & Dawson, 2003). The problem statement must directly relate to the program, so it should represent the issues the program will address. A community may have more problems than are identified in the problem statement. The grant writer has to focus on one main problem in the problem statement, and then support this statement with data and literature. Similarly, a problem statement cannot be too narrow. Funders want to provide funds to address an encompassing issue in a community and not a trivial problem.

BEST PRACTICE HINT

Use the term used in the RFP— either *problem statement*, *statement of need*, or *needs statement*—to title this section. Using the RFP terms helps grant reviewers understand the proposal.

Reviewers will explore the problem or needs statement thoroughly. One strategy for success in writing this section is to ensure that the needs or problem statement aligns with the mission and outcomes of the funding agency. When reviewers understand a community's challenge the review process goes more smoothly. Any questions or confusion in a proposal can affect the grant proposal's review. Ensuring that reviewers understand the need or problem is crucial in garnering funds (Bordage & Dawson, 2003).

TABLE 8-8 SAMPLE GRANT PROBLEM/NEEDS STATEMENT

Problem Statement: According to the Douglas County Health Department, racial and ethnic disparities exist for many health indicators including heart disease, stroke, and cancer. The leading causes of death among African Americans in Douglas County include heart disease, cancer, diabetes, and stroke. The statistics for African Americans in Douglas County are astounding, with 25% higher death rate for heart disease than whites, 53% higher death rate for stroke than whites, and blacks have lower rates of health insurance than do whites. According to the Health Department, blacks represent the highest minority group with an estimated population of approximately 12.2% within Douglas County, calling on the community to address these significant health disparities. The Heart Ministry Center, a local nonprofit focused on addressing the needs of Omaha's predominantly African American community, is faced with the challenges of meeting multiple community needs. A recent needs assessment completed by the Heart Ministry Center revealed that the local African American population is in need of primary care services including basic health screenings and hypertension and diabetes education. We propose to address these health concerns and work to eliminate disparities by educating and empowering African Americans in our community regarding health status and connecting them to resources and supports that can lead to appropriate healthy behavior changes.

Source: Voltz, J. D., Ryan Haddad, A., Hohnstein, S., & Martens Stricklett, K. (2007). *A Heart for Health: The Health Report Card Project.* Nebraska Minority Public Health Association, $500.

Incorporating Capacity into the Background

As discussed throughout this book, grant writers should also identify community assets and strengths because needs and problems can be addressed only through capacities and the community's desire to change. Including facts and data about capacity is important. Capacities and assets can establish the viability of addressing the community issue (Wilken, 2008). Identifying resources can help strengthen the proposal's case because it also highlights gaps in resources that the program seeks to fill.

For example, in a rural community 85% of the population wants to improve the nutrition of its youth, but the local convenience store where the youth go sells only soda and no milk (D. Parker, personal communication, August 2007). This issue of access to milk is a real challenge to the community. However, the need is also affected by community capacity. The capacity is the community's commitment to improving the health of the youth, and the challenge is the lack of accessibility to healthy foods. Another example is in a tribal community, 75% of the patients seen in physical and occupational therapy indicate that they want to exercise, but there are no sidewalks in the community and wild dogs run around in packs (Stabler &

Doll, 2009). The community identified the desire of community members and wrote grants to fund the sidewalk installation and to build and run an animal shelter. With these two barriers eliminated, more people in the community began participating in walking programs.

Grant reviewers want to know and understand the challenges faced by the community and also the community's capacities. Including this information in the background demonstrates a focus on capacity building and establishes the program as more viable for funding.

BEST PRACTICE HINT

Explore and identify community capacity through a community assessment.

Theoretical Foundation

As outlined in some RFPs, some grant agencies require the applicant to identify a theoretical approach upon which the program will be based (Gitlin & Lyons, 2004). Many grantors now require a program to follow an evidence-based approach, similar to the demands of medical interventions. This is especially the case for federal funding agencies such as the Substance Abuse and Mental Health Services Administration (SAMHSA). Funders want to know that the approaches proposed in the program are proven to be effective and have been demonstrated to produce community change. The description of the theoretical foundation may be required in the background as part of the program justification.

The theoretical framework used depends on the program being proposed. For example, if the occupational therapy practitioner is writing a grant to fund a sensory room, the grant writer can explain and share the evidence as proven by the sensory integration theory. In the grant proposal, the practitioner would include literature and research studies that demonstrate the evidence of sensory integration. The grant writer needs to justify the use of a sensory room model through proven theoretical evidence. A review and citation of the literature are also important in this section (Gitlin & Lyons, 2004). Not all grants require a theoretical foundation or evidence-based approach, but including a description of one is a strategy that grant writers can use to strengthen a grant proposal.

Goals, Objectives, Activities, and Outcomes

The goals, objectives, activities, and outcomes section of the grant proposal is extremely important because it describes to grant reviewers the proposed program outcomes (Coley & Scheinberg, 2008). The key to a successful grant proposal is a well-designed program. The purpose of this book is to demonstrate the importance of the integration of the two. So,

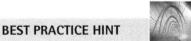

BEST PRACTICE HINT

Include only two or three goals in a grant proposal.

with proper program planning, writing this section of the grant proposal should be simple, as long as the grant writer follows the guidelines outlined in the RFP. Grant writers should know exactly what the program plans to achieve and how the funding will help the program achieve it. This information should be conveyed clearly in the proposal.

The goals and objectives section of the grant proposal is where the grant writer outlines exactly what the program plans to achieve. In other words, in this section the grant writer outlines exactly what will be done and how these activities will effect community change. In grant writing, **goals** are matched with objectives. **Objectives** describe the program outcomes that will be measured in the evaluation plan. **Activities** outline exactly what will be done to reach the goals and objectives. The activities are the specifics of the program and are the description of actual programmatic activities to be completed as part of the program. **Outcomes** are the impacts the program will make.

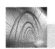

BEST PRACTICE HINT

Goals should always refer to the needs identified earlier in the proposal.

Occupational therapy practitioners should be familiar with goal writing from treatment planning. Goal writing in grants is a little different because the focus is on a program and not an individual client. Goals describe the overall purpose of the proposed program (Gitlin & Lyons, 2004). Goals are a basic overview of what the program aims to accomplish. The goals for a program grant should relate to community change and are often more general than objectives. Goals must tie directly back to the proposal's background and/or needs/problem statement. Goals should always be written to be feasible and should include the proposed number of participants or community members the proposed program plans to reach. Goals should also always relate directly to the needs or problems discussed. If a disconnection occurs between the needs and the goals, the grant proposal will be disjointed and reviewers will not be clear on the proposed program's purpose. This section of the grant proposal provides the opportunity to describe the purpose of the program and what benefits the program will have on the community. Making the tie between the two is essential in good grant writing.

LET'S STOP AND THINK

Write down a potential program goal. Share it with a peer and evaluate one another's program goal based on what you have learned thus far.

In general, it is recommended that a grant proposal include no more than two or three specific goals for a project (Falk, 2006). Smaller grant projects will have fewer goals than larger ones will. In a successful grant proposal, goals are feasible with the funding to be received. Drafting goals that reach beyond the funding or scope of the granting agency is inappropriate and reviewers will deny funding.

LET'S STOP AND THINK

Write down a potential grant objective that ties into the grant goal written earlier. Share it with a peer and evaluate one another's grant objective based on what you have learned thus far.

After drafting the overall goals, objectives come next. Objectives are specifically what the program team hopes to accomplish that will contribute to achieving the overall goals and will be measured and evaluated (Gitlin & Lyons, 2004). When drafting the evaluation plan, the objectives need to be reviewed and can actually drive the evaluation plan. For objectives, grant writers need to think practically and identify what

---

TABLE 8-9 GRANT GOAL EXAMPLES

- The overall goal of this project is to promote health education and empower the residents of North City, a predominantly African American community, to become more aware of their health status (Voltz, Ryan Haddad, Hohnstein, & Martens Stricklett, 2007).

- By the end of the program, the program team will create and offer a unique health fair and monthly educational learning modules to students at the Faith School (Begley, Doll, Ryan Haddad, & Martens Stricklett, 2008).

- By the end of the program, the program team convenes a leadership institute for leaders in health information distribution in minority communities (Goulet et al., 2006).

TABLE 8-10 GRANT OBJECTIVE EXAMPLES

- By the end of year 1 of the program, the program team will provide primary care assessments to a minimum of 40 community members (i.e., hypertension checks and education, diabetes screenings, skin cancer screenings, osteoporosis screenings, drug information, healthy walking approaches, cholesterol checks, calcium and vitamin D counseling, etc.) at a local community health fair.

- By the end of the program, the program team will train health professions students in providing health screenings to an underserved, minority population, emphasizing the development of community leaders and civic responsibility as both students and future health professionals.

- By the end of year 1 of the program, the program team will engage occupational therapy students in self-reflection to assess attributes of professional development.

---

the program hopes to accomplish. Objectives should be feasible and align with the goals appropriately. Objectives should also tie directly to addressing the needs and capacities outlined earlier in the grant proposal.

As discussed previously, goals and objectives need to be feasible for a grant proposal to garner funding. Grant objectives should be measurable and contain a timeline for completion and a project number outcome. One of the challenges of writing a grant proposal is predicting the number of community members that will be served or affected by a program (Bliss & Savik, 2005). However, most granting agencies want a specific number of

BEST PRACTICE HINT

Each goal should have two or three objectives.

community members affected to be identified in the proposal. These numbers are usually identified in the description of the grant objectives.

Grant writers should avoid overestimating the number of participants that the program will affect. If a grant proposal is funded, grantees have to report the progress of outcomes to the funding agency, and the funding agency expects the grantee to reach its objectives. Not reaching the stated objectives in a grant can reflect poorly on the program in grant reports and can actually affect funding and future funding. For example, if an objective identifies how many people the program will serve, these estimates need to be close to accurate. Once funded, grantees have to report the progress of outcomes to granting agencies.

Activities are specifically what will be done in the program and include the day-to-day tasks that will accomplish the goals and objectives (Gitlin & Lyons, 2004). In the activities section of the grant proposal, the grant writer should outline who will do what and when it will be completed. The activities include the simple everyday things that help a program along. Some granting agencies will not want to know these details, but some require specific activities to be discussed. When developing a program, drafting activities helps with organization and accountability.

Outcomes are what the program proposes to complete through its implementation. Outcomes are not just what happens at the end of the program but should occur throughout the implementation. Outcomes should tie directly to the goals and objectives in the proposal. The outcomes are demonstrated through evaluation methods used in the evaluation plan described in more detail in Chapter 10. They identify the impact of the program on the community and are really the purpose of the grant funding and the program. For community practice, outcomes usually relate to health behavior changes (Edberg, 2007; Brownson, 2001).

The goals, objectives, activities, and outcomes outline the program and what will be done to affect the community needs. This section must be well written with

goals, objectives, and activities complementing one another and should follow the grant guidelines. In this section, the grant reviewers will come to understand exactly what the program proposes to do and what the grant money will actually fund. Therefore, the grant writer should be thoughtful in the development of this section and thoroughly review this section. Grant writers can refer back to program development principles for help in the development of this section, which will lead to a program that fits nicely into a grant application and, most important, meets community needs.

TABLE 8-11 GRANT ACTIVITIES EXAMPLES

- The program coordinator will provide a sign-in sheet for all activities.
- The program will team develop and utilize a database to track community member use of the facility and individual programs.
- The grant coordinator will submit monthly program reports, including statistics, programming conducted, and future plans.

TABLE 8-12 GRANT OUTCOMES EXAMPLES

- An average of at least 30 community members per month will utilize services provided by the Community Health Educator.
- A minimum of three programs that target aspects of diabetes and cardiovascular disease prevention will be developed and conducted by June 30.
- More than 1000 minutes of educational coding will be submitted per year by appropriate Wellness Center staff.

Source: Cross, P., & Voltz, J. D. (2005). *Four Hills of Life Wellness Center Nebraska Native American Public Health Grant.* Nebraska Health and Human Services.

Implementation Plan

The **implementation plan** is the who, what, where, when, and how of the program (Chambless, 2003). This section outlines how the program will be implemented. Sometimes in grant guidelines the implementation plan is called the methodology, especially in the case of research grants. In this section of the proposal, the grant writer must identify who will be served by the project, what exactly will be done, where it will be done, and when it will be completed (Coley & Scheinberg, 2008). Some granting agencies require this section to be very detailed and others allow it to be more open ended.

In the implementation plan section, the grant writer must identify who will be served and how the individuals being served will be recruited, including who qualifies for the program and how they enter the program. The number served and strategies for ensuring that at least the minimum number proposed receives services should be covered in this section.

The implementation plan also discusses policies and procedures. Although these may or may not be required as part of the grant proposal, they should be a part of the program planning. The staff and members responsible for implementation should also be covered. Some grants require the inclusion of biosketches, but, if

TABLE 8-13 SAMPLE IMPLEMENTATION PLAN

Step	Assigned to	Start Date	Completion Date
Step 1: Research treatment centers	Program Director	January	February
Step 2: Perform needs assessment of treatment centers	Program Director	January	March
Step 3: Create database of treatment centers	Program Director	January	March
Step 4: Share database with planning committee	Program Director	March	March
Step 5: Contact treatment centers	Program Director and Committee Members	March	April
Step 6: Meet with treatment center contacts if necessary	Program Director	April	May
Step 7: Seek experts from treatment centers as speakers	Program Director	April	May
Step 8: Create an invitation list from treatment centers	Program Director and Committee Members	May	June

BEST PRACTICE HINT

Some granting agencies allow the inclusion of appendices. The appendices provide a place to include additional relevant information such as policies and procedures. Make sure to follow the RFP guidelines on appendices regarding what and how much can be included.

not, it is important for grant writers to identify the program team and why the individuals are qualified to implement the program. The grant writer can place this information in different sections of a proposal depending on the guidelines.

An implementation plan should also account for changes or challenges that arise and identify how the grant team will address these challenges. The implementation plan should focus on opportunities that may arise to change or enhance the program along the way (Weil, 2005). The program team can develop policies and procedures to prepare for both challenges and opportunities.

TABLE 8-14 SAMPLE GRANT TIMELINE

Activity	Dates	Participants
Create planning team	June 2006	Community members and project team
Develop course requirements for students	July 2006	Project planning team
Prepare syllabi for student projects	July 2006	Project planning team
Send out letters to schools	August 2006	Project planning team
Students complete projects	September 2006	Interprofessional students
Implement Brain Bash	October 2006	Project planning team and students

Timeline

A timeline is an important tool to use in a grant proposal because it helps both the writer and the reviewer understand the program in greater context. Some grants require a timeline, but in program development it is relevant to develop a timeline whether one is required or not. Timelines should tie directly to the program goals, objectives, and activities.

The timeline is quite simple to develop and requires the grant writer to consider how long activities can take to implement (Inouye & Fiellin, 2005). If the program is newly developed, the timeline will be estimated and may include more flexibility. If the program has been previously implemented, the timeline may be more concrete in nature. The length of time for implementation is considered in the timeline as well as the chronological order in which events and activities will take place (Ingersoll & Eberhard, 1999). This can help reviewers visualize the program more clearly. The timeline is also a valuable tool in implementation because it can keep the program team on task.

Evaluation Plan

All grant proposals require an evaluation plan. Because evaluation plans require specific skills and methods, they are discussed in more depth in Chapter 10.

Dissemination Plan

Every grant program should include a dissemination plan, whether formalized in the proposal or not. Some granting agencies require dissemination as part of the grant proposal and designate funding in the budget to support it. All grants have outcomes from their implementation, and the project team should make plans to disseminate these outcomes to a variety of populations (Bordage & Dawson, 2003). Dissemination is a crucial piece of the grant proposal because it advances the program and the profession of occupational therapy through the building of evidence (Holtzclaw et al., 2009). Engaging in scholarship surrounding the dissemination of a successful program also promotes professional development and career advancement for occupational therapy practitioners (Holtzclaw et al., 2009).

First, the project team should share the outcomes of the program with the community (Israel, Eng, Schulz, & Parker, 2005). They should disseminate the outcomes of a program or research study funded by a grant to the community in a format that is both appropriate and respectful. The team must consider factors such as literacy levels and culture in dissemination. Information should also be disseminated in a format that is useful to the community, and the community should have a voice in the dissemination of information from their programs. Dissemination occurs at multiple levels including individual community members, community organizations, the community as a whole and beyond, including political officials (Parker et al., 2005).

| LET'S STOP AND THINK |
Brainstorm where and how occupational therapy practitioners could disseminate best practices garnered from a successful grant-funded community program.

The project team can disseminate outcomes to the community using a variety of methods such as annual reports, newsletters, media campaigns, program websites, press releases, public presentations, and community forums (Parker et al., 2005). One strategy for sharing outcomes with the community outlined by Parker and associates (2005) includes developing a dissemination committee of community members and program team members who collectively decide how outcomes will be distributed to the community.

The grant project team should share outcomes with those directly involved in and served by the program and the community in which the program exists. In community programs, the community owns the data and the outcomes as much as the program team does. Efforts to share program outcomes are also strategic in maintaining community partnerships and lead to building trust and facilitating openness and communication among community partners and community members (Israel et al., 2005). In program development and implementation, it is very easy for the project team to forget to report outcomes to the community, especially when a funding agency requires a certain reporting structure. However, it is important that the team share this information with the community in an appropriate and relevant format.

TABLE 8-15 IDEAS FOR DISSEMINATION

- Present at a state association conference.
- Present at a national association conference.
- Draft a newspaper article about the program.
- Write an article for a practice magazine.
- Submit a manuscript to a professional journal.
- Share best practices at networking or professional meetings.
- Provide trainings or continuing education to other practitioners.

The project team should share community programs and successes not only with community members but also other communities and practitioners. A program that could easily be replicated saves time and resources for another underserved community and can lead to positive community change beyond a single community. Furthermore, replication justifies and strengthens existing programs. Project teams can share their best practices and program descriptions in a variety of venues such as conference presentations, manuscripts, television interviews, newsletters, and websites (Parker et al., 2005). Occupational therapy practitioners working in community settings should take advantage of these opportunities to promote professional development and expand the impact of the program. Some grantors even require dissemination of program details at conferences or professional meetings and may even designate which meetings. In this case, more formalized presentations such as poster or panel presentations may be appropriate.

For practitioners in an academic setting, dissemination is crucial for promotion and tenure (Holtzclaw et al., 2009). The principal investigator and grant team should develop a plan for disseminating to certain scholarly journals, professional organizations, and conferences. Funding for travel to conferences for program dissemination can often be included in the grant budget to support such endeavors.

Budget

The budget is another important part of any grant proposal and should not be skimmed over. When creating a budget, the grant writer needs to consider what resources are needed for program implementation and the guidelines required by both the granting agency and the agency receiving funding (Gitlin & Lyons, 2004). According to Ingersoll and Eberhard (1999), grant writers should consider all the pieces of the program that require time, space, and resources when drafting the grant budget. A budget in a grant proposal acts as a map for funding and aids in the implementation process when the money will be spent.

The proposed budget should follow all the guidelines outlined in the RFP. The budget must accurately match and complement the proposal's goals, objectives, and activities. Errors in the budget can cause the entire proposal to be dismissed by grant reviewers. The grant writer also must develop a budget justification describing why items are needed for program implementation (Holtzclaw et al., 2009).

BEST PRACTICE HINT

Get help from individuals experienced in budgeting to create a realistic grant budget.

Some RFPs are very specific about what the grant will fund and what it will not fund (Holtzclaw et al., 2009). For example, some grants will not fund salary or travel expenses. The grant writer must be aware of what is allowed and what is prohibited to ensure prohibited items are not included in the budget. Grant writers should address any confusing or conflicting items in the RFP about the budget with the grant program manager early in the grant writing process. Some RFPs require additions to a traditional grant budget such as copies of quotes on pricing for specific items. Any exceptions or anything unique should be noted and recognized. These details will be outlined specifically in the RFP.

BEST PRACTICE HINT

Have budget questions? Always contact the program manager because an error in the budget can prevent a program from receiving funding.

Grant writers must note any institutional requirements that the agency seeking funding requires or has in place (Gitlin & Lyons, 2004). Many academic institutions have a centralized grant office with staff trained to assist with these aspects of the grant proposal (Holtzclaw et al., 2009). In such cases, regulations exist related to the budget and what can be purchased with grant funding. Grant writers also need to consider details that are required in any grant budget. For example, if the grant budget includes salary, then the fringe benefit rate utilized by the institution needs to be included in the budget.

Components of a Grant Proposal Budget

Budgets usually consist of two major components: direct costs and indirect costs (Gitlin & Lyons, 2004). **Direct costs** are those items in the budget that will be funded by the grant money such as salary, benefits, equipment, consultants, and travel expenses. **Indirect costs** include those costs not directly tied to the project or program implementation such as "rental fees, payment of utilities, equipment depreciation, providing security, and general maintenance of workspace" (Ingersoll & Eberhard, 1999, p. 133).

In many situations, grant money does not cover the full salaries of personnel. In such cases, the percentage of effort the individual contributes to the proposed program must be calculated so that that certain percentage can be covered by the grant (Holtzclaw et al., 2009). The percentage of effort is based on the individual's current pay and the percentage of time the person will spend on the grant activities. For example, if an employee is paid $50,000 a year and will engage in grant activi-

TABLE 8-16 DIRECT AND INDIRECT BUDGET COSTS

Direct Costs	Indirect Costs
• Personnel	• Institutional space
• Equipment	• Utilities
• Supplies	• Insurance
• Trainings	• Maintenance
• Travel	• Administrative costs
• Renovations	
• Contracts	
• Food	

ties one day a week, or will expend 20% effort in the proposed program, the salary in the budget would be $10,000. Grant writers should consult with supervisors or a grant office for advice on appropriateness of calculating salaries. The budget needs to clearly identify personnel commitment and the amount of funding provided to the staff member. In some cases, the budget must be approved by the parent applying institution prior to grant submission, especially when job responsibilities go beyond the grant.

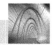

BEST PRACTICE HINT

When calculating salaries, do not forget to calculate the cost of benefits.

Other important information to consider prior to drafting the budget is the latest federal mileage rate. If mileage reimbursement is written into a grant proposal, it is standard protocol to use the federal reimbursement rate. Also, if travel is included in the grant budget, the grant writer must be aware of the costs of airfare and other expenses of travel. These details can assist in developing a realistic and fundable budget.

Indirect costs are lumped as a sum of money that can be used to pay for the aforementioned costs and are not specifically listed in the budget (Holtzclaw et al., 2009). Indirect costs are based on rates established by the federal government or the organization. In federal grants, rates vary by agency and can be as high as 45%. The grant writer needs to be aware of indirect rates prior to developing the budget to accurately include the indirect costs. Indirect rate information is outlined in the RFP, but if any questions arise, the grant writer should contact the program manager. Some institutions also have an established indirect rate for any grant received whereas others do not identify an indirect rate. Not all granting agencies allow for indirect costs. If not, this information needs to be articulated if an organization typically charges an indirect rate.

BEST PRACTICE HINT

To find the current federal mileage rate, visit the Internal Revenue Service at http://www.irs.gov/tax pros/article/0,,id=156624,00.html.

When working in communities, occupational therapy practitioners need to explore the impact of indirect costs. In some cases, practitioners may need to educate community partners on agency regulations and identified costs that affect the budget. A community partner can be puzzled or offended when a significant amount of the budget goes to indirect costs of an institution and not directly to the community. When partnering with community agencies, the factors that affect the budget need to be negotiated. Occupational therapy practitioners should take time to become educated on these factors to avoid problems with a community partner (Suarez-Balcazar, Hammel, & Helfrich, 2005). As described in Chapter 7 on community partnerships, trust and rapport building are important to program implementation. Misunderstandings about the budget should not get in the way of addressing community needs.

BEST PRACTICE HINT

Determine whether an indirect rate is required prior to developing the budget to save time and assign accurate funding amounts to budgeted items.

Basic Grant Budget Knowledge

When building the budget, detail is important. The grant writer should include as much detail as possible while still following the budget requirements outlined in the RFP. Some funding agencies provide a template for creating the budget that outlines what needs to be included. If one is provided by the funding agency, the grant writer should always follow the budget template (Ingersoll & Eberhard, 1999).

If a grant will be funded over a period of more than a year, important factors must be considered in the budgeting process, such as rising costs. If the grant budget includes salary, (if allowed by the granting agency) a raise should be included each year, so the budget may not be equal over subsequent funding years. The budget may differ across multiyear grants also because of equipment purchases at the beginning of the program where the budget includes more funding in year 1 and then funding decreases in subsequent years.

If it is necessary to purchase equipment, the budget should include funding for technical support or repairs. Maintenance of equipment is necessary in some form or other, and the grant budget should include preparations for these instances. The grant team might consider seeking a service agreement or building in contracted services to cover these expenses. They can base this decision on the amount and type of equipment purchased along with the amount of funding sought.

BEST PRACTICE HINT

Find out the amount of available rollover allowed each year to ensure that funds are not lost. Spending may need to accelerate or decelerate to ensure that requirements are met.

Most grantors allow a certain percentage of funding to roll over for multiyear grants. However, usually only a certain amount is allowed to do this. If a grant is received, this information should be well known by the staff and whoever manages the budget. If the money is not spent appropriately, the program can be cited and forced to give money back to the fund-

---

TABLE 8-17 SAMPLE SUBCONTRACT

STATEMENT OF INTENT TO ESTABLISH A CONSORTIUM AGREEMENT

Date:

Application Title: Suicide Prevention Plan

Proposed Project Period: October 1, 2008–September 30, 2011

The appropriate programmatic and administrative personnel of each institution involved in this grant application will establish written interinstitutional agreements that will ensure compliance with all pertinent federal regulations and policies in accordance with the "PHS Grants Policy Statement," PHS 398 "Application for Public Health Service Grant," and the NIH "Guidelines for Establishing and Operating Consortium Grants."

_____ _____

Signature   Signature

---

ing agency, which is never a favorable move. The project team should know all the details of the budget requirements upon receiving funding.

In some cases, a grant budget may include contracted services. In this case, the grantee has proposed to contract some of the program's services or needs to an external source (Coley & Scheinberg, 2008). In grant proposals, it is common to contract for an evaluator or other expert consultant. Contracts are also common if two agencies are working in collaboration. In most cases, grantors allow only one primary agency to apply for funds. But in cases of collaboration, some grantors allow contracts to be added to the budget. In this case, the grant money is still awarded to the main agency, and the agency awarded the funding distributes the money to the partner agency for the contract services. This aspect is usually worked out through a subcontract.

BEST PRACTICE HINT

Find out about no-cost extensions prior to the end of funding to allow time to apply and determine the amount of leftover funds.

In some cases, funding not spent has to be sent back to the funder following a specific timeline. In other cases, federal grantors allow what is called a no-cost extension. This occurs when the program has been implemented and there is grant money left over and the grantor awards to the grantee a period of time in which to spend the rest of the funds. No-cost extensions can last from a couple of months to a year (Youngblut & Brooten, 2002).

Some grant budgets require matching funds. Matching funds demonstrate a commitment to the program in the form of a match of the budget funds provided

TABLE 8-18 SAMPLE GRANT BUDGET				
Budget Category	Year 1	Year 2	Year 3	Year 4
A. Personnel	$31,200	$31,200	$32,136	$32,136
126,672				
B. Fringe Benefits	$8,112	$8,112	$8,355	$8,355
32,934				
C. Travel	$5,934	$3,153	$3,153	$3,153
15,393				
D. Equipment	$3,100	$ -0-	$ -0-	$ -0-
3,100				
E. Supplies	$4,401	$3,801	$3,801	$3,501
15,504				
F. Construction	$ -0-	$ -0-	$ -0-	$ -0-
0				
G. Consultants/Contracts	$10,750	$7,750	$5,750	$5,750
30,000				
H. Other	$7,560	$7,560	$7,560	$7,560
30,240				
Total Direct Costs	$71,057	$61,576	$60,755	$60,455
253,843				
I. Indirect Costs	$12,862	$11,115	$10,997	$10,942
45,946				
Total Project Costs	$82,919	$72,721	$71,752	$71,397
Federal Request	$299,789			
Non-Federal Amt.	$ -0-			

by the funded organization. Some matches call for a straight-up cash match and the organization receiving funding must fund a certain percentage of the budget. Other matches call for in-kind matches, which include pro bono services, services already being paid for by the agency (for example, power, phone, Internet) that support the program, and/or use of facilities without charge to the budget. Information on the specifics of a match will be outlined in the RFP. The details of the match may be included in the budget or other section depending on the grant.

TABLE 8-19 SAMPLE BUDGET ON SMALL GRANT		
Program Item	**Funds Requested**	**Budget Justification**
Program supplies/office supplies	$500.00	Folders, paper, posterboard
Printing	$400.00	Posters, letters to schools, evaluation forms, etc.
Event T-shirts	$1000.00	Promotes prevention and event within community
Transportation	$1000.00	Bus rental to transport students to rural communities (80 miles one-way)
Food	$1000.00	Healthy snacks served to participants, lunch served to students
Travel	$200.00	Gas mileage reimbursement for coordinator to meet with community members to plan event
Total requested	$4200.00	

Determining matching funds is an important part of the budget drafting process (Baker, Payne, & Smart, 1999).

Budget Justification

Each budget requires a **budget justification**. A budget justification describes each budget item requested and the rationale for its inclusion in the budget (Holtzclaw et al., 2009). Depending on the grant requirements, budget justifications can be very short and simple or complex. The budget justification is simply a written summary of what is being funded and why these items are necessary to the program. The budget justification is another area in the grant proposal where the grant writer can make a case for the program. According to Ingersoll and Eberhard (1999), the budget justification provides "compelling evidence for why the cost requested is necessary" (p. 133). The budget justification also provides the opportunity to explain where estimated costs come from and why they are essential to the program.

In some agencies, a fiscal specialist drafts the grant budget and budget justification (Klein, Foley, Legault, Manuel, & Schumaker, 2006). Academic institutions usually have individuals with expertise in drafting grant budgets in the institution's grant office. Funding specialists are a resource to any grant writer because they can save time and because of their expertise in developing grant budgets.

Line Item	Grant Year 8 Budget	Carryover Allocation from 2003–2004	Carryover Allocation from 2004–2005	Total Budget
Personnel Cost	32,500.00	5,000.00	6,000.00	43,500.00
Benefits	9,100.00	1,400.00	1,680.00	12,180.00
Utility Services	7,000.00	500.00	500.00	8,000.00
Community Activities	3,000.00	1,332.00	668.00	5,000.00
Maintenance	6,000.00	1,053.40	1,000.00	8,053.40
Telephone/Communication	3,500.00	0.00	500.00	4,000.00
Supplies	3,000.00	500.00	500.00	4,000.00
Equipment	3,250.00	0.00	0.00	3,250.00
Transportation	300.00	100.00	0.00	400.00
Travel	400.00	300.00	300.00	1,000.00
Continuing Education	200.00	200.00	200.00	600.00
Indirect Costs	15,083.30	3,163.72	2,507.91	20,754.93
Total	83,333.30	13,549.12	13,855.91	110,738.33

TABLE 8-20 SAMPLE BUDGET ON MEDIUM-SIZED GRANT

Funding specialists are often aware of all the "ins and outs" of grants and know the proper procedures for drafting the budget and justification. These individuals can also assist in figuring out budget specifics, such as salary information and the benefits rate, and are aware of government regulations that affect grant budgets such as the government rate for mileage reimbursement.

When working with a funding specialist, the grant writer should send the RFP to him or her, and then set up a meeting. The funding specialist will read the RFP to become familiar with what is and is not allowed in the budget. In a meeting, the grant writer and the funding specialist should discuss what is needed to implement the program successfully. Then, the funding specialist can draft a relevant and applicable grant budget. The grant writer should always review the budget and justification prior to grant submission to ensure that all guidelines and necessary items are included in the budget. If the grant writer creates the budget independently, in most organizations that have a funding specialist, the funding specialist will be required to review the grant budget and justification to ensure that it is compliant with the grant requirements (Holtzclaw et al., 2009).

TABLE 8-21 SAMPLE BUDGET ON LARGE GRANT

Grant Budget

Budget Detail Worksheet/Budget Narrative

A. Personnel:

YEAR ONE

Name/Position	Computation	Cost
Project Manager	$15.00 ph × 2080 hrs.	$31,200

Personnel cost includes a salary for an FTE Project Manager at $31,200 annually. This individual will provide 100% of their time to the project. (Position Description is attached in the Appendix.)

	Year 1 Total:	**$31,200**

YEAR TWO

Name/Position	Computation	Cost
Project Manager	$15.00 ph × 2080 hrs.	$31,200

Personnel cost includes a salary for an FTE Project Manager at $31,200 annually. This individual will provide 100% of their time to the project. (Position Description is attached in the Appendix.)

	Year 2 Total:	**$31,200**

YEAR THREE

Name/Position	Computation	Cost
Project Manager	$15.45 ph × 2080 hrs.	$32,136

Personnel cost includes a salary for an FTE Project Manager at $31,200 annually. This individual will provide 100% of their time to the project. This salary includes a 3% Cost of Living Increase of $963 during the third year of the project.

	Year 3 Total:	**$32,136**

YEAR FOUR

Name/Position	Computation	Cost
Project Manager	$15.45 ph × 2080 hrs.	$32,136

Personnel cost includes a salary for an FTE Project Manager at $32,136 annually.

	Year 4 Total:	**$32,136**

Continues

TABLE 8-21 SAMPLE BUDGET ON LARGE GRANT (CONTINUED)

Budget Detail Worksheet/Budget Narrative

B.   **Fringe Benefits:**

YEAR ONE

Name/Position	Computation	Cost
Employer's FICA	($31,200 × 7.65%)	$2,387
Health Insurance	($31,200 × 11.45%)	$3,572
Workers' Compensation	($31,200 × 1.1%)	$ 343
Unemployment Insurance	($31,200 × 5.8%)	$1,810

Fringe benefit rate of 26% includes FICA @ 7.65%; workers' compensation @ 1.1%; unemployment insurance @ 5.8%; and health insurance @ 11.45%.

                                      Year 1 Total: <u>**$8,112**</u>

YEAR TWO

Name/Position	Computation	Cost
Employer's FICA	($31,200 × 7.65%)	$2,387
Health Insurance	($31,200 × 11.45%)	$3,572
Workers' Compensation	($31,200 × 1.1%)	$ 343
Unemployment Insurance	($31,200 × 5.8%)	$1,810

Fringe benefit rate of 26% includes FICA @ 7.65%; workers' compensation @ 1.1%; unemployment insurance @ 5.8%; and health insurance @ 11.45%.

                                      Year 2 Total: <u>**$8,112**</u>

YEAR THREE

Name/Position	Computation	Cost
Employer's FICA	($32,136 × 7.65%)	$2,458
Health Insurance	($32,136 × 11.45%)	$3,680
Workers' Compensation	($32,136 × 1.1%)	$ 353
Unemployment Insurance	($32,136 × 5.8%)	$1,864

Fringe benefit rate of 26% includes FICA @ 7.65%; workers' compensation @ 1.1%; unemployment insurance @ 5.8%; and health insurance @ 11.45%.

                                      Year 3 Total: <u>**$8,355**</u>

TABLE 8-21 SAMPLE BUDGET ON LARGE GRANT (CONTINUED)

YEAR FOUR

Name/Position	Computation	Cost
Employer's FICA	($32,136 × 7.65%)	$2,458
Health Insurance	($32,136 × 11.45%)	$3,680
Workers' Compensation	($32,136 × 1.1%)	$ 353
Unemployment Insurance	($32,136 × 5.8%)	$1,864

Fringe benefit rate of 26% includes FICA @ 7.65%; workers' compensation @ 1.1%; unemployment insurance @ 5.8%; and health insurance @ 11.45%.

Year 4 Total: **$8,355**

Budget Detail Worksheet/Budget Narrative

C. Travel:

YEAR ONE

Purpose of Travel	Location	Item	Computation	Cost
New Grantee	Washington, D.C.	Airfare	($600 × 2 people)	$1,200
National Training		Lodging	($190 × 2 nights × 2 people)	$ 760
		Per Diem	($11.50 × 24 qtrs. × 2 people)	$ 552
		Taxi/Parking	($100 × 2 people)	$ 200
		Mileage	(170 miles × .40.5 per mile)	$ 69
Regional	To Be Determined	Airfare	($400 × 2 people)	$ 800
Training		Lodging	($140 × 2 nights × 2 people)	$ 560
		Per Diem	($11.50 × 24 qtrs. × 2 people)	$ 552
		Taxi/Parking	($100 × 2 people)	$ 200
		Mileage	(170 miles × .40.5 per mile)	$ 69
Local Transportation		Mileage	(2400 miles × .40.5 per mile)	$ 972

Travel costs for two persons to attend a mandatory, one-time, national orientation meeting in year one in Washington, D.C., estimated at $2781; two persons to attend a mandatory regional meeting in year one (TBD), estimated at $2181; and local transportation, which includes transporting youth to and from project activities and attending meetings, home visits, and court hearings, calculated at .40.5 per mile × 12,400 miles = $972.

Year 1 Total: **$5,934**

Continues

TABLE 8-21 SAMPLE BUDGET ON LARGE GRANT (CONTINUED)

YEAR TWO

Purpose of Travel	Location	Item	Computation	Cost
TYP Regional	To Be Determined	Airfare	($400 × 2 people)	$ 800
Training		Lodging	($140 × 2 nights × 2 people)	$ 560
		Per Diem	($11.50 × 24 qtrs. × 2 people)	$ 552
		Taxi/Parking	($100 × 2 people)	$ 200
		Mileage	(170 miles × .40.5 per mile)	$ 69
Local Transportation		Mileage	(2400 miles × .40.5 per mile)	$ 972

Travel costs for two persons to attend one annual regional cluster meeting at a location to be determined, estimated at $2181; and local transportation, which includes transporting youth to and from project activities and attending meetings, home visits, and court hearings, calculated at .40.5 per mile × 2,400 miles = $972.

Year 2 Total: <u>$3,153</u>

YEAR THREE

Purpose of Travel	Location	Item	Computation	Cost
TYP Regional	To Be Determined	Airfare	($400 × 4 people)	$ 800
Training		Lodging	($140 × 2 nights × 2 people)	$ 560
		Per Diem	($11.50 × 24 qtrs. × 2 people)	$ 552
		Taxi/Parking	($100 × 2 people)	$ 200
		Mileage	(170 miles × .40.5 per mile)	$ 69
Local Transportation		Mileage	(2400 miles × .40.5 per mile)	$ 972

Travel costs for two persons to attend one annual regional cluster meeting at a location to be determined, estimated at $2,181; and local transportation, which includes transporting youth to and from project activities and attending meetings, home visits, and court hearings, calculated at .40.5 per mile × 1,200 miles = $486.

Year 3 Total: <u>$3,153</u>

TABLE 8-21 SAMPLE BUDGET ON LARGE GRANT (CONTINUED)

YEAR FOUR

Purpose of Travel	Location	Item	Computation	Cost
TYP Regional	To Be Determined	Airfare	($400 × 2 people)	$ 800
Training	Lodging		($140 × 2 nights × 2 people) $ 560	
	Per Diem		($11.50 × 24 qtrs. × 2 people)$ 552	
	Taxi/Parking		($100 × 2 people)	$ 200
	Mileage		(170 miles × .40.5 per mile) $ 69	
Local Transportation		Mileage	(2400 miles × .40.5 per mile) $ 972	

Travel costs for two persons to attend one annual regional cluster meeting at a location to be determined estimated at $2,181 and local transportation, which includes transporting youth to and from project activities and attending meetings, home visits, and court hearings, calculated at .40.5 per mile × 1,200 miles = $486.

Year 4 Total: **$3,153**

Budget Detail Worksheet/Budget Narrative

D. Equipment:

YEAR ONE

Item	Computation	Cost
Dell Computers w/CD-ROM	($1,000)	$1,000
Dell Laptop Computer ($1,800) $1,800		
Video/Digital Camera	($300)	$ 300

The project will purchase of one Dell computer system with Internet access and e-mail capability to be dedicated to project operations, calculated at $900, and a Dell laptop computer for evaluation process and meetings. The two computers will be provided for staff to complete reports, collect and analyze data, write grants, and perform daily functions for the project. The video camera at $300 will be used for family and youth groups, film trainings and meetings, to record activities for assessments, and to make videos for future grants. The organization has obtained prices for each of the requested equipment items.

Year 1 Total: **$3,100**

Continues

TABLE 8-21 SAMPLE BUDGET ON LARGE GRANT (CONTINUED)

YEAR TWO

Item	Computation	Cost
N/A		
	Year 2 Total:	$ -0-

YEAR THREE

Item	Computation	Cost
N/A		
	Year 3 Total:	$ -0-

YEAR FOUR

Item	Computation	Cost
N/A		
	Year 4 Total:	$ -0-

Budget Detail Worksheet/Budget Narrative

E. Supplies:

YEAR ONE

Supply Items	Computation	Cost
Office Supplies	($100/mo. × 12 mo plus $600 start up)	$1,800
Postage	($50/mo. × 12 mo.)	$ 600
Copy/Printing	($100/mo. × 12 mo.)	$1,200
Computer Supplies (ink cartridges, software, etc)	($66.75/mo. × 12 mo.)	$801

Office supplies include typical expendable items related to everyday use, including pens, staples, calculators, paper clips, etc., and are calculated at $100 per month or $1,200 for the year with $600 start-up. Postage has been calculated at $50 per month and $600 for the year. Copy/printing costs are estimated at $100 per month and $1,200 for the year. Computer supplies are estimated $66.76 per month for a year for computer-specific supplies.

	Year 1 Total:	**$4,401**

TABLE 8-21 SAMPLE BUDGET ON LARGE GRANT (CONTINUED)

YEAR TWO

Supply Items	Computation	Cost
Office Supplies	($100/mo. × 12 mo.)	$1,200
Postage	($50/mo. × 12 mo.)	$600
Copy/Printing	($100/mo. × 12 mo.)	$1,200
Computer Supplies (ink cartridges, software, etc.)	($66.75/mo. × 12 mo.)	$801

Office supplies include typical expendable items related to everyday use, including pens, staples, calculators, paper clips, etc., and are calculated at $100 per month or $1,200 for the year. Postage has been calculated at $50 per month and $600 for the year. Copy/printing costs are estimated at $100 per month and $1,200 for the year. Computer supplies are estimated $66.76 per month for a year for computer-specific supplies.

Year 2 Total: **$3,801**

YEAR THREE

Supply Items	Computation	Cost
Office Supplies	($100/mo. × 12 mo.)	$1,200
Postage	($50/mo. × 12 mo.)	$600
Copy/Printing	($100/mo. × 12 mo.)	$1,200
Computer Supplies (ink cartridges, software, etc.)	($66.75/mo. × 12 mo.)	$801

Office supplies include typical expendable items related to everyday use, including pens, staples, calculators, paper clips, etc., and are calculated at $100 per month or $1,200 for the year. Postage has been calculated at $50 per month and $600 for the year. Copy/printing costs are estimated at $100 per month and $1,200 for the year. Computer supplies are estimated $66.76 per month for a year for computer-specific supplies.

Year 3 Total: **$3,801**

Continues

TABLE 8-21 SAMPLE BUDGET ON LARGE GRANT (CONTINUED)

YEAR FOUR

Supply Items	Computation	Cost
Office Supplies	($100/mo. × 12 mo.)	$1,200
Postage	($50/mo. × 12 mo.)	$600
Copy/Printing	($75/mo. × 12 mo.)	$900
Computer Supplies (ink cartridges, software, etc.)	($66.75/mo. × 12 mo.)	$801

Office supplies include typical expendable items related to everyday use, including pens, staples, calculators, paper clips, etc., and are calculated at $100 per month or $1,200 for the year. Postage has been calculated at $50 per month and $600 for the year. Copy/printing costs are estimated at $75 per month and $900 for the year. Computer supplies are estimated $66.76 per month for a year for computer-specific supplies.

Year 4 Total: **$3,501**

Budget Detail Worksheet/Budget Narrative

F. Construction:

YEAR ONE

Purpose	Description of Work	Cost
N/A		
	Year 1 Total:	$ -0-

YEAR TWO

Purpose	Description of Work	Cost
N/A		
	Year 2 Total:	$ -0-

YEAR THREE

Purpose	Description of Work	Cost
N/A		
	Year 3 Total:	$ -0-

YEAR FOUR

Purpose	Description of Work	Cost
N/A		
	Year 4 Total:	$ -0-

TABLE 8-21 SAMPLE BUDGET ON LARGE GRANT (CONTINUED)

Budget Detail Worksheet/Budget Narrative

G. Consultants/Contracts

YEAR ONE

Name of Consultant	Service Provided	Computation	Cost
Evaluator	Evaluation Leadership	($3,750 per year)	$3,750
Cultural expert	Cultural Evaluation	($5,000 per year)	$5,000
University	Programmatic Evaluation	($2,000 per year)	$2,000

Dr. Evaluator will contract to provide evaluation leadership at $3,750 per year plus; University will provide programmatic evaluation and sustainability plan training at $2,000 per year; and Cultural expert will contribute cultural evaluation expertise and additional capacity-building training at $4,000 per year plus $500 expenses × 2 trips ($1,000).

Year 1 Total: **$10,750**

YEAR TWO

Name of Consultant	Service Provided	Computation	Cost
Evaluator	Evaluation and Data	($3,750 per year)	$3,750
Cultural expert	Training	($2,000 per year)	$2,000
University	Sustainability	($2,000 per year)	$2,000

Dr. Evaluator will contract to provide evaluation leadership at $3,750 per year; University will provide programmatic evaluation and sustainability plan training at $2,000 per year; and Cultural expert will contribute cultural evaluation expertise and capacity-building training follow-up at $1,000 per year plus $500 expenses × 2 trips ($1,000).

Year 2 Total: **$7,750**

YEAR THREE

Name of Consultant	Service Provided	Computation	Cost
Evaluator Evaluation and Data		($3,750 per year)	$3,750
University Sustainability ($2,000 per year) $2,000			

Dr. Evaluator will contract to provide evaluation leadership at $3,750 per year; University will provide programmatic evaluation and sustainability plan training at $2,000 per year.

Year 3 Total: **$5,750**

Continues

TABLE 8-21 SAMPLE BUDGET ON LARGE GRANT (CONTINUED)

YEAR FOUR

Name of Consultant	Service Provided	Computation	Cost
Evaluator Evaluation and Data		($3,750 per year)	$3,750

University Sustainability ($2,000 per year) $2,000

Dr. Evaluator will contract to provide evaluation leadership at $3,750 per year; University will provide programmatic evaluation and sustainability plan training at $2,000 per year.

	Year 4 Total:	**$5,750**

Budget Detail Worksheet/Budget Narrative

H. Other Costs

YEAR ONE

Description	Computation	Cost
Rental Space	(400 sq. ft. × $15/sq. ft.)	$6,000
Telephone	($100/mo. × 12 mo.)	$1,200
Internet/E-Mail	($30/mo. × 12 mo.)	$ 360

Rental space includes a 20 × 20 ft. room to hold Youth Court hearings and activities. No space is currently available in tribally owned facilities. Telephone and e-mail services are vital to day-to-day operations.

	Year 1 Total:	**$7,560**

YEAR TWO

Description	Computation	Cost
Rental Space	(400 sq. ft. × $15/sq. ft.)	$6,000
Telephone	($100/mo. × 12 mo.)	$1,200
Internet/E-Mail	($30/mo. × 12 mo.)	$ 360

Rental space includes a 20 × 20 ft. room to hold Youth Court hearings and activities. No space is currently available in tribally owned facilities. Telephone and e-mail services are vital to day-to-day operations.

	Year 2 Total:	**$7,560**

TABLE 8-21 SAMPLE BUDGET ON LARGE GRANT (CONTINUED)

YEAR THREE

Description	Computation	Cost
Rental Space	(400 sq. ft. × $15/sq. ft.)	$6,000
Telephone	($100/mo. × 12 mo.)	$1,200
Internet/E-Mail	($30/mo. × 12 mo.)	$ 360

Rental space includes a 20 × 20 ft. room to hold Youth Court hearings and activities. No space is currently available in tribally owned facilities. Telephone and e-mail services are vital to day-to-day operations.

	Year 3 Total:	**$7,560**

YEAR FOUR

Description	Computation	Cost
Rental Space	(400 sq. ft. × $15/sq. ft.)	$6,000
Telephone	($100/mo. × 12 mo.)	$1,200
Internet/E-Mail	($30/mo. × 12 mo.)	$ 360

Rental space includes a 20 × 20 ft. room to hold Youth Court hearings and activities. No space is currently available in tribally owned facilities. Telephone and e-mail services are vital to day-to-day operations.

	Year 4 Total:	**$7,560**

Budget Detail Worksheet/Budget Narrative

I. Indirect Costs

YEAR ONE

Description	Computation	Cost
Current indirect cost rate = 18.1%.	18.1% × $69,582	$12,594

A copy of the organization's current indirect cost agreement is attached to this document.

	Year 1 Total:	**$12,594**

YEAR TWO

Description	Computation	Cost
Current indirect cost rate = 18.1%.	18.1% × $61,401	$11,114

A copy of the organization's current indirect cost agreement is attached to this document.

	Year 2 Total:	**$11,114**

Continues

TABLE 8-21 SAMPLE BUDGET ON LARGE GRANT (CONTINUED)

YEAR THREE

Description	Computation	Cost
Current indirect cost rate = 18.1%.	18.1% × $61,580	$61,580
A copy of the organization's current indirect cost agreement is attached to this document.		
	Year 3 Total:	<u>$11,146</u>

YEAR FOUR

Description	Computation	Cost
Current indirect cost rate = 18.1%.	18.1% × $61,280	$11,092
A copy of the organization's current indirect cost agreement is attached to this document.		
	Year 4 Total:	<u>$11,092</u>

Project Team

Writing a grant proposal is not a solitary project, especially in the case of a grant to fund community initiatives. Just as developing a program requires the input of many, so too does the grant proposal. The individuals who will implement the program are part of the grant team. In a grant proposal, the grant writer must describe the team members and their qualifications for implementing the project, including past experience and expertise. In some grant applications, the members of the team and their past experiences affect the grant proposal, so choosing a committed and expert team is essential (Holtzclaw et al., 2009). In this section, the grant writer needs to outline the team's successes and expertise, along with the specific skills members bring to the project. For example, the grant writer might discuss how the team members have worked together previously or other programs that have been successfully implemented by the team.

Some grant applications require biosketches of team members and will provide formats for these in the grant application. Some funding agencies have very strict requirements for grant team members including a past track record of program implementation, publications, and other documented scholarship. However, other granting agencies may want to fund a team who has little experience. All the requirements for the grant team are outlined in the RFP.

References

Grant proposals include a literature review or facts in the problem or needs statement and/or literature review. The grant writer must cite references properly

TABLE 8-22 COMMON ITEMS TO INCLUDE IN GRANT APPENDICES
• Internal Revenue Service (IRS) determination letter • Biosketches of the program team • Memorandums of understand (MOUs) or support letters • Job descriptions • Paperwork forms for program

throughout the grant proposal according to the RFP guidelines and include a reference list of all sources cited in the grant proposal (Gitlin & Lyons, 2004; Holtzclaw et al., 2009). The grant writer can include the references in the narrative or as an appendix. The grant writer should follow the citation requirements recommended by the granting agency. If none are listed, the grant writer can default to a personally preferred format. Questions regarding this should be directed to the grant program manager.

Appendices

Each grant proposal differs in what can be included in appendices and how many pages are allowed for these attachments. Common inclusions in the appendices are documents such as the Internal Revenue Service (IRS) determination letter that confirms nonprofit status, biosketches of the program team, and memorandums of understand (MOU) or support letters from community partners. Support letters and MOUs from community partners can be a method to demonstrate collaboration and desire by the community for the program. The appendices may also include samples of forms or paperwork that are going to be used in the program and copies of job descriptions of the project team.

Developing a Logic Model

Logic models are preferred by some funders as a framework for mapping out the grant program (Schultz et al., 2000; Keener, Snell-Johns, Livet, & Wandersman, 2004). According to the Kellogg Foundation (2004), **logic models** are a "systematic and visual way to present and share your understanding of the relationships among the resources you have to operate your program, the activities you plan, and the changes or results you hope to achieve." Logic models provide for grant reviewers a visual of the whole program in flow chart format. Logic models can be a valuable method for establishing program planning, an implementation plan, and the program evaluation plan (Kellogg Foundation, 2004). Some grant writers prefer logic models and others do not. However, if it is required, the grant writer must

TABLE 8-23 SAMPLE SUPPORT LETTER

Date

Dear Sir or Madam,

I am writing in support of the Suicide Prevention Plan as outlined in the grant proposal.

When I reviewed the Suicide Prevention Plan developed previously by community members, I felt a passion to implement the culturally relevant and community-driven ideas to prevent further devastation to the community. Through our discussions, I brought forth what services community-based practitioners could provide to prevent suicide and grieve if one does occur. With the shortages of healthcare practitioners to meet the needs of the youth, I commit the expertise and services of representatives from the School of Health Professions in occupational therapy, physical therapy, and pharmacy. To build reserves and impact, health professions students will assist in the development and implementation of services and trainings to youth in the community focused on stress management and coping skills. At the same time, these students will have the invaluable opportunity to learn the culture and develop the professional skills to interact with diverse and underserved populations throughout their careers.

At University, we believe in the value of providing treatment to the whole person. Our faculty and students believe in addressing issues with a holistic frame of mind with consideration for cultural values and beliefs. We fully support the Suicide Prevention Plan, which outlines and addresses the issue of suicide on multiple levels. As an individual who believes wholeheartedly in community capacity building and change, I am committed to this project and affecting the youth of the community, promoting a full, happy life. Furthermore, our long-standing partnership with the community has led to much collaboration addressing health issues and success in educating the community on topics such as diabetes and obesity. Therefore, I fully support this project and look forward to addressing this new topic and a further developed partnership with the community.

Sincerely,

Joy D. Doll, OTD, OTR/L
Assistant Professor, Clinical Education
Department of Occupational Therapy

include a logic model in the grant proposal. The requirements for the logic model will be outlined in the RFP. A logic model may sometimes replace an implementation plan in a grant proposal.

Logic models have several components including inputs, processes, outputs, and outcomes. Inputs and processes represent the planned work of the program whereas outputs and outcomes represent the proposed results of the program (Kellogg Foundation, 2004). Inputs are simply what the organization or community plans to invest or put into the program. The input section may discuss resources and capacities needed to implement the program. These resources and capacities may exist in the community and need to be garnered prior to program implementation. Processes are the policies and procedures the team plans to put into place to implement the program effectively.

Outputs are divided into two sections: activities and participation. Activities are what the grant team plans to do (i.e., the goals, objectives, and activities). Participation includes whom the program plans to reach with each activity. Outcomes, also sometimes called impact, are viewed in the short term, medium term, and long term. Short-term outcomes focus on learning that occurs from the program; medium-term outcomes focus on actions that have resulted from the program; and long-term outcomes focus on the conditions that have changed as a result of the program (McNamara, 2000). In many logic models, other factors are considered such as the program's priorities, assumptions, external factors, and the evaluation plan.

The grant writer should not be intimidated by logic models. Instead of writing out all the components of the proposal, the logic model requires the grant writer to think in a visual or table format. Logic models can be simple or complex depending on the grant requirements and the program. Multiple methods for developing a logic model exist across the literature (Kellogg Foundation, 2004). The grant writer should explore grant requirements and then follow the model that fits best with describing the program. See Table 8-24 for a sample logic model, and Process Worksheet 8-9 for a framework for developing a logic model.

Institutional Review Boards

Even community practice and program grants require research. Actually, all community programs should include some data collection, analysis, and distribution to identify the worthiness of an occupational therapy program. Reports and outcomes from the grant program should be disseminated both to the community and professional organizations (Israel et al., 2005). If a dissemination plan is in place, then the grant team will need to apply to an institutional review board (IRB) for approval to disseminate program outcomes.

Institutional review boards (IRBs) exist in academic institutions and hospitals. Some communities have IRBs, such as Native American tribes, which have their own tribal IRBs. Human subjects research requires IRB approval. For IRB forms

TABLE 8-24 SAMPLE GRANT LOGIC MODEL: THE SACRED CHILD LOGIC MODEL

Resources (Inputs) ➡	Program Components (Focused Activities) ➡	Outputs (Objectives) ➡	Outcomes (Goals)
Leadership: • Community response team **Partners:** • Tribal council • Alcohol program • Tribal court • Public school **Approach Philosophies:** • Evidence-based design • Cultural relevance • Community integration • Data use and monitoring	**Activity 1: Walking in Beauty on the Red Road (WBRR)** • Outpatient treatment (5 per week) • Family treatment sessions (10–15 youth ages each session) • Court-ordered and walk-ins • Extensive aftercare (for a minimum of 1 year) **Activity 2: Youth Outreach Efforts** • Community-based outreach • Includes after-school programs • Community trainings and forums • Mandatory aftercare component **Activity 3: Youth Services Center** • Extensive peer-to-peer services • Services hosted at the center • Assist those in recovery • Coordinate youth involvement • Coordinate youth mentoring	<u>**Objective 1:**</u> To undertake the culturally relevant, evidence-based substance abuse program Walking in Beauty on the Red Road (WBRR) for youth ages 12–18 on the reservation. Utilize the GAIN-Quick Assessment to identify eligibility and need for substance abuse and mental health treatment. Utilize the CESA to identify cultural strengths and needs • *100 youth directly participate* • *400 community members assist* <u>**Objective 2:**</u> To integrate WBRR into new and existing youth and family outreach programs to provide a comprehensive approach to building participant awareness, recruitment, and referral into this substance abuse program. • *100 youth directly participate* • *400 community members assist*	**Project Overall Goal:** An effective and comprehensive recovery support infrastructure on the reservation that: • Assists youth in attaining sobriety • Prevents relapse • Provides a framework to change community norms • Is culturally relevant • Has core values of teachings

Source: Penn, J., Grandgenett, N., & Voltz, J. D. (2007). *Omaha Tribe's Ten Clans Intervention Initiative Tribal Youth Project.* Department of Justice.

TABLE 8-25 IMPORTANT QUESTIONS TO CONSIDER WHEN DEVELOPING A RESEARCH DESIGN IN A GRANT PROPOSAL
• How much is known and understood about the topic? • Will there be an intervention? • If there is an intervention, will all subjects get it? • Does the researcher control who gets the intervention? • If there is an intervention and the investigator controls who receives it, is it feasible to randomly assign subjects to get or not get the intervention? • How many times will data be collected from subjects and when? • To what extent can factors that potentially interfere with the relationship between the intervention and outcome variable(s) be minimized or controlled?

and further information, the grant writer should contact the IRB office to ensure compliance (Holtzclaw et al., 2009). Staff in the IRB office can help the grant writer draft the IRB proposal and follow the steps needed to comply with the IRB. Training required by the IRB may be necessary for staff to maintain compliance and should be done prior to the grant implementation.

In the case of research grants, the grant writer needs to determine the research design to be utilized for the project. Colwell and associates (2005) outline key questions to ask when considering the design to be used for research. See Table 8-25 for these questions.

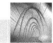

BEST PRACTICE HINT

Obtain IRB approval prior to receiving notification of grant funds so that you are ready to implement when funds arrive.

Grant Visuals

Rarely, grant proposals require that a visual that demonstrates a community partnership or the grant project be included. Grant visuals act as branding of the program and also help reviewers understand the context of the grant proposal (Jensen & Royeen, 2001). Requirements for visuals will be described in the RFP. Grant writers can consult graphic artists to develop grant visuals, but most visuals need not be extremely complex. As always, if questions arise about this requirement, the grant writer needs to review the RFP and contact the program manager as necessary.

Conclusion

Grant proposals can be complex and lengthy to draft and include many different components. Although grants come in all shapes and sizes, this chapter covers many of the components common to most grant applications. Grant writers should always follow the guidelines put forth in the RFP, which outline all the necessary components required for a successful grant proposal. By following the tips given in this chapter, occupational therapy practitioners can create quality grant applications.

Glossary

Abstract Abbreviated description of the proposed program

Activity Outline of which specific steps will be taken to reach the goals and objectives in a grant proposal

Budget justification Description of each budget item requested and the rationale for its inclusion in the budget

Cover letter A letter that describes to reviewers the intent to apply for the grant funding, the organization applying for funding, and also the proposed program

Direct cost Items in the budget that will be funded by the grant money such as salary, benefits, equipment, consultants, and travel

Goal Description of the overall purpose of the proposed program in the grant proposal

Grant narrative The section of the grant proposal that includes the goals, objectives, activities, proposed outcomes, background, needs statement or problem statement depending on the RFP, literature review, theoretical foundation, methodology or implementation plan, timeline, and dissemination plan

Grant proposal An "agreement between the proposal developers and the funding agency and serves as the blueprint for the project" (Ingersoll & Eberhard, 1999)

Implementation plan A plan included in a grant proposal that describes the who, what, where, when, and how of the program

Indirect cost Items not directly tied to the project or program implementation such as "rental fees, payment of utilities, equipment depreciation, providing security, and general maintenance of workspace" (Ingersoll & Eberhard, 1999, p. 133)

Letter of intent A letter to the funding agency informing it of the applying agency's intent to apply for a grant

Logic model A visual representation of the whole program in flow chart format

Objective Description of the proposed program outcomes that will be measured in the evaluation plan in a grant proposal

Outcome Description of what the program proposes to complete through its implementation

Problem statement or needs statement A statement in a grant proposal that describes the community and the problem or need that affects the community

References

Baker, M., Payne, A. A., & Smart, M. (1999). An empirical study of matching grants: The "cap on CAP." *Journal of Public Economics, 71*(2), 269–288.

Barnard, J. (2002). Keys to writing a competitive grant. *Journal of Pediatric Gastroenterology and Nutrition, 35,* 107–110.

Begley, K., Doll J. D., Martens Stricklett, K., & Ryan Haddad, A. (2008). *What's in Your Future? A Health Education and Health Professions Program for Community Youth.* Grant provided by the Omaha Urban Area Health Education Center.

Beitz, J. M., & Bliss, D. Z. (2005). Preparing a successful grant proposal. Part 1: Developing research aims and the significance of the project. *Journal of Wound, Ostomy, and Continence Nursing, 32*(1), 16–18.

Berg, K. M., Gill, T. M., Brown, A. F., Zerzan, J., Elmore, J. G., & Wilson, I. B. (2007). Demystifying the NIH grant application process. *Journal of General Internal Medicine, 22*(11), 1587–1595.

Bliss, D. Z., & Savik, K. (2005). Writing a grant proposal—part 2: Research methods—part 2. *Journal of Wound, Ostomy and Continence Nursing, 32*(4), 226–229.

Bordage, G., & Dawson, B. (2003). Experimental study design and grant writing in eight steps and 28 questions. *Medical Education, 37,* 376–385.

Brownson, C. A. (2001). Program development: Planning, implementation, and evaluation strategies. In M. Scaffa (Ed.), *Occupational therapy in community-based practice settings.* Philadelphia: F. A. Davis.

Chambless, D. L. (2003). Hints for writing a NIMH grant. *Behavior Therapist, 26,* 258–261.

Cochran, T. M., Goulet, C., Voltz, J. D., Jensen, G. M., Ryan Haddad, A., & Wilken, A. (2006). *Brain Bash—An Interactive Interprofessional Educational Outreach for the Prevention of Youth Substance Abuse and the Promotion of Healthy Living.* Omaha Urban Area Health Education Center.

Coley, S. M., & Scheinberg, C. A. (2008). *Proposal writing: Effective grantmanship.* Thousand Oaks, CA: Sage Publications.

Colwell, J. C., Bliss, D. Z., Engberg, S., & Moore, K. N. (2005). Preparing a grant proposal—part 5: Organization and revision. *Journal of Wound, Ostomy, and Continence Nursing, 32*(5), 291–293.

Cross, P., & Voltz, J. D. (2005). *Four Hills of Life Wellness Center Nebraska Native American Public Health Grant.* Nebraska Health and Human Services.

Dahlen, R. (2001). Fundamentals of grant writing: Lessons learned from the process. *Nurse Education, 26*(2), 54–56.

Edberg, M. (2007). *Essentials of health behavior: Social and behavior health in public health.* Sudbury, MA: Jones and Bartlett.

Environmental Protection Agency. (2007). Tips on writing a grant proposal. Retrieved July 21, 2008, from http://www.epa.gov/ogd/recipient/tips.htm

Falk, G.W. (2006). Turning an idea into a grant. *Gastrointestinal Endoscopy, 64*(6), S11-S13.

Flecky, K., & Doll, J. D. (2008). *Engaging Students: The Community as Classroom.* Midwest Consortium for Service Learning Grant.

Gitlin, L. N., & Lyons, K. J. (1996). *Successful grant writing: Strategies for health and human service professionals.* New York: Springer.

Gitlin, L. N., & Lyons, K. J. (2004). *Successful grant writing: Strategies for health and human service professionals* (2nd ed.). New York: Springer.

Goulet, C., Cochran, T. M., Jensen, G. M., Coppard, B. M., Chapman, T., Ryan Haddad, A., et al. (2006). *"Against the Current"—Bridging the Gap to eHealth Information for the Omaha Tribe of Nebraska.* National Library of Medicine.

Hocking, C., & Wright St. Clair, V. (2007). Writing for publication: Tips and reflections for busy therapists. *New Zealand Journal of Occupational Therapy, 54*(1), 26–32.

Holtzclaw, B. J., Kenner, C., & Walden, M. (2009). *Grant writing handbook for nurses* (2nd ed.). Sudbury, MA: Jones and Bartlett.

Ingersoll, G. L., & Eberhard, D. (1999). Grants management skills keep funded projects on target. *Nursing Economics, 17,* 131–141.

Inouye, S. K., & Fiellin, D. A. (2005). An evidence-based guide to writing grant proposals for clinical research. *Annals of Internal Medicine, 142,* 274–282.

Israel, B. A., Eng, E., Schulz, A. J., & Parker, E. A. (2005). Introduction to method in community-based participatory research for health. In *Methods in Community-Based Participatory Research for Health.* San Francisco: Jossey-Bass.

Jensen, G. M., & Royeen, C. B. (2001). Analysis of academic–community partnerships using the integration matrix. *Journal of Allied Health*, 30, 168–175.

Keener, D. C., Snell-Johns, J., Livet, M., & Wandersman, A. (2004). Lessons that influenced the current conceptualization of empowerment evaluation: Reflections from two evaluation projects. In D. M. Fetterman & A. Wandersman (Eds.), *Empowerment evaluation principles in practice* (pp. 73–91). New York: Guilford Press.

W. K. Kellogg Foundation. (2004). Using logic models to bring together planning, evaluation, and action: Logic model development guide. Battle Creek, MI: Author.

Klein, K. P., Foley, K. L., Legault, L., Manuel, J., & Schumaker, S. A. (2006). Creation of a grant support service within a Women's Health Center of Excellence: Experiences and lessons learned. Journal of Women's Health, 15(2), 127–134.

Lusk, S. L. (2004). Developing an outstanding grant application. Western Journal of Nursing Research, 26(3), 367–373.

McNamara, P. (2000). Guidelines and framework for designing basic logic model. Retrieved July 21, 2008, from http://www.managementhelp.org/np×progs/np×mod/org×frm.htm

Mosey, A. C. (1998). The competent scholar. American Journal of Occupational Therapy, 52, 760–764.

Mu, K., Bracciano, A., Goulet, C., & Voltz, J. D. (2007). Chinese Study in Health Care: An Innovative Approach for Teaching Health Care Professionals. Submitted to the United States Department of Education.

National Registry of Evidence-Based Programs and Practices. (2008). What is NREPP? Retrieved October 29, 2008, from http://www.nrepp.samhsa.gov/about.asp

Non-Profit Guides. (2008). Welcome to non-profit guides. Retrieved October 29, 2008, from http://www.npguides.org/

Notario-Risk, N., & Ottenwess, K. (2000). Nonprofits and data: A how-to series: Using data to support grant applications and other funding opportunities. Retrieved October 29, 2008, from http://www.cridata.org/Publications/supportinggrantapps.pdf

Parker, E. A., Robins, T. G., Israel, B. A., Brakefield-Caldwell, W., Edgren, K. K. & Wilkins, D. J. (2005). Developing and implementing guidelines for dissemination: The experience of the Community Action Against Asthma Project. In B. A. Israel, E. Eng, A. J. Schulz, & E. A. Parker (Eds.), *Methods in community-based participatory research for health* (pp. 285–306). San Francisco: Jossey-Bass.

Penn, J., Grandgenett, N., & Voltz, J. D. (2007). *Omaha Tribe's Ten Clans Intervention Initiative Tribal Youth Project.* Department of Justice.

Reeves, T. J., & Bennett, C. E. (2004). We the People: Asians in the United States: Census 2000 Special Reports. Retrieved March 24, 2009, from http://www.census.gov/prod/2004pubs/censr-17.pdf

Ryan Haddad, A., Koenig, P., & Voltz, J. D. (2007). *Caring for the Caregiver: An Outreach Program for Caregivers.* Take Action: Healthy People, Places, and Practices in Communities Project. United States Office of Disease Prevention and Health Promotion.

Schultz, J. A., Fawcett, S. B., Francisco, V. T., Wolff, T., Berkowitz, B. R., & Nagy, G. (2000). The community tool box: Using the Internet to support the work of community health and development. *Journal of Technology in Human Services*, *17*(2/3), 193–215.

Stabler, W., & Doll, J. D. (2009). "Against the Current": Strategies for success in health care—A case example of a rural, Native American community. In C. B. Royeen, G. M. Jensen, & R. A. Harvan (Eds.), *Leadership in interprofessional health education and practice* (pp. 249–262). Sudbury, MA: Jones and Bartlett.

Suarez-Balcazar, Y., Hammel, J., & Helfrich, C. (2005). A model of university–community partnerships for occupational therapy scholarship and practice. *Occupational Therapy in Health Care, 19*, 47–70.

Voltz, J. D., Ryan Haddad, A., Hohnstein, S., & Martens Stricklett, K. (2007). *A Heart for Health: The Health Report Card Project.* Nebraska Minority Public Health Association, $500.

Weil, V. (2005). Standards for evaluating proposals to develop ethics curricula. *Science and Engineering Ethics, 11*, 501–507.

Wilken, M. (2009). Health Report Card Project: Building community capacity. In C. B. Royeen, G. M. Jensen, & R. A. Harvan (Eds.), *Leadership in interprofessional health education and practice* (pp. 413–426). Sudbury, MA: Jones and Bartlett.

Writing Center—University of North Carolina at Chapel Hill. (2007). Grant proposals. Retrieved January 22, 2009, from http://www.unc.edu/depts/wcweb/handouts/grant×proposals.html

Youngblut, J. M., & Brooten, D. (2002). Institutional research responsibilities and needed infrastructure. *Journal of Nursing Scholarship, 34*(1), 159–164.

PROCESS WORKSHEET 8-1 **PRESS RELEASE WORKSHEET**

Instructions: This worksheet provides a basic template and instructions for completing a press release. Press releases are a format to let the community know about a program or grant.

FOR IMMEDIATE RELEASE

Contact Person

Organizational Name

Contact Information (Phone and E-mail)

Title of Press Release

City, State (Date) – Press releases can be used for two purposes. Press releases can be used to advertise an upcoming event or share the occurrence of a past impacting event.

A press release should include information about the event such as the location, time, number of participants, and the overall impact. Press releases should not be more than a page and should provide an overall description of an event.

Press releases are an effective method for letting local media agencies and partners know about the success of a program.

PROCESS WORKSHEET 8-2   **BUDGET WORKSHEET 1**

Instructions: Use this template for drafting a grant budget if no grant forms are provided with the RFP.

Category	Amount	Budget Justification
Personnel		
Fringe benefits		
Travel		
Equipment		
Supplies		
Consultants		
Contracts		
Other		
Other		
Indirect cost rate		
Total direct costs		

PROCESS WORKSHEET 8-3 **BUDGET WORKSHEET 2**

Instructions: Use this template for drafting a grant budget if no grant forms are provided with the RFP.

Item	Year 1	Year 2	Year 3	TOTAL	Justification
Educational Budget					
Mileage					
Copying/ Printing					
Promotional materials					
Office supplies					
Educational supplies					
Food supplies					
Travel					
Salary					
TOTAL					

PROCESS WORKSHEET 8-4 **GRANT PROPOSAL CHECKLIST**

Instructions: Use this checklist to develop a timeline for completion of a grant proposal and a review for a developed grant proposal for completed components.

Proposal Component	Timeline for Completion	Completed
Title		
Abstract		
Introduction		
Goals		
Objectives		
Activities		
Outcomes		
Background/Needs statement/Problem statement		
Theoretical foundation		
Implementation plan		
Evaluation plan		
Timeline		
Dissemination plan		
Institutional paperwork		
Team biographies		
Budget		
Budget justification		
Reference list		
Appendices		

Instructions: Use this worksheet to begin to develop the grant proposal's needs/problem statement.

Problem/Need	Sources That Describe Need/Problem	Community Capacities to Address Need/Problem

PROCESS WORKSHEET 8-6 GRANT TIMELINE WORKSHEET

Instructions: Use the following table to develop a grant proposal timeline.

Activity	Dates	Participants

PROCESS WORKSHEET 8-7 **DISSEMINATION PLAN WORKSHEET**

Instructions: Use this worksheet to develop a dissemination plan for a grant. Circle which strategies will work for each targeted dissemination.

Community	Annual report Newsletter Media campaign Program website Press releases Public presentations Community forums Other: _____
Professional	Presentation at a state association conference Presentation at a national association conference Newspaper article about the program Article for a practice magazine Manuscript to a professional journal Networking or professional meetings Trainings or continuing education to other practitioners Other: _____

PROCESS WORKSHEET 8-8 PROGRAM TEAM WORKSHEET

Instructions: Use this worksheet to develop a grant program team.

Name of Team Member	Credentials	Expertise/Skills

PROCESS WORKSHEET 8-9 **LOGIC MODEL WORKSHEET**

Instructions: Use the chart to create a grant logic model.

Resources (Inputs) ➡	Program Components (Focused Activities) ➡	Outputs (Objectives) ➡	Outcomes (Goals)

Perform a SWOT analysis of your program or project. SWOT stands for Strengths, Weaknesses, Opportunities, and Threats. Identify current strengths, weaknesses, opportunities for growth, and threats to the community project or program. You can use this analysis as a tool to get you thinking about the program in a broad sense. SWOTs can be used for individual analysis or can be performed by a group of people who then come together to compare and contrast analyses. The SWOT is a tool that is unique to each program and can be used to analyze current infrastructure, strategize future steps, or even simply to explore the feasibility of beginning a program.

Strengths	Weaknesses
Opportunities	**Threats**

PROCESS WORKSHEET 8-11 IMPLEMENTATION PLAN WORKSHEET

Instructions: Complete the following worksheet to identify the implementation plan for the grant proposal.

Goal 1:

Objective 1:				
Outcome(s):				
Strategy(ies):				

Activities	Who Is Responsible	Timeline:		Status
		Start Date	End Date	

Instructions: Complete the logic model based on the grant project.

INPUTS ➡	OUTPUTS ➡		OUTCOMES – IMPACT		
	Activities	Participation	Short	Medium	Longer term
What we invest	What we do	Who is reached	Short-term changes we expect	Medium-term changes we expect	Long-term changes we expect

ASSUMPTIONS   **EXTERNAL FACTORS**

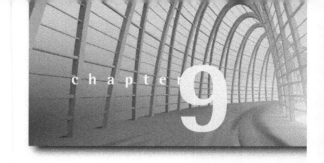

Making a Case: Using Data to Maximize a Grant Proposal

LEARNING OBJECTIVES

By the end of this chapter, the reader will be able to complete the
following:
1. Identify data sources for a community program.
2. Discuss techniques for using data to justify a community need.

Overview

This chapter provides information on finding and integrating appropriate
data into a grant proposal.

Introduction

Writing a grant proposal requires the grant writer to make a robust case for
why the community or program deserves the funding provided by the granting agency. Including relevant and appropriate data enhances the program
and makes a case for a need or needs in a grant proposal. Most grant proposals require a literature review and inclusion of community demographics that
paint a picture of the community to be served by the grant funding. However,
conducting a literature review and exploring demographic data can be overwhelming, and the process of determining which data are most appropriate
for a grant proposal can be confusing to the novice.

259

The Purpose of Data Gathering

In a grant proposal, the grant writer has to make a case for why the funder should provide money for the proposed program. Justifying the necessity for funding a program is often made in the literature review and problem or needs statement sections of the grant proposal. The **background or literature review** lays a foundation for the grant proposal and is directly tied to the **problem statement or statement of need**. Community needs should be supported in a quantitative and very clear manner in a grant proposal to make the need explicit to grant reviewers (Inouye & Fiellin, 2005).

As mentioned, data can be included in two sections of the grant. First, data are used in the background/literature review section of a grant proposal. In this section, the grant writer describes the community using supporting data and begins to introduce the community needs that the proposed program will address. Second, data are required in the problem statement or statement of need section of the grant proposal. In this section, the grant writer specifically identifies the community need and uses complementary data to support and describe the need to grant reviewers.

A literature review can accomplish multiple tasks. First, the literature review can be used to identify data and statistics to be used for a community profile (Fazio, 2008). In the grant proposal, these data can be used to describe the community and discuss why the community should receive funding. A community profile and need profile are important because the grant funder may not be familiar with the community and its needs; therefore, data provide a glimpse of the needs and capacities of the community for grant reviewers who may never even visit the community.

Second, grant writers can use the literature review to explore the evidence from and existence of programs similar to the proposed program (Gitlin & Lyons, 2004). A literature review in a grant proposal "should summarize and synthesize all relevant studies done to date, while clearly identifying knowledge gaps that remain" (Falk, 2006, S11). Grant writers can use information from a literature review to strengthen the case for the proposed program. A literature review can also exemplify programs that have a demonstrated record of success related to a specific health issue. A grant proposal can use information about an existing successful program, such as data and outcomes, to demonstrate that program's impact and how best practices from the successful program can be used to address the need in the community seeking assistance in the grant proposal.

BEST PRACTICE HINT

Be sure to follow the structure provided by the request for proposals and place data in the appropriate sections according to the grant requirements. Some RFPs require a specific problem statement while others only desire a literature review. Follow the guidelines discussed in the RFP.

BEST PRACTICE HINT

Think of a literature review for a grant proposal as similar to one you would write for a scholarly paper except with a focus on a program related to a grant instead of on disseminating scholarly information. The goal is to describe what the literature says to support your point.

TABLE 9-1 PURPOSE OF DATA GATHERING

- Provides a community profile.
- Describes community need.
- Identifies best practices.

A new grant writer might question why it is relevant to include sound data in a grant proposal. The inclusion of strong and reliable data points can make the difference between receiving funding and not receiving funding. The data included in a grant proposal should be well thought out prior to inclusion. A successful grant proposal includes data that support the community need and describe the community, along with a summary of the literature that describes the issue and supports the proposed program. Both elements are necessary to justify to grant reviewers why a need is relevant and why a program should receive funding.

Data are more than just numbers. Data can validate that the community's perceptions of an issue are real and legitimate (Community Research Institute [CRI], 2007a). Demonstrating the reality of the need helps the community and the grant writer discuss the issues and need in an objective manner when presenting them in a grant proposal. Data also lay a foundation for monitoring the impact of a program on a need and facilitating community change (CRI, 2007a).

> **LET'S STOP AND THINK**
>
> Identify some important data points crucial to any grant proposal.

Types of Data

Grant proposals should include a variety of data to describe the target population and the community needs and capacities. Different types of data can be included in a grant proposal.

Demographic Data

Demographic data are simply information that describes a group or community. Demographic data include items such as ethnicity, age, gender, family composition, and socioeconomic status (U.S. Census Bureau, 2008). Grant writers can use demographic data in a grant proposal to describe the community and the target population to be served by the proposed program. In some cases, grant reviewers know little about the community, so demographic data can paint a picture of the community. In other instances, demographic data describe a target population more specifically when the target population is a subset of the community that will be served by the program. Examples of target populations are individuals with cerebral palsy or community members who have documented mental health disorders.

TABLE 9-2 TYPES OF DEMOGRAPHIC DATA

- Ethnicity
- Age
- Gender
- Family composition
- Marital status
- Socioeconomic status
- Total population
- Education levels

BEST PRACTICE HINT

Brainstorm what you already know about the community and how you know it. Data may be close at hand in reports or information you already have on file, which will save you time in the search process.

LET'S STOP AND THINK

Identify some demographic data you know about your own community. How do you know this? Where would you go to find more information?

Grant writers can also use demographic data to demonstrate their knowledge and understanding of the target population. The inclusion of such data is important because funding agencies want to provide funding to organizations that truly understand the communities they plan to serve. Community knowledge demonstrates expertise and promotes success in a program, which grant reviewers view favorably.

As mentioned, demographic data include information such as census data (U.S. Census Bureau, 2008). Census data can be valuable in describing the community and completing a community profile in a grant proposal. Census data can describe everything from the ages and jobs of community members to details such as languages spoken at home and access to transportation (U.S. Census Bureau, 2008). Census data can be retrieved both from the United States Census Bureau and regional offices across the United States. Local offices such as the Office on Aging or the state Department of Health and Human Services may also have such data.

Social Indicators

Social indicators provide data on subpopulations of a community (CRI, 2007b). Examples include religious affiliation, health status, and criminal behavior. These data describe the values of the population and also challenges that the community may face. This information is valuable to a grant proposal for multiple reasons. Because community programs should be developed on the premise of understanding the community's values, grant writers must know and understand the community and demonstrate this knowledge by including social indicators in the grant proposal.

TABLE 9-3 EXAMPLE OF DEMOGRAPHIC DATA IN GRANT PROPOSAL

"Currently, there are over 35,000 occupational therapy professionals and students, and over 275,000 physical therapy professionals practicing in the US in various settings including hospitals, schools, skilled nursing facilities treating individuals across life span, from infants to dwelling elders."

The preceding example describes the demographics of occupational and physical therapy practitioners in the United States. This information demonstrates the types of practitioners and the disparity between the numbers of OT and PT practitioners.

Source: Mu, K., Bracciano, A., Goulet, C., & Voltz, J. D. (2007). *Chinese Study in Health Care: An Innovative Approach for Teaching Health Care Professionals.* Submitted to the United States Department of Education.

TABLE 9-4 EXAMPLE OF SOCIAL INDICATORS IN GRANT PROPOSAL

"As identified by the Institute of Medicine, diversity in the health care workforce improves patient access, increases culturally appropriate health care, and provides greater patient satisfaction. Health disparities exist in minority populations making them underserved and traditionally research shows that minorities suffer from higher rates of chronic disease and disability."

The preceding example describes the social issue of a lack of minority practitioners, which has been shown to increase the likelihood of disparity in quality of health care. These data were used in a grant application to provide health professions education to minority youth at an alternative school.

Source: Goertz, H., Ryan Haddad, A., Lee, T., & Voltz, J. D. (2006). *Developing Minority Health Professionals/Researchers for Tomorrow.* Sociological Initiatives Foundation Grant.

Furthermore, social indicators can highlight a need or a challenge in the community by identifying factors that influence quality of life. Social indicators can also be used to describe community capacity because the grant writer may be able to identify collective community values that can promote positive change.

Rate, Prevalence, and Incidence

Besides data related to demographics and social indicators, **epidemiological data** are relevant to a community grant proposal. Epidemiological data focus on the impact of a health

LET'S STOP AND THINK

Identify some social indicators you know about your own community. How do you know about them? Where would you go to find more information?

> **TABLE 9-5 ANOTHER EXAMPLE OF SOCIAL INDICATORS IN GRANT PROPOSAL**
>
> "Nationally, suicide is the second leading cause of death among American Indian adolescents and young adults in the 15- to 24-year-old age group and is the third leading cause of death in the 10 to 14 age group."
>
> The preceding example describes the prevalence of suicide among American Indians and was used in a suicide prevention grant proposal.
>
> *Source:* Penn, J., Grandgenett, N., & Voltz, J. D. (2007). *Omaha Tribe's Ten Clans Intervention Initiative Tribal Youth Project.* Department of Justice.

problem on a specific population or group (Edberg, 2007). Epidemiological data provide insight into the trends of specific health issues in a given population (Edberg, 2007; CRI, 2007b). Rate, prevalence, and incidence are statistics that indicate a community's issues in context. **Rate** is simply how often a disease or health issue occurs among a certain population (Abramson & Abramson, 2001). Rates are divided into either prevalence or incidence.

LET'S STOP AND THINK

Identify the rate, prevalence, and incidence of a health issue in your own community. How do you know this? Where would you go to find more information?

Prevalence is the rate of cases of disease or a health issue in a certain population (Edberg, 2007). Prevalence describes how much the problem affects the community and its population. **Incidence** describes the current rate of a disease or health issue in a community (Edberg, 2007). Incidence indicates the current status of the issue. These elements can demonstrate how large an issue is or how much a community need has decreased as a result of a program.

Where to Find the Right Data

After deciding what data are important to include in the grant proposal, the grant writer must find relevant data. Two types of data are common to program development and grant writing. **Primary data** are data directly collected from the community partner in the community assessment using a variety of approaches such as surveys, interviews, focus groups, and community forums. These data come directly from the community, and methods for collecting this type of data are described in Chapter 6. **Secondary data** are data from sources that describe the community and are typically found in archives (Brownson, 2001). Secondary data can be used to describe a community and its needs. Secondary data include demographic data, social indicators, and epidemiological data.

Data can come from a variety of sources. The proposed program will indicate which type of data is relevant to support the grant proposal. Data can be found in

TABLE 9-6 SOURCES OF SECONDARY DATA FOR A GRANT PROPOSAL

- Local hospitals
- School districts
- Health departments
- Other local programs
- Chambers of commerce
- Local library
- Office on aging

public databases, in the literature, and in the community (CRI, 2007c). A community assessment is one method of gathering data specific to the community. Supplemental data from secondary sources can also describe the community and its needs. These sources are appropriate for use in the background/literature review section of a grant proposal.

Public databases contain census information, health statistics, and epidemiological data. For general demographic data, the main resource is the United States Census Bureau. The Census Bureau can provide data on a variety of topics including population status, population projections, housing, health insurance rates, economic status, poverty rates, and much more. Data from the Census Bureau provide a quick glimpse of valuable information that can help paint the picture required in a grant proposal.

BEST PRACTICE HINT

Keep data sources handy for grant writing and grant reporting. Create both a digital and paper-based file to store data for quick retrieval.

Another location for data is the local chamber of commerce (CRI, 2007d). Often, the local chamber has data on everything from population to local economics to health and education challenges. Sometimes the data the grant writer seeks is located on the chamber website; otherwise, grant writers can contact the local chamber personnel, who are usually more than happy to assist. The focus of a chamber of commerce is to enhance the local community, so it should be supportive of any agency seeking grant funding.

There are many other sources of health statistics that are reliable and relevant to a grant proposal. Any agency that maintains records in the community can be a resource, including local hospitals, school districts, health departments, the Office on Aging, area health education centers (AHECs), and other local programs (CRI, 2007d). For example, if the program's focus is on safety, the grant writer can check with the local safety council to see whether it maintains a database of information that would

BEST PRACTICE HINT

Bookmark websites where data are readily retrievable for quick access.

TABLE 9-7 FEDERAL RESOURCES FOR DATA	
Type of Data	**Federal Source**
Mental health issues	Substance Abuse and Mental Health Services Administration (SAMHSA)
Health professions shortages	Health Resources and Services Administration (HRSA)
Health statistics	Centers for Disease Control and Prevention (CDC)
Census information	U.S. Census Bureau

prove useful for a grant proposal. Many of these resources can be found online or by contacting the agency. For example, health departments complete reports on specific topics, and the reports are public information. These reports provide a wealth of data that can support a grant proposal. In many cases, these reports are published and made available to the public through websites and the public library.

To find national health statistics, the grant writer can search reliable federal agencies such as the Centers for Disease Control and Prevention (CDC) and the National Center for Health Statistics. The National Library of Medicine (NLM) is also an excellent and reliable source with a multitude of health information that can support a grant proposal. Grant writers can also search professional organizations' websites. For example, if the proposal focuses on rural health issues, the grant writers check whether the team can use the National Rural Health Association (NRHA) as a resource. If the proposed program focuses on diabetes, the project team explores the American Diabetes Association (ADA) website and literature. Focused data are usually available on the websites of these federal and professional organizations in the form of reports.

BEST PRACTICE HINT

Use the National Library of Medicine, which funds resource librarians who can provide you with data on health issues, health disparities, and culturally appropriate educational materials. This information can be a great way to supplement a program.

Grant writers should never underestimate the value of the local library. Often librarians are more than happy to help grant writers find relevant data to support a grant proposal. Searching through journal articles may provide insight into similar programs that have been successful. By using these data, grant writers can strengthen any grant proposal. Journals are often reliable sources for finding best practices, which, when included in the grant proposal, enhance the validity of the proposed program.

Challenges to Data Gathering

Searching for data can be time consuming, yet it is essential to find data that sufficiently support the proposal (CRI, 2007e). Grant writers should always use reliable sources for data. Some requests for proposals outline specific requirements for data to be included. Some grant RFPs require data from specific sources or from both local and national sources. If questions arise, grant writers should contact the grant program manager for clarification.

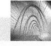

BEST PRACTICE HINT

Always include data from both local and national sources, if possible, to describe the issue's relevance locally and nationally.

The data included in a grant proposal should always be used to help describe a population or community and the challenges faced by that population or community. Sometimes it may be challenging to find supportive data. For example, if a health problem is newly identified or little research has been conducted on it, it might be difficult for the grant writer to find relevant data. In some cases, the population or community may have little specific data that relate to the group. Data might also be outdated, which can hinder a proposal rather than help it. When data are outdated, irrelevant, or nonexistent, the project team must conduct some sort of community assessment to create usable data.

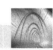

BEST PRACTICE HINT

Use your resources. Community members or students at local universities may be available to help you access data. Furthermore, students may have access to library databases beyond the scope of a practitioner.

Other challenges to data collection include issues with access to relevant databases to conduct a literature review. Also, the grant writer or project team may have little experience in data collection or literature reviews, so may be unable to determine whether data are appropriate for a grant proposal (CRI, 2007e). All of these challenges can affect a grant proposal in a negative way.

Strategies for Incorporating Data into a Grant Proposal

The grant writer or project team should ensure that the data included in the proposal are current and relevant. The team should be critical of data and explore sources thoroughly to ensure that the data are reliable. Using poor or irrelevant data reflects poorly on a grant proposal (CRI, 2007a). For example, if the grant reviewers are familiar with the community and its need, errors in supportive data included in a proposal can be detrimental to garnering funds.

A grant writer should always avoid making assumptions when it comes to data. Data can be interpreted differently from different viewpoints. The grant writer needs to ensure that the data included in a grant proposal are clearly tied to the proposal and describe the community, the need, or the capacity (CRI, 2007f). Grant writers should also be cautious

LET'S STOP AND THINK

Brainstorm about which data sources might not be appropriate resources for a grant proposal. (Hint: Wikipedia!)

about the picture the data paint of the community and its challenges. If the problem appears impossible to address, then the chances for funding are likely to be reduced. Grant writers should use data not only to describe the problems and needs but also to highlight the capacities and strengths of the community (Kretzmann & McKnight, 1993).

Data should support the local need and the community (CRI, 2007f). Providing data that are broad may not show clear ties to the community and its needs. As mentioned earlier, grant writers should include community information to demonstrate their knowledge of the community and its needs. Furthermore, the inclusion of local data helps grant reviewers know and understand the community problem in context. Each community is unique, so application of data to the specific community demonstrates to grant reviewers how the proposed program will be successful in the specific community discussed in the proposal.

Data should come from more than one data point, meaning that the project team should include more than one type of data from multiple sources (CRI, 2007a). If possible, the grant writer should discuss the community need and support it with multiple data points. This approach ensures a comprehensive discussion of the need. Grant writers can do this by describing the problem in the context of the community and then comparing it to national statistics. Data should also support the historical context of the need and the community, identifying factors such as the time frame of the problem and the community members who have addressed the issue previously (CRI, 2007b). When including data from literature reviews, the data should be from academic, peer-reviewed journals (CRI, 2007a). Data from these sources have been well researched and reviewed so that they are reliable and can support a need or problem in a grant proposal. Some RFPs specifically request certain data sources be used, and it is important for the grant writer to follow these requests.

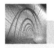

BEST PRACTICE HINT

Have someone review your grant proposal, and ask for specific feedback about the data and their representation of the community need.

Although data tell objective information about a community, its needs, and its capacities, data can fall short in telling the story of the community (CRI, 2007f). Qualitative accounts can provide insight into the challenges a community faces. Although grant proposals should be straightforward and focused on the community profile and health issues, the power of examples can enhance a grant proposal. Personal stories and reports from community members can be valuable in a grant proposal to describe a need in a community. Even though qualitative data are not measurable, this information can be used to support the proposed program and its potential impact. Qualitative information can be gathered through interviews, focus groups, and other qualitative means.

Although data are important in a grant proposal, they are not the only important component required to make a grant proposal viable. Community capacity, including team member capacity and past programmatic successes, is also important to include in the grant proposal. Especially, if past programs had relevant outcomes, including data about them can strengthen the current proposal.

Conclusion

The grant writer should use sound data throughout a grant proposal. Often data are used in the background/literature review and the needs or problem statement sections of the grant proposal. Data lay the foundation and "sell" the program to grant reviewers. Grant writers can also use literature and background support to rationalize the program and demonstrate the program's evidence-based approaches. A grant proposal without support demonstrates a lack of effort and knowledge of the community on the part of the grant writer. Therefore, grant writers must accurately integrate and utilize data that support the grant proposal.

> **LET'S STOP AND THINK**
>
> Think of a personal story in your community that could help paint the picture of the community and its needs in a grant proposal.

Glossary

Background/literature review Section of a grant proposal in which the grant writer describes the community using supporting data and begins to introduce the community needs that the proposed program will address

Demographic data Description of a group or community that includes information such as ethnicity, age, gender, family composition, and socioeconomic status

Epidemiological data Data representing the impact of a health problem on a specific population or group

Incidence The current rate of a disease or health issue in a community

Prevalence The rates of cases of disease or health issues in a certain population

Primary data Data directly collected from the community partner in the community assessment using a variety of approaches such as surveys, interviews, focus groups, and community forums

Problem statement or statement of need Section of a grant proposal in which the grant writer identifies the community need and complementary data that support and describe the need to grant reviewers

Rate Represents how often a disease or health issue occurs among a certain population

Secondary data Data from sources that describe the community and that are typically found in archives

Social indicators Data on subpopulations focused on the characteristics of a community including religious affiliation, health status, and criminal behavior

References

Abramson, J. H., & Abramson, Z. H. (2001). *Making sense of data.* Oxford: Oxford University Press.

Brownson, C. A. (2001) Program development: Planning, implementation, and evaluation strategies. In M. Scaffa (Ed.), *Occupational therapy in community-based practice settings.* Philadelphia: F. A. Davis.

Community Research Institute. (2007a). Monitoring trends and identifying emerging problems. Nonprofits and data: A how-to series. Retrieved November 3, 2008, from http://www.cridata.org/tutorials.aspx

Community Research Institute. (2007b). Using data to characterize disparities across sub populations/communities. Nonprofits and data: A how-to series. Retrieved November 3, 2008, from http://www.cridata.org/tutorials.aspx

Community Research Institute. (2007c). Using data to disseminate information to engage community and policymakers. Nonprofits and data: A how-to series. Retrieved November 3, 2008, from http://www.cridata.org/tutorials.aspx

Community Research Institute. (2007d). Using data to establish priorities and plan programs. Nonprofits and data: A how-to series. Retrieved November 3, 2008, from http://www.cridata.org/tutorials.aspx

Community Research Institute. (2007e). Using data to evaluate progress in meeting goals. Nonprofits and data: A how-to series. Retrieved November 3, 2008, from http://www.cridata.org/tutorials.aspx

Community Research Institute. (2007f). Using data to support grant applications and other funding opportunities. Nonprofits and data: A how-to series. Retrieved November 3, 2008, from http://www.cridata.org/tutorials.aspx

Edberg, M. (2007). *Essentials of health behavior: Social and behavior health in public health.* Sudbury, MA: Jones and Bartlett.

Falk, G. W. (2006). Turning an idea into a grant. *Gastrointestinal Endoscopy, 64*(6), S11–S13.

Fazio, L. S. (2008). *Developing occupation-centered programs for the community* (2nd ed.). Upper Saddle River, NJ: Prentice Hall.

Gitlin, L. N., & Lyons, K. J. (2004). *Successful grant writing: Strategies for health and human service professionals.* New York: Springer.

Goertz, H., Ryan Haddad, A., Lee, T., & Voltz, J. D. (2006). *Developing Minority Health Professionals/Researchers for Tomorrow.* Sociological Initiatives Foundation Grant.

Inouye, S. K., & Fiellin, D. A. (2005). An evidence-based guide to writing grant proposals for clinical research. *Annals of Internal Medicine, 142,* 274–282.

Kretzmann, J. P., & McKnight, J. L. (1993). *Building communities from the inside out: A path toward finding and mobilizing a community's assets.* Skokie, IL: ACTA Publications.

Mu, K., Bracciano, A., Goulet, C., & Voltz, J. D. (2007). *Chinese Study in Health Care: An Innovative Approach for Teaching Health Care Professionals.* Submitted to the United States Department of Education.

Penn, J., Grandgenett, N., & Voltz, J. D. (2007). *Omaha Tribe's Ten Clans Intervention Initiative Tribal Youth Project.* Department of Justice.

U.S. Census Bureau. (2008). Finding census data for grant writing and community needs assessment. Retrieved November 3, 2008, from http://www.census.gov/field/www/faith/

PROCESS WORKSHEET 9-1 **SECONDARY DATA**

Instructions: Track secondary data that describe the community.

Type of Data	Data	Source
Demographic data		
Social indicators		
Rate		
Prevalence		
Incidence		
Other		

PROCESS WORKSHEET 9-2 **LITERATURE REVIEW**

Instructions: Use this form to track literature review for grant proposal.

Journal	Article	Relevant Data

PROCESS WORKSHEET 9-3 **DATA SOURCES**

Instructions: Use this worksheet to track data sources for the grant proposal.

Source	Data Sought	Contact Person

PROCESS WORKSHEET 9-4 **OVERCOMING CHALLENGES**

Instructions: Use this worksheet as a format for brainstorming on how to overcome challenges with data collection for the grant proposal.

Challenge	Strategy	Person Responsible

PROCESS WORKSHEET 9-5 **CHECKLIST FOR DATA COLLECTION**

Instructions: Use this checklist as a way to check for quality control of data used in the grant proposal.

Descriptor	Checklist
Data are current.	
Data are from multiple sources.	
Data describe the community.	
Data describe need thoroughly.	
Data come from reliable sources.	
Literature review data are from peer-reviewed journals.	
Data clearly support community.	
Data clearly support community need.	
Data describe community capacity.	
Data are from local sources.	
Data are from national sources.	
Qualitative data are included.	
Other: _____	
Other: _____	

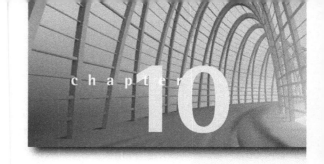

chapter 10

Program Evaluation

LEARNING OBJECTIVES

By the end of this chapter, the reader will be able to complete the following:
1. Discuss the importance of an evaluation plan for a grant proposal and/or program.
2. Compare and contrast evaluation methods.
3. Identify evaluation methods relevant to a program.
4. Draft a sample evaluation plan.

Key Terms

Comparative
   evaluation approach
Evaluation plan
External evaluation
Focus group
Formative evaluation
Impact evaluation
Internal evaluation
Outcome evaluation
Participatory
   evaluation
Process evaluation
Summative evaluation

Overview

This chapter discusses the importance of evaluation planning for program development and grant writing. Evaluation planning is a crucial component of both program development and grant writing. This chapter covers methods for developing an evaluation plan along with worksheets to help the project team develop an evaluation plan.

Introduction

Evaluation is a critical portion of any program and should be included even in a small program. In occupational therapy practice, the evaluation is the initial encounter to assess challenges and develop a treatment plan (American

Occupational Therapy Association [AOTA], 2008). In the context of a community program, the evaluation focuses on the outcomes and is completed throughout the process of implementation to track whether outcomes match proposed goals and objectives (Timmreck, 2003; Edberg, 2007). The evaluation process used in programs transcends individual results to assess the results or outcomes of a program, which makes it different from traditional occupational therapy evaluation (Brownson, 2001).

The steps and processes of program evaluation are usually included in a formal **evaluation plan**. Evaluation plans outline how a program will evaluate its effectiveness (Fazio, 2008). In their most simple form, evaluation plans reveal the basics of a program such as what works, what does not work, what to improve, and sometimes how to improve it (Edberg, 2007). Evaluation results describe how proposed goals were met and what outcomes arose from the program. Occupational therapy practitioners should remember that an evaluation plan is simply a way of assessing the progress and outcomes of a program instead of an individual client. Occupational therapy practitioners already think like this when documenting patient progress in a clinical situation.

In the context of grants, the evaluation plan can act as the resource for tracking outcomes that must be reported to funding agencies. The project team should develop evaluation plans to meet the needs of the program or grant but can expand beyond these parameters. The results from evaluation plans can make a larger impact and provide insight and information that can influence policy development and implementation (Suarez-Balcazar, 2005).

Need for Program Evaluation

An evaluation plan is an infrastructure developed to provide feedback on a program (Fazio, 2008). A well-built evaluation plan reveals which components of a program worked and which did not, what went well during program implementation and what did not. Evaluation plans account for outcomes and specifically program implementation. In a sense, evaluation plans offer a framework for ensuring quality of a program by providing a lens through which the project team can view program challenges as well as program successes (Edberg, 2007).

Ultimately, in community practice, the goal of evaluation is to determine the change made by the implemented program (Edberg, 2007). The ultimate goal of community programming is to facilitate positive change in the community to address a gap in services based on the community's capacity (Kretzmann & McKnight, 1993). For grant funders, the goal is to change behavior or to address a gap in services. In any case, change is meant to occur to fill the gap or facilitate healthy living through behavior modification. The evaluation plan measures and shows that change occurred, and possibly how and why it occurred. Furthermore, grant funding agencies want to know how their funding made an impact and require grantees to demonstrate accountability, often through the results of an evaluation plan (Voltz, 2007).

In addition to measuring change, the evaluation plan holds the program accountable to produce the outcomes it proposes to accomplish (Edberg, 2007). Community programs are accountable on several levels. First, programs are accountable to those they serve. Results from community programs are owned by the community because they are the community's experience. The project team should always share program outcomes with community participants to demonstrate effectiveness and maintain relationships (Israel, Lantz, McGranaghan, Kerr, & Guzman, 2005). If a program is funded by a grant, then the funding agency also requires accountability of the program. Funding agencies have requirements for reporting outcomes and may outline requirements for evaluation methods, driving the evaluation plan.

BEST PRACTICE HINT

When writing the grant proposal, the program planning team should include plans for sharing evaluation results with community members through newsletters, public forums, and/or town hall meetings.

Evidence-based practice is a theme important not only in traditional occupational therapy practice but also in community practice (Hammel, 2001; Holm, 2000). Community programs are called to demonstrate effectiveness, identify best practices, and develop model programs that can affect the health of communities (Edberg, 2007). Federal agencies, including the Substance Abuse and Mental Health Services Administration and the Centers for Disease Control and Prevention, identify model community programs as evidence-based practice and publish these programs for communities to use (Edberg, 2007). The evaluation plan results can demonstrate and make a case for a program's impact by developing the evidence necessary to prove program effectiveness.

Occupational therapy practitioners may question what role they can play in the evaluation process. In many cases, the evaluation plan is carried out by more than one individual and uses a participatory approach in community practice. Suarez-Balcazar (2005) outlines several roles for occupational therapy practitioners in the evaluation process including participating in the identification of community capacities and facilitating or providing training. Occupational therapy practitioners may also be involved in development and implementation of the actual evaluation plan, depending on their comfort level with data collection and analysis.

Developing and implementing a program is very time intensive, and it is important for the project team not to let the evaluation piece get lost. An evaluation plan with a timeline and specific guidelines facilitates program review and modification and ensures ongoing success (Brownson, 2001; Edberg, 2007). Besides monitoring program progress, the evaluation plan also ensures that communication with collaborators and community members is ongoing. Engaging in assessment can send a message to community members that the program coordinators are interested and

LET'S STOP AND THINK

What roles can the occupational therapy practitioner play in the evaluation process?

TABLE 10-1 INFORMATION IN EVALUATION PLANS
• What data will be collected
• When the data will be collected
• How the data will be collected
• Who will collect the data

vested in feedback from the community (Israel et al., 2005). This process alone can promote an environment in and relationship with the community that builds capacity and further collaboration. Research has shown that if the community is involved in the evaluation planning and implementation, the community feels a "sense of ownership over the evaluation, the credibility and trust in the process, and participants' level of involvement in brainstorming sessions" increases (Suarez-Balcazar, 2005; Cousins & Earl, 1995; Wandersman et al., 2004).

In the context of a grant proposal, the evaluation plan measures specifically what the funder wants to know. But evaluation plans should not be limited by grant requirements. An evaluation should be part of a program whether external funding requires it or not. Evaluation plans should be comprehensive for the organization and not solely meet the needs of the grant.

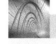

BEST PRACTICE HINT

Involve the community in the evaluation planning process, both in development and implementation of the plan.

So, what exactly does evaluation reveal about a program? Depending on the evaluation plan, evaluation data can provide information regarding how many people were reached by the program, the program's effectiveness, knowledge gained from participation in the program, and even behaviors changed by the program. Multiple measures are available to explore all these aspects of a program.

Evaluation Methods: Internal vs. External Evaluation

Evaluation can be conducted either internally or externally. **Internal evaluation** is when the evaluation is conducted by members on the project team (Huffman et al., 2002). **External evaluation** is completed by an external evaluator, usually an expert consultant focused solely on performing evaluation duties (Worley, Silagy, Prideaux, Newble, & Jones, 2000). Pros and cons exist with each method of the program or grant. The project team needs to weigh all the pros and cons when choosing an evaluation approach.

Internal evaluation has the risk of carrying bias because those involved in the evaluation are involved in the program implementation and possibly the program planning and development. This approach is viewed as having low objectivity and does not have the credibility of an external approach (Huffman et al., 2002). Participants may not feel comfortable providing data to a person directly involved with program implementation. In this case and if possible, it may be advisable to have a person on the team who focuses solely on program evaluation (Timmreck, 2003). Furthermore, the internal evaluator may not be well trained or an expert in evaluation, which can affect the outcomes or value of the results (Rush & Lord, 2002).

> **LET'S STOP AND THINK**
>
> What benefits are there for internal evaluation? What challenges exist to internal evaluation? Brainstorm some of your thoughts.

External evaluation usually incurs more cost because it entails hiring or buying out the time of an evaluator. Yet, there are benefits to this cost. Most evaluators are formally trained in statistics, data analysis, and producing written evaluation reports (Edwards, Jumper-Thurman, Plested, Oetting, & Swanson, 2000). An external evaluator may also be a resource in writing the evaluation plan to help determine the best approaches for evaluation of the program. Participants may feel more comfortable providing feedback to an external evaluator, and feedback can be obtained anonymously (Worley et al., 2000).

Besides a grant mandate, another reason for choosing an external evaluation may be that communication within an organization or a community is not very strong. When this occurs, the project team may feel like the outcome of the evaluation may not be reliable and may decide to hire an external evaluator. Another reason for using external evaluation is time constraints. Some grants have a short funding period, yet still require an evaluation. In a short grant period, it may be difficult to implement participatory evaluation approaches. When an evaluation is needed in a short amount of time, an external evaluator can save the day. External evaluators have expertise focused on evaluation, and when the project team is in a time crunch, an external evaluator can move quickly and with efficiency and proficiency.

> **LET'S STOP AND THINK**
>
> What are the benefits of external evaluation? What challenges exist to external evaluation? Brainstorm some of your thoughts.

Research on evaluation in community health programs identifies the fact that the evaluator does not fully understand the community as one barrier of external evaluation (O'Sullivan & O'Sullivan, 1998; Judd, Frankish, & Moulton, 2001). Furthermore, the evaluator and the community may have different opinions on the necessary outcomes for the evaluation plan based on their perspectives and expertise. If this occurs, the participants may not provide the evaluator with appropriate or relevant data during evaluation (Meagher & Healy, 2003).

BEST PRACTICE HINT

Always review the funding availability when exploring evaluation. If possible, it is always helpful to hire an external evaluator. Seek experts in evaluation from local universities who may charge significantly lower fees than other professionals do.

As part of this process, the project team should identify who will be involved in the evaluation process. Ultimately, everyone involved in the program provides assistance in data collection. But the team needs to determine who will collect and collate data, who will analyze the data, and who will complete

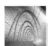

BEST PRACTICE HINT

If possible, hire an external evaluator who knows the community and can help ensure that the evaluation data relates to the community.

reports from the data results. Like program development and grant writing, evaluation planning and implementation are collaborative processes. The project team should explore different evaluation methods to identify which would work best for the qualifications of the team, and which provides the most cost benefit and required program outcomes to report to funders. Worksheets at the end of the chapter can help the project team develop an evaluation plan.

Participatory Evaluation

In community programs, a valuable evaluation method is participatory evaluation. Participatory evaluation is closely associated with participatory action research models (Stoecker, 2005). According to Cousins and Whitmore (2007), **participatory evaluation** "implies that, when doing an evaluation, researchers, facilitators, or professional evaluators collaborate in some way with individuals, groups, or communities who have a decided stake in the program, development project, or other entity being evaluated" (p. 87). In other words, the participants involved in the program contribute to the evaluation (Suarez-Balcazar, Orellena-Damacella, Portillo, Lanum, & Sharma, 2003).

The principles of participatory evaluation are similar to the asset-based approaches identified by Kretzmann and McKnight (1993), as discussed earlier in this book. In participatory evaluation, community members or program participants are involved throughout the evaluation process and develop a sense of ownership of the evaluation plan (Fawcett et al., 2003). This approach promotes empowerment and accountability of all involved in the program. Outcomes are focused on what the community identifies as relevant and important. Throughout this book, the concept of collaboration with the community has been emphasized. It should be no different in the evaluation process. Program participants should be considered the experts in the program and should work closely with the evaluator (Stoecker, 2005), even if an external evaluator is employed.

LET'S STOP AND THINK

What benefits do you think come with following a participatory evaluation approach? What challenges do you think arise in following a participatory evaluation approach?

Participatory evaluation can come with significant obstacles to implementation. In participatory evaluation, community members are highly engaged, which usually means that they must be provided with some training to ensure that they understand the process (Cousins & Whitmore, 2007). Providing training can be a challenge, but it is also a part of collaboration. Also, in participatory evaluation, time must be taken to listen to community members. The project team can use focus groups and interviews, which can be time consuming, to analyze versus surveys.

Ultimately, in participatory evaluation, the community determines which approaches work best for them.

Choosing an Evaluation Method

The project team must choose the evaluation method early in the program planning phase and outline it in the grant proposal. Choosing an evaluation method can be difficult, and the project team should review all methods thoroughly to ensure that the chosen method matches well with the program and the community's needs. Although participatory evaluation provides a community-centered model, sometimes an external evaluation is the best approach. Some grants require an external evaluation—making deciding on evaluation approach easy. In the past, external evaluation used to be the main model employed by grant agencies. But in the recent past, grant agencies have come to understand the value of participatory evaluation and some are allowing programs to determine which model works best for them (Aubel, 1999; Checkoway & Richards-Schuster, 2008). Some programs opt for an evaluation plan that is considered a hybrid of participatory evaluation and external evaluation (Stoecker, 2005). In this model, the external evaluator focuses on the needs of the community during evaluation. In other words, the external evaluator utilizes all the methods of participatory evaluation but is not involved in the implementation of the program.

BEST PRACTICE HINT

Include community members on the evaluation team to ensure that data are collected and distributed in a way meaningful to the community.

BEST PRACTICE HINT

Review the RFP to see whether the grant guidelines outline requirements for the type of evaluation to be used. If any questions arise, contact the project director to clarify.

LET'S STOP AND THINK

Describe some benefits of following a hybrid model that uses an external evaluator with participatory evaluation.

Types of Evaluation Data

After choosing an evaluation method, the project team must determine which types of evaluation will be included in the evaluation plan. In this process, the team considers the pros and cons of different evaluation approaches, and then creates a plan that takes into consideration what type of data will be collected during the evaluation. It is important to distinguish between these steps in evaluation planning. Choosing a method allows the project team to determine which method will be best for collecting evaluation data, whereas choosing the type of evaluation conducted determines which types of data will be collected to evaluate the program effectively.

For the team to decide what data will be collected, it is important that they understand the types of evaluation. Evaluation can be either formative or summative in nature (Timmreck, 2003). **Formative evaluation** is used when a problem exists and solutions to the problem need to be explored. In the case of community programs, it might be used as a tool when a program is not reaching its goals. For-

---

TABLE 10-2 EXAMPLES OF PROCESS EVALUATION

- Procedures
- Policies
- Program performance

---

mative evaluation can help find a solution to the problem. **Summative evaluation** explores the program's impact and efficiency (Timmreck, 2003). Most community programs will employ an evaluation plan based on a summative model to monitor the program's progress.

Three main types of evaluation serve as methods for program outcomes data collection: process evaluation, impact evaluation, and outcome evaluation. **Process evaluation** looks at basic program implementation (Edberg, 2007). For example, if a program offers a seminar, a form of process evaluation would be to find the number of attendees, which can be measured simply by having a sign-in sheet. This alone is evaluation data that indicate information about the program. The data retrieved from a process evaluation describe whether the program was implemented as planned (Edberg, 2007). Process evaluation can be either quantitative or qualitative. In the preceding example, the number of attendees is a quantitative measure, but after the seminar, the seminar leader may seek feedback from the participants. This data may be how people felt about the seminar including their impressions of its implementation, the speaker, and so forth; these are qualitative data.

The second type of evaluation is **impact evaluation**. Impact evaluation explores both the benefits and resources and the cost of implementing the program (Timmreck, 2003). The focus of this type of evaluation is to explore the impact of the program itself. It monitors the program throughout program implementation, not just at the final outcome. This approach is commonly used in collaboration with the PRECEDE-PROCEED Model discussed in Chapter 2 (Timmreck, 2003; Edberg, 2007).

The third type of evaluation is **outcome evaluation**. Outcome evaluation provides information related to the program's outcomes, including knowledge gained and/or behavior changed (Fazio, 2008). Basically, the outcome evaluation focuses on what happens when the program is over (Timmreck, 2003). An example is *Matter of Balance*, a program developed to assist community-dwelling older adults address their fear of falling. Research conducted after the program demonstrated that older adults who participated in the program had decreased fear and an increase in activity engagement resulting from decreased fear (Tennstedt, Peterson, Howland, & Lachman, 1998). This example demonstrates how outcome evaluation can be used to determine whether a program affects the behavior of the participants.

TABLE 10-3 EVALUATION APPROACHES

- Record keeping
- Inventory
- Comparative design
- Quasi-experimental design
- Controlled experimental design
- Comprehensive research design

Outcome evaluation can also be quantitative or qualitative. An example of outcome evaluation is a pretest and posttest model. A preassessment is given to assess participants' knowledge before they participate in the program, and then after the intervention, a postassessment is given to assess what participants learned. Furthermore, outcome evaluation can focus on both short- and long-term outcomes of the program (Timmreck, 2003; Edberg, 2007).

LET'S STOP AND THINK

Brainstorm how each type of evaluation can be used in a community practice setting.

Types of Evaluation Design

No evaluation plan will be the same as any other, and there are no standardized approaches to choosing and developing an evaluation plan. Evaluation plans should be designed based on the "situation, the program and the kinds of evidence needed" (Edberg, 2007, p. 159). However, definitive approaches for collecting the information needed for the evaluation plan exist and should be identified in the evaluation plan.

An evaluation calls upon the project team to collect data on the program. Multiple procedures exist for data collection; some are fairly simple and others are more complex. The first approach to demonstrating a program's success through data is to maintain records of the program (Timmreck, 2003; Edberg, 2007). These records include tracking participation of community members including the number of participants. Other information to track can be how many times a training was implemented; number of healthcare services delivered; and number of hits on the program website. The data tracked for record keeping is based on the goals of the program and the measurements required by the evaluation plan.

Inventories explore the progress made toward the program's goals (Timmreck, 2003; Edberg, 2007). When focused on a health-related community program, examples include how many individuals increased participation in exercise or how the number of falls was reduced because of the intervention. This information is measured through exploring behavior change usually in the form of participant surveys or questionnaires.

TABLE 10-4 EXAMPLES OF EVALUATION METHODS

- Tracking numbers of participants
- Observation
- Satisfaction surveys of program participants
- Pre- and posttests of program information
- Focus groups
- Individual interviews
- Content analysis of agendas, trainings, and meeting minutes
- Participant and staff reflections
- Case analysis
- Photography as a data point

Source: Durrance, J. C., & Fisher, K. E. (2008). Outcomes toolkit version 2.0 [software]. Retrieved July 31, 2008, from http://ibec.ischool.washington.edu/static/ibeccat.aspx@ subcat=outcome%20toolkit&cat=tools%20and%20resources.htm

---

In a **comparative evaluation approach**, the evaluation plan explores how the program compares to others (Timmreck, 2003). The project team might use this approach if they are implementing a program in multiple communities or if the program was previously implemented and baseline data exist. The project team might then compare the data using case analysis across the programs.

Quasi-experimental designs compare different groups or communities using the same tools (Timmreck, 2003; Edberg, 2007). For example, the project team uses the same questionnaires and instruments on both groups. In this approach, the project team collects data from a control group, for whom the program was not implemented. This approach determines the effectiveness of the program on a specific group of people and the impact of not implementing the program.

The most complex evaluation approach is a comprehensive research design. In this case, the program has a well-designed research plan that uses multiple evaluation methods (Timmreck, 2003; Edberg, 2007). This approach requires the project team to have expertise in data collection, instrumentation, administration, and data analysis. For a research-based grant program, this approach will most likely be required.

For each approach, multiple methods exist for collecting the data needed. The methods the project team chooses for data collection depend on the requirements of the evaluation plan and which evaluation approach they chose. Some examples include pre and post surveys, questionnaires, focus groups, and interviews (Fazio, 2008).

Techniques for Data Collection for an Evaluation Plan

After determining which approach or approaches are most useful and relevant for the evaluation, the team needs to identify which techniques to use to gather the evaluation data. The team should include the chosen techniques in the evaluation plan and describe them in the evaluation plan in the grant proposal. Some of the techniques require more time and expertise, whereas others are fairly simple and require little training or understanding of evaluation.

Every grant evaluation plan should include a mechanism for tracking basic program information. Tracking includes counting the number of participants, number of trainings, and other relevant figures that demonstrate program outcomes. During program development, the project team must create an infrastructure for information tracking and decide which measures will be tracked. In some cases, the RFP outlines tracking requirements, which are submitted in grant reports, and these should be included in the evaluation plan.

Program implementers and grant funders want to know how many people participated in the program and also how much the program affected the participants. The evaluation team can measure the impact of the program in a variety of ways. The program team can find out how participants feel about the program by using satisfaction surveys, interviews, and/or focus groups. To assess what participants learned from the program, they can use pretests and posttests about relevant program information. Pretests and posttests need to be developed and pilot tested before use.

Surveys can be a viable evaluation technique; however, a challenge to using a survey for evaluation includes developing or finding a reliable questionnaire (Timmreck, 2003). Some things to consider when designing a survey is the method of implementation including how the survey will be distributed, collected, and analyzed. The project team should also consider the reading level and primary language of the community to ensure that all community members are assessed accurately. The team should determine a sample population prior to survey distribution. Then, they must collect, enter, and analyze the survey results to develop the evaluation program results. This sometimes requires staff expertise and unique software, which the team should plan for in the grant proposal.

Focus groups are small groups of people pulled together to answer a collection of questions (Timmreck, 2003; Sharpe, Greaney, Lee, & Royce, 2000; Clark et al., 2003). These groups can provide feedback on a program and allow evaluators to assess a program's impact and the perceptions of participants. The team needs to determine how many participants should be involved in a focus group, how many and how often focus groups will be run, along with the targeted focus group questions. Some challenges with focus groups include the time it takes to implement and analyze the focus group results. To conduct focus groups, a member of the team should be aware of how to run the group and ask questions to keep the group on task (Clark et al., 2003). The focus group should also be an open forum where members feel free to express their opinions openly (Timmreck, 2003). By providing food or another incentive, the project team can increase participation.

Interviews offer the opinions of a small group of participants (Timmreck, 2003). The team can conduct interviews in person or via phone. Phone interviews allow participants to be interviewed from any location, which assists in compliance. One benefit to an interview is the opportunity the team has to probe individuals based on their unique experiences with the program, which can provide valuable evaluation data. Interviews are also an effective method to use with participants who have any kind of sensory disability including vision problems or individuals who may be illiterate (Brownson, 2001). Staff working on the program can also be interviewed to assess the program's inner workings. Staff interviews can be another valuable data point in an evaluation plan.

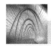

Evaluation plans need not be limited and can employ a variety of techniques. Some evaluation plans might employ creative approaches such as life narratives or photography, from which the team interprets the results. Evaluation techniques most relevant to the program and that collect the evaluation data needed to express the program's outcomes should be used.

Challenges to Evaluation Plans

Evaluations are important and necessary, but can be associated with challenges. A significant obstacle to implementing an evaluation plan is the fact that evaluation is time consuming and requires extensive resources. Small programs that receive insufficient grant funding are challenged even more by time and resource constraints. Some grants allot money for evaluation as a certain percentage of the budget. Other grants require a minimum percentage of the budget be used for the evaluation. Still other grants do not describe this aspect and some do not allow funds for this process even though evaluation is still required. The project team needs to address these challenges when developing the evaluation plan to ensure that they can handle all aspects of the evaluation.

In community settings, evaluation planning raises unique issues. The right balance of evaluation is essential. Evaluation can be interruptive or even inappropriate to a community. Participants can easily become "overassessed," which can damage outcomes or overwhelm participants so that completing a component of the evaluation is too cumbersome. Furthermore, evaluation results should be community-centered and focused on results that the community wants. As discussed earlier, community members and evaluators can have different priorities for evaluation

(Lantz, Viruell-Fuentes, Israel, Softley, & Guzman, 2001). The project team should thoughtfully consider such aspects as the amount of evaluation and the community's direction of evaluation to facilitate a positive evaluation experience. If a grant requires evaluation that does not match with community desires, then the team must consider an evaluation plan that addresses the needs of both parties.

Community health can be difficult to measure, and the evaluation plan needs to be comprehensive to capture this evidence. Measuring some aspects of change resulting from a program can provide its own unique concerns. According to Merzel and D'Afflitti (2003),

> Regardless of whether an experimental or quasi-experimental design is employed, identification of communities with comparable characteristics is difficult to achieve, especially given the complexity of communities as social units and the limited ability to obtain accurate and complete measures of the environmental influences that can affect program outcomes. (p. 563)

Some types of behavior change are difficult to track and measure. To fully investigate this information in an evaluation plan can require intensive research and expertise in research design. Teams must be sure to avoid assuming that a single program facilitated change when many other factors could be at play. Also, if information is going to be publicly disseminated, it is important for the team to receive approval from an institutional review board (IRB) for research. The IRB will determine whether and what type of approval is required based on the program.

The evaluation team must have the appropriate expertise to conduct evaluations. The team may be intimidated by the process, may lack the expertise to conduct an evaluation or may not be capable of administering the kind of evaluation required to measure the impact of the program (Merzel & D'Afflitti, 2003). In such cases, the project team might need to ensure that staff are trained to be involved in the program. Sometimes training can be included and funded through a grant proposal. Nevertheless, the evaluation plan must consider the expertise and willingness of the project evaluation team. It must be developed based on the expertise of the team and the community needs.

One pitfall is developing a complex evaluation plan that no one on the team can articulate or complete. This can create a major problem and can lead to issues with grantors. If the grant proposal outlines an evaluation plan, that plan needs to be followed. If the team anticipates difficulty following the proposed plan, they must contact the grantor's staff immediately to determine the procedures to change the plan. It is better to plan for the capacity of the organization and staff to avoid such challenges. The grant writer can explain the team's capacity to the funder in a grant proposal to ensure that the program's resources match the funding requirements.

The project evaluation team can overcome difficulties in evaluation planning and implementation with planning and thoughtful development. The team can also document the problems they encountered in grant reports to demonstrate the compromises they made in the evaluation plan. Ultimately, the project team must meet grant requirements and the program may need to compromise to achieve these standards. The project team should not let challenges such as these prevent them from including and implementing an evaluation plan. The time it takes them to implement an evaluation plan can be made up by using the collected data in the future, which makes it easier to draft new grants or seek donations.

BEST PRACTICE HINT

Evaluation data from a current program can be used to write a future grant and can serve as future community assessment data or other data needed in a proposal.

One strategy to overcome issues with evaluation is for the team to be creative and to problem solve with community members. The project team can also seek resources such as academicians, college students, or community members with evaluation expertise who are willing to assist. Sometimes support staff from the grantor can assist or answer questions regarding evaluation. If this resource is available, the project team should take advantage of it as needed.

Drafting the Evaluation Plan

Evaluation plans are meant to be very objective documents that identify the who, what, when, where, and how of program evaluation. A comprehensive evaluation plan includes the following: evaluation questions, program aspects being measured/evaluated, processes for tracking goal and objective outcomes, process for gathering evaluation data, data collection and analysis methods, a timeline, personnel completing evaluation components, budget, and reports to be completed (Timmreck, 2003). The project team can use a logic model to describe the evaluation plan. Logic models are discussed in Chapter 8 in detail.

According to Suarez-Balcazar (2005), an evaluation plan "usually specifies the link between the program elements, including program goals, activities, inputs, outputs (process evaluation), and impact indicators (outcome evaluation) within the contextual characteristics of the community" (p. 135). Evaluation plans should be ongoing and integrated into every component of the program to view outcomes (Stoecker, 2005). It is important in drafting the evaluation that the project team makes this objective clear and evident. Grant reviewers also need to understand the evaluation plan as described in the grant, so a clear plan can help garner funding.

The project team should develop the evaluation plan in the program planning stage. As mentioned, evaluation should be ongoing, and a proficient program manager should continually evaluate the program's success and explore ways to improve the program. The grant proposal specifies times for evaluation and subsequent reports on the evaluation data. Evaluation should be built in as part of the ongoing program implementation, integrating multiple forms of evaluation such as process, impact, and outcome evaluation (Edberg, 2007). Furthermore, the project team should conduct evaluation for the sake of the program and not for the sake of a grant.

By following a few steps when drafting the evaluation plan, the project team can ensure that the plan is comprehensive, meets grant requirements, and aligns with the program and community needs. The first step is to decide on what information the evaluation plan will provide or what information the program and community needs (Timmreck, 2003). The evaluation plan structure may be driven by the grant requirements, but programs are never limited to solely what the grant requires. In other words, the evaluation plan identifies what will be included in the grant reports, if necessary, so it is essential that the plan aligns with grant requirements, but it should not limited by the requirements. Beyond grant requirements, the team should gather information relevant to the community or program.

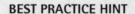

BEST PRACTICE HINT

Evaluation results must include information required by the grantor. However, in the grant reports or as an appendix to the report include other relevant evaluation data that positively represent the program.

As the processes and required evaluation data are determined, the project team must identify the evaluation team. The team needs to decide whether they will use internal or external evaluation, who will track evaluation data, who will draft reports, and what community members will be involved. Training staff and community members may be necessary at this time to help them fully understand the concept of an evaluation plan. Also, the team can identify experts and resources needed for evaluation.

The project team should start evaluation planning by determining the questions that need to be answered (Stoecker, 2005). Evaluation plans for grants should answer the questions funders want answered but can also expand beyond these requirements. To discover the question or questions that the evaluation plan will address, the team must look back at the initial assessment of the community and mission or goals of the program (Timmreck, 2003). The results from community assessment should provide insight into the answers the evaluation is looking for and provide a baseline for the evaluation plan. For example, if the program focuses on reducing obesity of local youth, then it would be helpful to identify the average baseline body mass index (BMI) of the local children using initial assessments. These data can then be used to form an evaluation related to the program and outcomes to reduce youth obesity.

Most often, the evaluation questions should target specific program outcomes. For example, if the community issue is teen suicide, then an evaluation question might be: Does this program reduce the number of teen deaths related to suicide? The outcome is measurable and relates to the community needs and the program goals and objectives. Another example is for the issue of older adult falls. The evaluation question might be: Does completing home safety assessments in the homes of community-dwelling older adults reduce falls? Outcome data could include the number of emergency room visits for falls and self-reporting by participants on their number of falls. Depending on the type of evaluation methods used and required, evaluation questions may be simpler, such as: How many people have been educated by the health education series on older adult falls? In this example, the goal of the program is to educate, and the number educated on the topic is the outcome.

The team should develop evaluation questions with a community-centered approach. Evaluation plans sometimes need to evolve to address the community and the program outcomes or the team's ability to collect data (Stoecker, 2005). Evaluation plans should always be flexible based on what is going on with the program and the community (Merzel & D'Afflitti, 2003). In the previous example of a teen suicide prevention program, the evaluation team needs to make sure information is tracked and available; otherwise, the question will go unanswered. Evaluation questions should remain close to the program goals and objectives to ensure that the team follows the plan.

Once the questions are determined, the next step is for the team to choose the methods to use in evaluation (Stoecker, 2005). Specific methods for gathering data are discussed earlier in this chapter. The team should collect data that can be measured and that relate to the evaluation questions. Building questions into an evaluation plan that cannot be measured is useless and can be damaging to the program. The team must remember that the purpose of evaluation is to demonstrate the program's effectiveness, so the evaluation questions and measures should always maintain focus on these factors (Timmreck, 2003; Edberg, 2007).

In many cases, the community can identify which outcomes and questions can be measured and may know what data already exist. For example, if a rural community has a critical access hospital, information on emergency room admissions might be easy to gather and focuses on the population served. In contrast, in a metropolitan area that includes many emergency rooms, it might be difficult to determine who goes to which emergency room, so tying outcomes to the program may be challenging.

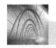

BEST PRACTICE HINT

Outline the entire evaluation plan and choose appropriate measures to ensure that the evaluation team does not face significant challenges during implementation.

Furthermore, evaluation data needs to be accessible. For example, private data such as participant medical records may be difficult to obtain, making it impossible to demonstrate an outcome. When reviewing evaluation questions, the project team should always consider whether there is a source of data that can demonstrate the outcome to answer the question.

At this point, it is helpful for the team to identify who will gather the data and the timeline for gathering this data. They must also consider data analysis, including which analysis methods will be used, who will conduct the analysis, and the timeline for completion. Data analysis depends on the methods chosen for data collection. There is no one correct method for analyzing data, and the community should determine the best approach (Fawcett et al., 2003). Last, the team must determine a timeline and method for presenting the evaluation results. The specifics of this topic are discussed later in the chapter.

Sometimes programs have outcomes that were not intended but that have a positive impact on the community. A crucial aspect of evaluation is to document these unintended successes (Cohen, Baer, & Satterwhite, 2002). This information can aid in garnering future support for the program and proving program viability.

An Evaluation Plan Model

Although there are multiple approaches to evaluation, Suarez-Balcazar and associates (2003) provide a model for implementing an evaluation plan in community practice that includes five phases. These phases include the following: developing partnerships and evaluation planning; developing a logic model using an outcomes framework; identifying the methodology and data collection strategies; interpreting and reporting findings; and gathering feedback, monitoring, and using findings (Suarez-Balcazar, 2005, p. 135).

The first step in this model, partnership development and evaluation planning, includes developing a collaborative partnership, engaging active participants of the community on the evaluation team, and gathering individuals together to plan the evaluation. All of these tasks align with the participatory evaluation model discussed earlier in the chapter. In community practice, partnerships aid in the development of programs that meet complicated community needs, and a strong partnership is required to complete a successful evaluation of a community program (Jensen & Royeen, 2001).

After developing and maintaining the collaborative evaluation team, the team can focus on developing a logic model as the format for the evaluation plan. At this point, the evaluation team engages in brainstorming to collaboratively identify systems to document program outcomes. The team can explore the literature for best practices and then identify which best practices suit the community and the program.

Next, the evaluation team identifies the methodology and data collection strategies for the evaluation plan. The model recommends using a mixed methods approach to gather both quantitative and qualitative evaluation data regarding the program. The team needs to garner approval from an institutional review board (IRB) and then identify both the participants and the measurement tools to be used in the evaluation plan.

Based on the evaluation plan and ongoing evaluation results, the evaluation team can begin to interpret and report findings from the evaluation plan. As part of this step in the model, the team needs to determine the timeline and structure of reporting the evaluation results. This includes identifying which members of the team will complete the reports and how the information will be disseminated.

The last step in this evaluation model is to provide feedback and monitor and utilize the evaluation plan's findings. At this stage, the evaluation team provides the community with feedback based on evaluation results. This feedback can include how well the program is reaching its outcomes and any health behavior changes

TABLE 10-5 EVALUATION PLAN MODEL PHASES AND ACTIONS

Phase	Actions
Develop a partnership and plan evaluation.	• Develop collaborative partnership. • Include active participants in community life on evaluation planning team. • Meet as a group to plan evaluation.
Develop a logic model.	• Brainstorm with evaluation team. • Identify systematic ways for documenting outcomes. • Conduct a literature review. • Establish best practices for the evaluation plan.
Identify the methodology and data collection strategies.	• Utilize a mixed methods approach. • Seek institutional review board (IRB) approval. • Identify participants/sample. • Determine measurement tools.
Interpret and report findings.	• Develop reporting structure and timeline. • Conduct data analysis.
Provide feedback; monitor and utilize findings.	• Determine how the data will be utilized. • Provide community with feedback based on evaluation results.

Source: Suarez-Balcazar, Y. (2005). Empowerment and participatory evaluation of a community health intervention: Implications for occupational therapy. *Occupational Therapy Journal of Research, 25*(4), 1–10.

BEST PRACTICE HINT

Following an evaluation model, ensure that all steps and pieces of the evaluation plan are included both for program development and in a grant proposal.

the program is beginning to effect. From this point, community members can provide feedback to the program on suggested program modifications to increase success and impact (Suarez-Balcazar, 2005).

Writing Up the Results

Evaluation plans usually contain a timeline for reports including types of reports and when they need to be completed. When writing reports, the evaluation team needs to consider the audience. In community practice, there may be more than one audience, which means that reports may need to be tailored to targeted audiences. For example, the team may need to provide a report to the grantor and one to the community advisory board. In this case, each entity may care about different outcomes and the reports should focus on each group's specific concerns. The team must write reports at the appropriate

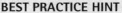

TABLE 10-6 METHODS FOR SHARING EVALUATION DATA
• Organizational annual report
• Executive summary
• Full report
• Oral presentation highlighting important outcomes

reading level for the audience, which can be different among groups. The key is to know the audience and provide them with the just-right report. Data reported in a format that is not relevant to the target audience will not make an impact.

In some cases, submitting an executive summary of evaluation results may be more appropriate than preparing an entire report. Again, this depends on the audience, and report writers must consider this thoughtfully when preparing the report format. The evaluation team can share reports in multiple ways and multiple formats. There are a lot of data to share in an evaluation report, but the team must consider which data are relevant to the target audience. The team will distribute reports to current funders and advisors, and also the outcome data from the evaluation plan might be used for future projects or even for fund-raising. Some strategies for enhancing a report are to use visuals such as charts and graphs or to use a case study (Timmreck, 2003). Profiling someone the program has served, also known as "sharing the story," can be an effective method for demonstrating the program's success.

An evaluation report should include the following sections: the program results and findings, evaluation methods used to complete the report, the program's history and background, the theoretical basis for the program, implications drawn from the evaluation, recommendations based on the outcomes, and barriers or reasons for unmet objectives (Timmreck, 2003). A report should always discuss reasons that objectives were not met. Grant funders specifically want to know this information because financial support was provided to ensure the proposed objectives were met. The evaluation results often reveal barriers to program implementation. The evaluation team should describe these barriers in the report along with plans to address them to increase program success.

There is always the concern that the evaluation plan could reveal that a program is ineffective (Stoecker, 2005). However, evaluation plans are meant to be carried

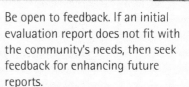

BEST PRACTICE HINT

Be open to feedback. If an initial evaluation report does not fit with the community's needs, then seek feedback for enhancing future reports.

BEST PRACTICE HINT

Create a community profile telling the stories of the impact of the program on community members by using photos of community members arranged in a creative and attractive format.

out throughout a program so that the team and community members can identify areas of ineffectiveness and can modify the program to ensure that positive outcomes occur. If the program proves to be ineffective, the project team should modify it, document the changes, and report them to funders and community members.

Conclusion

Evaluation planning is a crucial component to program development and grant writing. No grant proposal should be written without a program evaluation plan, even if the grant funder does not require one. Furthermore, what is the purpose of implementing a program without the ability to demonstrate its outcomes? The need for an evaluation plan is clear. The project team should not let challenges or fear prevent them from including an evaluation plan in any program. Occupational therapy practitioners can lead or be a part of an evaluation team, as evidenced in this chapter. After all, evaluation is what occupational therapists do!

Glossary

Comparative evaluation approach An evaluation approach that explores how the program compares to others

Evaluation plan An infrastructure developed to provide feedback on a program

External evaluation Evaluation is completed by an external evaluator, usually an expert consultant focused on solely performing evaluation duties.

Focus group Method of garnering evaluation data that pulls together small groups of people to answer a collection of questions

Formative evaluation A type of evaluation focused on determining an existing problem and identifying potential solutions to the problem

Impact evaluation A type of evaluation that explores the benefits, resources, and cost of implementing the program

Internal evaluation Evaluation is conducted by an individual on the program team.

Outcome evaluation A type of evaluation that provides information related to the program's outcomes including knowledge gained and/or behavior changed.

Participatory evaluation A type of evaluation that "implies that, when doing an evaluation, researchers, facilitators, or professional evaluators collaborate in some way with individuals, groups, or communities who have a decided stake in the program, development project, or other entity being evaluated" (Cousins & Whitmore, 2007, p. 87).

Process evaluation A type of evaluation that explores basic program implementation

Summative evaluation A type of evaluation focused on exploring the program's impact and efficiency

References

American Occupational Therapy Association. (2008). Occupational therapy practice framework: Domain and process, 2nd edition. *American Journal of Occupational Therapy*, *62*(6), 625–683.

Aubel, J. (1999). *Participatory program evaluation manual: Involving program stakeholders in the evaluation process* (2nd ed.). Calverton, MD: Catholic Relief Services.

Brownson, C. A. (2001). Program development: Planning, implementation, and evaluation strategies. In M. Scaffa (Ed.), *Occupational therapy in community-based practice settings*. Philadelphia: F. A. Davis.

Checkoway, B., & Richards-Schuster, K. (2008). *Facilitators guide for participatory evaluation for young people*. Ann Arbor: University of Michigan.

Clark, M. J., Cary, S., Diemert, G., Ceballos, R., Sifuentes, M., Atteberry, M., et al. (2003). Involving communities in community assessment. *Public Health Nursing, 20*(6), 456–463.

Cohen, L., Baer, N., & Satterwhite, P. (2002) Developing effective coalitions: An eight step guide. In M. E. Wurzbach (Ed.), *Community health education and promotion: A guide to program design and evaluation* (2nd ed., pp. 144–161). Gaithersburg, MD: Aspen.

Cousins, J. B., & Earl, L. M. (1995). The case for participatory evaluation: Theory, research, practices. In J. B. Cousins & L. Earl (Eds.), *Participatory evaluation in education: Studies in evaluation use and organizational learning* (pp. 3–17). London: Falmer Press.

Cousins, J. B., & Whitmore, E. (2007). Framing participatory evaluation. *New Directions for Evaluation, 80*, 87–105.

Durrance, J. C., & Fisher, K. E. (2008). Outcomes toolkit version 2.0 [software]. Retrieved July 31, 2008, from http://ibec.ischool.washington.edu/static/ibeccat.aspx@subcat= outcome%20toolkit&cat=tools%20and%20resources.htm

Edberg, M. (2007). *Essentials of health behavior: Social and behavior health in public health*. Sudbury, MA: Jones and Bartlett.

Edwards, R. W., Jumper-Thurman, P., Plested, B. A., Oetting, E. R., & Swanson, L. (2000). Community readiness: Research to practice. *Journal of Community Psychology, 28*(3), 291–307.

Fawcett, S. B., Boothroyd, R., Schultz, J. A., Francisco, V. T., Carson, V., & Bremby, R. (2003). Building capacity for participatory evaluation within community initiatives. *Journal of Prevention and Intervention in Community, 26*(2), 21–36.

Fazio, L. (2008). *Developing occupation-centered programs for the community* (2nd ed.). Upper Saddle River, NJ: Prentice Hall.

Hammel, K. W. (2001). Using qualitative research to inform the client-centered evidence-based practice of occupational therapy. *British Journal of Occupational Therapy, 64*(5), 228–234.

Holm, M. B. (2000). Our mandate for the new millennium: Evidence-based practice, 2000 Eleanor Clarke Slagle lecture. *American Journal of Occupational Therapy, 54*, 575–585.

Huffman, L., Koopman, C., Blasey, C., Botcheva, L., Hill, K. E., Marks, A. S., et al. (2002). A program evaluation strategy in a community-based behavioral health and education services agency for children and families. *Journal of Applied Behavioral Science, 38*(2), 191–215.

Israel, B. A., Lantz, P. M., McGranaghan, R. J., Kerr, D. L., & Guzman, J. R. (2005). Documentation and evaluation of CBPR partnerships. In B. A. Israel, E. Eng, A. J. Schulz, & E. A. Parker (Eds.), *Methods in community-based participatory research for health* (pp. 255–277). San Francisco: Jossey-Bass.

Jensen, G. M., & Royeen, C. B. (2001). Analysis of academic-community partnerships using the integration matrix. *Journal of Allied Health, 30*, 168–175.

Judd, J., Frankish, C. J., & Moulton, G. (2001). Setting standards in the evaluation of community-based health promotion programs—A unifying approach. *Health Promotion International, 16*(4), 367–380.

Kretzmann, J. P., & McKnight, J. L. (1993). *Building communities from the inside out: A path toward finding and mobilizing a community's assets*. Skokie, IL: ACTA Publications.

Lantz, P. M., Viruell-Fuentes, E., Israel, B. A., Softley, D., & Guzman, R. (2001). Can communities and academia work together on public health research? Evaluation results from a community-based participatory research partnership in Detroit. *Journal of Urban Health, 78*(3), 495–507.

Meagher, G., & Healy, K. (2003). Caring, controlling, contracting, and counting: Governments and non-profits in community services. *Australian Journal of Public Administration, 62*(3), 40–51.

Merzel, C., & D'Affliti, J. (2003). Reconsidering community-based health promotion: Promise, performance and potential. *American Journal of Public Health, 93*(4), 557–574.

Office of Disease Prevention and Health Promotion. (2008). *Healthy people 2020: The road ahead.* Retrieved July 31, 2008, from http://www.healthypeople.gov/hp2020/

O'Sullivan, R. G., & O'Sullivan, J. M. (1998). Evaluation voices: Promoting evaluation from within programs through collaboration. *Evaluation and Program Planning, 21*(1), 21–29.

Rush, B., & Lord, J. (2002). Disseminating a model for internal evaluation of supported employment programs for people with developmental disabilities. *Journal of Developmental Disabilities, 9*(1), 35–51.

Sharpe, P. A., Greaney, M. L., Lee, P. R., & Royce, S. W. (2000). Assets-oriented community assessment. *Public Health Reports, 115*, 205–211.

Stoecker, R. (2005). *Research methods for community change.* Thousand Oaks, CA: Sage.

Suarez-Balcazar, Y. (2005). Empowerment and participatory evaluation of a community health intervention: Implications for occupational therapy. *Occupational Therapy Journal of Research, 25*(4), 1–10.

Suarez-Balcazar, Y., Orellana-Damacela, L., Portillo, N., Lanum, M., & Sharma, A. (2003). Implementing an outcomes model in the participatory evaluation of community initiatives. *Journal of Prevention and Intervention in the Community, 26*, 5–20.

Tennstedt, S., Peterson, E., Howland, J., & Lachman, M. (1998). *Matter of balance.* Boston: Boston University Royal Center Consortium.

Timmreck, T. C. (2003). *Planning, program development and evaluation* (2nd ed.). Sudbury, MA: Jones and Bartlett.

Voltz, J. D. (2007). Grant writing guide. *Advance for Occupational Therapy Practitioners, 23*(11), 29–32.

Wandersman, A., Keener, D., Snell-Johns, J., Miller, R., Flaspohler, P., Livet-Dye, M., et al. (2004). Empowerment evaluation: Principles and action. In L. A. Jason, C. B. Keys, Y. Suarez-Balcazar, R. R. Taylor, M. I. Davis, J. Durlak, et al. (Eds.), *Participatory community research: Theories and methods in action* (pp. 139–156). Washington, DC: American Psychological Association.

Worley, P., Silagy, C., Prideaux, D., Newble, D., & Jones, A. (2000). The Parallel Rural Community Curriculum: An integrated clinical curriculum based in rural general practice. *Medical Education, 34*, 558–565.

PROCESS WORKSHEET 10-1 **EVALUATION PLANNING**

Instructions: Identify each component in the table to begin evaluation planning.

Title of Program: _____

Program Goals: _____

Program Objectives: _____

Evaluation Question	Evaluation Outcome	Evaluation Method	Data Collector	Data Analyzer	Timeline

PROCESS WORKSHEET 10-2 **DETERMINING EVALUATION DATA COLLECTION METHODS**

Instructions: Use this worksheet to determine the methods for collecting data in the evaluation plan.

Title of Program: _____

Program Goals: _____

Program Objectives: _____

Evaluation Questions: _____

Answer the following questions to help determine what data will be relevant to the evaluation plan and where this data will come from.

What data do we already have that can help us answer our evaluation question(s)?

_____

_____

_____

Where can we gather data regarding our evaluation question(s)?

_____

_____

_____

What data can we gather from existing community records?

_____

_____

_____

What data will we need to collect?

_____

_____

_____

What methods will we use to collect needed data?

_____

_____

_____

PROCESS WORKSHEET 10-3 **DETERMINING EVALUATION DATA COLLECTION METHODS**

Instructions: Complete the following table to identify the best evaluation methods for the program.

Method	Pros	Cons
Tracking numbers of participants		
Observation		
Satisfaction surveys of program participants		
Pre- and posttests of program information		
Focus groups		
Individual interviews		
Content analysis of agendas, trainings, and meeting minutes		
Participant and staff reflections		

PROCESS WORKSHEET 10-4 **FACING EVALUATION CHALLENGES**

Instructions: Use this worksheet to tackle evaluation challenges.

Challenge	Action Plan
Time	
Funding	
Staff expertise	
Other: _____	
Other: _____	

PROCESS WORKSHEET 10-5 **PARTICIPATORY EVALUATION**

Instructions: Use this worksheet to analyze the evaluation plan using a participatory evaluation process.

Questions	Methods
How will we listen and learn from community members?	
What training will be provided to community members involved in the evaluation?	
How will the evaluation data be distributed?	
What are the selection criteria for participant members on the evaluation team?	
What cross-cultural issues need to be considered in evaluation planning?	

PROCESS WORKSHEET 10-6 **EVALUATION PLAN CHECKLIST**

Instructions: Use this checklist to ensure that the evaluation plan is complete.

Evaluation Plan	Description	YES	NO
Evaluation questions			
Program aspects being measured/evaluated			
Processes for tracking goal and objective outcomes			
Process for gathering evaluation data			
Data collection			
Data analysis			
Timeline			
Personnel			
Budget			
Reports			

Instructions: Use this worksheet to begin the evaluation plan.

Evaluation Plan	Description
Who will complete the evaluation?	
What will be evaluated?	
When will the evaluation occur?	
Where will the evaluation occur?	
How will the program be evaluated?	

PROCESS WORKSHEET 10-8 **EVALUATION REPORT CHECKLIST**

Instructions: Use this checklist to ensure that the evaluation report is complete.

Evaluation Plan	Description	YES	NO
Program results			
Evaluation methods used			
Program background/history			
Theoretical basis of program			
Future implications			
Program recommendations			
Barriers to unmet objectives			

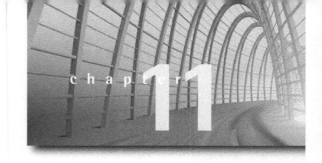

chapter 11

Sustainability

LEARNING OBJECTIVES

By the end of this chapter, the reader will be able to complete the
following:
1. Discuss the importance of sustainability planning for communities.
2. Identify strategies for supporting a program without grant funding.
3. Plan for sustainability related to a program.

Key Terms

Individual
    sustainability
Institutional
    sustainability
Sustainability
Sustainability planning

Overview

This chapter discusses the all-important topic of sustainability in community
programs. Sustainability planning is a crucial component of community
practice and must be included in all grant proposals. Not all programs need
to last forever, but a program should not cease when grant funding ends,
especially if the community need still persists. This chapter discusses the
importance and relevance of sustainability planning along with strategies for
sustainability related to program development and grant writing.

Introduction

Sustainability should be the first thing the project team considers before even
engaging in program planning! Although thinking of sustainability during

program development seems challenging, **sustainability planning** is essential in community practice (Edberg, 2007). If an idea for community programming is not sustainable, then it needs to be reevaluated. Creating a program or attempting to address a need for a short time is inappropriate unless the issue itself is short term. For most health issues and programs developed and facilitated by occupational therapy practitioners, short-term solutions do not apply.

Sustainability is important to consider in all community programs for multiple reasons. First, programs that lack sustainability can do more harm than good by making a community aware of a problem but then addressing it only temporarily (Edberg, 2007) or incompletely. Although it seems unlikely and unfortunate that a program might be created and then dissolve when grant funding ends, this practice is quite common (Edberg, 2007). Relying solely on grant funding and not planning for sustainability trap a program into a downward spiral that leaves the program always playing catch up to survive. When communities have significant needs, a sustainable program is necessary and crucial.

Second, funders want to know about a program's impact and also its sustainability. Rarely do funders support programs that do not promise to make a lasting impact on a community and its needs. A grant is an investment in an idea that addresses a need. Most grantors do not want to invest in an idea that will not make an impact past a short grant period. Therefore, sustainability planning is necessary and required for a successful grant proposal.

> **LET'S STOP AND THINK**
>
> Why do you think sustainability is so important to community programming?

What Is Sustainability?

Sustainability has multiple definitions. In its most basic sense, sustainability is the continuation of something (Shediac-Rizkallah & Bone, 1998). For the purposes of this book, **sustainability** is defined as the continuation of a community program modified as necessary to meet community needs (Paine-Andrews, Fisher, Campuzano, Fawcett, & Berkely-Paxton, 2000). Sustainability is not static and is ever evolving (Shediac-Rizkallah & Bone, 1998). Sustainability is more than simply having funding to continue a program. It includes other factors that influence the program's ongoing success. Program sustainability in communities means that the project team goes beyond program implementation to connect with the community and build capacity to engrain the program into the community (Edberg, 2007). Sustainable community programs are "endurable, livable, adaptable, and supportable" (Akerlund, 2000, p. 354).

Sustainability occurs at multiple levels including the institutional and the individual levels. On the individual level, sustainability relies on the buy-in of community members and individuals who benefit from the program services. Individuals must carry on the activities and participate in an ongoing basis (Shea,

Basch, Wechsler, & Lantingua, 1996). An example of **individual sustainability** is a community coalition formed and implemented by community members (Community Anti-Drug Coalitions of America, 2008); the individual community members come together to mobilize the community for change. **Institutional sustainability** relies on how "organizations are brought together to create networks that reinforce program goals and promote coordinated efforts" (Lefebvre, 1990; Shediac-Rizkallah & Bone, 1998, p. 92). Community partnerships between agencies represent an approach to sustainability at the organizational level (Faulk, Farley, & Coker, 2001). An example includes academic–community partnership models in which an academic institution and a community work together to address each other's needs.

The Importance of Sustainability

Occupational therapy practitioners need to recognize that grants are meant to be a jumpstart to a program, and that the money never lasts forever. According to Akerlund (2000), "If a program is truly making a difference, grantees have a responsibility to their community and to program recipients to put as much effort into program sustainability as they do in the program itself" (p. 354). A grant is never meant to fund programs permanently. Grant money is meant to be used to begin funding a programmatic idea, and the intentions are for the organization or agency to find ways to sustain the program by the time funding dissipates (Akerlund, 2000). However, this fact is often misunderstood about grants, and project teams often use grants as a method to fund activities continuously.

A community faces tragedy when the program is making a difference but the grant program team has not planned ahead for sustainability. In this situation, when grant funding ends, a community is left without methods for addressing a need. Shediac-Rizkallah and Bone (1998) state strongly and firmly the truth about many community programs:

> Throughout the world, considerable resources are spent implementing community-based health programs that are discontinued soon after initial funding ends . . . the primary focus of many community-based programs has traditionally been on determining program efficacy, while the long-term viability of potentially successful programs has been a "latent" concern. (p. 87)

The focus on program efficacy rather than community need is one reason that community programs face demise. If community programs are meant to effect change in healthy behaviors, the focus of a program should move beyond simply being effective and also look at how change has occurred in the community. Community change is a factor that promotes program sustainability (Edberg, 2007). Program efficacy and effectiveness are measured through the evaluation plan, and that is why evaluation focuses on outcomes instead of program efficiency in community programs to promote sustainability (Timmreck, 2003).

TABLE 11-1 REASONS FOR PROGRAM TERMINATION

- No sustainability plan
- Sustainability not a program priority
- Community buy-in not strong
- Fiscal barriers

Major problems exist when a program lacks sustainability. In some underserved and culturally rich communities, mistrust of outside individuals and sometimes mistrust of health care in general are a part of the community's dynamics. Developing a program that suddenly ends when funding ends sends a message to the community that the program was not really for their benefit (Jensen & Royeen, 2001). This can lead to further mistrust and make it difficult to forge future partnerships. For example, if a program that runs a mobile health van offering health screenings to those in the community without insurance disappears when grant funding goes away, the damage to an individual's health can be very serious. Diseases are not identified and treated early and costs for health care rise. Health screenings are not a temporary need, and therefore the program should not provide a temporary solution to an ongoing community need.

According to Glaser (1981), "Not all innovations should last or endure for long periods of time" and community programs should be flexible enough to transform to meet new needs. However, there are many reasons why a program should go beyond a funding period. The first is that most health-related programs take significant time to demonstrate impact (Edberg, 2007). Community change and behavior change are not quick processes, and thus, programs need to be longer to really produce results (Resnicow & Botvin, 1993; Prasad & de L Costello, 1995).

Not all programs are sustainable, and some fail to continue after grant funding ends. Typically, programs that end did not plan for sustainability, did not make sustainability a priority, the community did not buy in to the program, and the program implementers did not engage in analyzing the fiscal aspects of continuation of the program (Akerlund, 2000). These factors leading to program termination demonstrate the importance of planning for sustainability early and on an ongoing basis.

LET'S STOP AND THINK

Identify other potential reasons that a program might terminate.

Strategies for Achieving Program Sustainability

When addressing significant health issues in communities, sustainability can appear nearly impossible to achieve because of barriers and lack of resources. Yet sustainability is possible. Sustainable programs are successful programs, meaning they are well designed and complement both the community and its needs and capacities (Akerlund, 2000). The project team must think like businesspeople and consider how the fiscal aspects of the program can be sustainable (Akerlund, 2000). Furthermore, successful programs that are sustainable are those that become integrated into the community and toward which the community feels a sense of ownership (Edberg, 2007).

Successful approaches to sustainability include ongoing evaluation, ongoing service development/modification to meet community needs and desires, effective program marketing, and use of capacity-building approaches (Gaines, Wold, Bean, Brannon, & Leary, 2004). Evaluation plans continually evaluate the effectiveness of a program, which provides valuable insight into barriers and strategies for sustainability. Ongoing evaluation should be built into the evaluation plan section of any grant proposal.

BEST PRACTICE HINT

Use evaluation to promote sustainability. These two factors are a good match because the evaluation plan can reveal what is working and what does not work. The program team can use evaluation data to alter the program so that it moves toward success and sustainability. The evaluation plan will infer the status of sustainability of the program.

Furthermore, the evaluation plan can reveal whether a program is struggling or not reaching its proposed goals. The project team can use this feedback to modify the program accordingly to ensure success. Because evaluation plans measure the outcomes and act as a method for quality improvement in community programs, they should focus on ensuring that program outcomes are accurately measured and also explore the feasibility of sustainability. Program success should be well documented so that it can be used to inform community members, funding agencies, and other potential supporters of the impact and importance of the community program (Akerlund, 2000).

Evaluation plans should also explore the program's ability to be replicated (Akerlund, 2000). A program that is capable of being replicated in another community or with another subset of the population is sustainable and likely to receive future external funding. Replicable programs can be published and disseminated to promote sustainability and application in other settings. Furthermore, when a program can be replicated, it demonstrates the strength of the program, which can lead to sustainability and ongoing support both within the community and from external funding sources.

As discussed extensively throughout this book, programs should be community-centered and the community should own the program (Akerlund, 2000; Edberg, 2007; Fazio, 2008). Community members should be involved in sustainability planning from the beginning, and grant writers should take the time to educate the community on the temporality of grants along with strategies for sustainability (Edberg, 2007). Community programs also need to be flexible to be successful. Community programs should not just respond to

BEST PRACTICE HINT

Disseminate information about a successful program at conferences or through publications to ensure its sustainability and ongoing impact.

community needs but also social, economic, and environmental conditions that affect the community and the program (Brennan Ramirez, Baker, & Metzler, 2008). Community programs are developed to address community needs, and sustainability is more likely to occur when services are modified as community needs and desires change. As mentioned, the evaluation process provides insight into what can be altered for ongoing success. Besides making program adjustments as necessary, the project team should educate community members about these changes. Changes that affect the program should be driven both by the community and the evaluation plan to ensure that community buy-in, a crucial aspect of sustainability, continues.

In one situation, a team of healthcare professionals developed a family exercise program for youth identified as at risk for obesity. The program team wrote grants to sustain the program, but when new funding was not secured and the current funding ended, the program ended. The community members had no idea why the exercise program stopped and were left to wonder (J. Furze, personal communication, July 2008). This example is not that unusual. If a program is going to end, the project team should at least inform the community members because doing so is respectful and important in the process of community practice.

Sustainability of grant-funded programs relies on marketing and recruitment. Marketing may seem like a minuscule aspect of a community program, but any program needs to be used in an ongoing manner to be successful; therefore, marketing and recruitment are critical for sustainability in the case of grants and fee-for-service models (Fazio, 2008). Just because there is an existing need in a community does not mean that community members automatically access services. In the case of a grant proposal, the grant writer must outline how many community members will be served, and the program must attain these numbers. In grant reports, grantees must demonstrate that the program served the proposed numbers of community members or describe why the proposed number were not served. Obviously, the grantee is accountable to the grant funder for sustainability of the program. In the same sense, in a fee-for-service program, recruiting the required number of community participants to cover costs is essential and crucial for sustainability.

BEST PRACTICE HINT

Develop and implement a marketing plan to ensure that program recruitment is ongoing and participants are retained.

For example, in the case of therapy services, a sustainable approach may be to develop a reimbursement system for services or a fee-for-service program. In some cases, some services provided by a community program may be billable (Paine-Andrews et al., 2000). Otherwise, it is appropriate to develop a fee-for-service model. The project team must look carefully at several factors, including the demand for the services and the ability of participants to pay for the services. Participants must want and desire the services at a high level to pay for them, especially if money is tight or the socioeconomic status of the community served is low.

Also, the team must consider the costs to run the program. The program team must ask: How much revenue does this program need to sustain itself? Mapping out the amount of money that needs to come in to balance the budget is important in creating a fee-for-service model. After determining that a fee is required for the program to be sustainable, the project team must determine a fee schedule. In some cases, a flat fee works, and in others, a sliding scale fee is better. The fee structure depends on the organization and the services being offered. The team must consider all these factors when establishing a fee-for-service program (Fazio, 2008). Simple issues such as charging too much or not enough can lead to a program's failure to sustain.

An example of a fee-for-service program is a nonprofit agency in a metropolitan area that saw a need for health equipment for individuals. This organization developed a health equipment loan program in which the organization accepts donations of used health equipment and then loans out the equipment to participants. The agency garnered a grant to buy a truck for delivery and pickup. When the equipment is donated, it is cleaned and repaired. Then, the health equipment is loaned to individuals in the community who are in need.

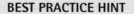

BEST PRACTICE HINT

Contact program directors of other programs and ask them about fees they charge to aid you in determining your program fees.

This program is sustainable and requires no ongoing grant funding because individuals are charged a loan fee of $10 to $100 per year based on the equipment they are borrowing. Recipients of the health equipment are allowed to keep the equipment as long as they need it and are asked to return the equipment when they no longer need it. The fees charged by the program are significantly lower than retail prices (for example: a standard wheelchair is loaned for $60), and the program meets individuals' temporary needs for equipment and recycles unused health equipment. The fees charged supply staff salary, rent for a showroom, and the supplies needed for cleaning and repairing the equipment. Also, the organization charges a delivery fee to cover the cost of gas and truck maintenance. This program exemplifies a community program that charges small fees but makes a large community impact (P. Koenig, personal communication, November 2008).

Another sustainability approach is for the project team to explore community resources. If a fee structure cannot provide funding for a program, the team must obtain external funding. Knowing sources for funding is very important. Establishing donors or corporate sponsors may be an approach that works (Paine-Andrews et al., 2000). Asking for money and resources is never an easy task, but if the community believes and needs the services, then it is less challenging. Finding funding through donors and sponsorships is similar to finding grant

LET'S STOP AND THINK

Can you think of a sustainable program? Reflect on why the program is sustainable and what lessons you can learn from its sustainability.

money. The project team should leave no stone unturned and should never be afraid to ask for funding to sustain a successful community program that is addressing community needs. The team should include a plan for garnering funds in the sustainability plan.

Corporations and individuals are often looking for successful community programs to donate to and want to support the local community. Besides corporate and individual financial donors, other potential financial resources may come from community foundations, civic organizations, government agencies, professional organizations, small businesses, and financial institutions (U.S. Department of Justice, 2005). The project team should choose to target specific organizations and communicate with one another to ensure that the appropriate contact procedures are followed and duplications do not occur.

Networking is an important way for the project team to find out about funding opportunities and to begin to seek donations. The local chamber of commerce may have contacts as might networking organizations such as the local Rotary. Corporations that provide donations to community programming usually have unique requirements for those seeking their support, so the project team needs to find out this information prior to solicitation and follow proper procedures.

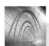

BEST PRACTICE HINT

Networking is not only about gathering resources but also about sharing. If you know about a grant that might fit for a colleague, share it with that person. This builds rapport and your colleague may reciprocate one day.

Resources beyond funding, such as volunteered time and service, are important to consider. If the goal is for the community to buy in to the program, then the resources and demands on the community need to be considered. The project team should consider valuable resources such as time commitment and supplies for ongoing growth and development. They can garner assistance to sustain the program through donated services such as accounting or billing services or by recruiting volunteers to help with program implementation.

If the program is part of a larger organization, the approach to sustainability may be through institutionalization. For example, some faculty at a university developed an infrastructure for interprofessional community engagement activities for students to underserved communities that were funded by grants from the Health Resources and Services Administration (HRSA). However, in 2004, HRSA changed its initiatives and the grant funding streams dissolved. The faculty addressed the university administration, demonstrating the impact such experiences had on the community, the students, and even the alumni. All of their data were able to demonstrate to the administration that the infrastructure was valuable and addressed the institution's mission so that the university began to support the infrastructure. This example also shows the importance of evaluation and data collection: Existing grant reports demonstrated the impact of the grant-funded projects on multiple levels, including the impact on the community, the students, the alumni, and proved the match between the program outcomes and the institutional mission (T. Cochran, personal communication, November 2008).

TABLE 11-2 STRATEGIES FOR PROGRAM SUSTAINABILITY

- Ongoing evaluation
- Ongoing service development/modification to meet community needs and desires
- Effective program marketing
- Services are reasonably priced
- Use of capacity-building approaches
- Replicability of program
- Community member involvement

Partnerships are another way to sustain a program (Jensen & Royeen, 2001). Perhaps one organization alone cannot fund an activity, but in partnership with another, the organizations can together support the program. Community collaborations can also reduce the competition among community organizations and maximize the impact of programs on the community. It is important for the project team to consider the feasibility of community partnerships in sustainability planning.

Sustainability also relies upon building community capacity. Capacities are unique to each community and each program. With sustainability planning, the opportunity for engaging in capacity building occurs (Edberg, 2007). The first step in building community capacity is to ensure that community members are included in sustainability planning (Wilken, 2008). Then, the team can develop objectives in the sustainability plan that are geared toward developing community capacity. By involving the community in this process, the project team can identify capacities and promote capacity building. Strategies for including community members in program sustainability include development and maintenance of a community advisory board and training and hiring community members to implement the program (Akerlund, 2000; Edberg, 2007).

Factors Influencing Sustainability Planning

Although no specific model exists that can guarantee sustainability of community programs, project teams can think about sustainability in multiple ways to lead to success. Sustainability requires planning, and the project team should engage in this planning early in the program development and grant writing processes. Sustainability is a complex process that involves multiple levels that call for individual change, organizational change, community action, and institutional change

TABLE 11-3 FACTORS TO CONSIDER IN SUSTAINABILITY PLANNING	
Factors	**Things to Consider**
Project design and implementation	• Effectiveness of program • Relationship with community • Length of program • Funding • Staff expertise
Organizational setting	• Strength of organization in which program exists • Opportunity for program integration • Organizational leadership
Broader community context	• Socioeconomic status of community members • Political priorities • Community participation

Source: Adapted from Shediac-Rizkallah, M. C. & Bone, L. R. (1998). Planning for the sustainability of community-based health programs: Conceptual frameworks and future directions for research, practice and policy. *Health Education Research, 13,* 87–108.

(Swerissen & Crisp, 2004). Shediac-Rizkallah and Bone (1998) propose that there are three levels a project team should explore when planning for sustainability: factors surrounding program design and implementation, factors within the organization where the program is held, and factors in the broader community context such as the political and social contexts.

Program Design and Implementation

During program design and implementation, the project team should consider the following factors related to sustainability: effectiveness of the program, the relationship with the community, the length of the program, funding, and staff expertise. Program effectiveness will be discovered in the evaluation, which reveals whether the program is really worth continuing, responds to community needs, or requires changes to be effective. When a program is ineffective or the need is short term, sustainability might not be relevant (Glaser, 1981).

The length of the program is an important factor to consider. With most health-related community issues, a short-term solution is not viable (Edberg, 2007; Timmreck, 2003;

BEST PRACTICE HINT

Just like all the other parts of program development and grant writing, be sure to include community members in the sustainability planning process.

Scaffa, 2001). However, some programs can be implemented and completed that do not make a long-standing impact but that do serve a need. Because all grants provide funding for a designated time period, it is possible that the team can develop a short-term program to fit a grant proposal's requirements. If so, the grant writer should also ensure that the program fits with the community and its needs. In this case, planning for sustainability is unnecessary and, potentially, a waste of time.

> **LET'S STOP AND THINK**
>
> Brainstorm an example of when sustainability planning is not relevant in community program development.

If the plan is to sustain the program for the long term, then goals and objectives need to be put into place that promote and suggest sustainability. If sustainability has not been considered in initial program development and grant writing, the project team may need to go back to the drawing board of basic program development and redevelop components of the program to be sustainable for the long term. Grant writers should plan and identify ongoing objectives for the program (Akerlund, 2000).

Community change occurs with community involvement. Sustainability of a program relies on the community, and programs have to have a good relationship with the community to continue (Edberg, 2007). Relationships with community partners and community members can be challenging, as discussed earlier in this book. If relations with the community are not strong or experience significant difficulties, then sustaining the program may be hard (Brennan Ramirez et al., 2008).

The expertise of staff is a very important factor in sustainability, especially because sustainability implies that programs change according to the evolving community. Having staff who are flexible and able to offer expertise in multiple areas related to community issues is important in maintaining a successful program. Involving stakeholders from the community or hiring community members to implement the program enhances this aspect (Edberg, 2007). If funding the salaries of staff is difficult, then the program may choose to move toward a volunteer model. This strategy will depend on the program, the access to volunteers, and the community needs (Akerlund, 2000).

Obviously, money plays a role in the ability of a program to sustain itself. Multiple strategies exist to explore financial sustainability of a program. If a program is grant funded, the program must remain sustainable either by garnering outside funds or by implementing a fee for services. A cost-benefit analysis should be done to demonstrate to funders and donors the impact of the program and its relevance (Akerlund, 2000). If seeking funds from external sources, the project team needs to have a plan in place to search for future grant funds or engage in fund-raising efforts. The strategies for fund-raising are many and differ based on a program's structure and needs. Fund-raising need not seek only funds but also services and supplies needed by the program. The program team should also be aware of in-kind services—those that are provided free of cost to the program. Seeking in-kind services can aid in balancing a program budget (Akerlund, 2000).

In a fee-structured program, program participants are required to pay a fee for services. Implementing a fee can reduce the number of people who seek the service but can also help balance out the budget because costs are reduced when demand is reduced (Paine-Andrews et al., 2000). The sustainability plan should consider and be prepared for a projected drop in number of participants. As previously mentioned, fees need to be realistic for what the community can afford and the services that are being offered. The program team needs to complete a careful analysis of costs and develop a fair and reliable fee structure (Shediac-Rizkallah & Bone, 1998). A sliding scale approach, which allows people to pay for services according to their ability to pay, may work well.

Another strategy that can affect the bottom line is the number of participants served. In some cases, it may be advisable to reduce the amount of services or the number served. Although this reduces impact, it also reduces cost and may also help with quality assurance. This strategy may not be an ideal option for tackling a major community issue, but it can be one strategy for moving forward with a sustainable program.

Organizational Setting

In regard to sustainability, the project team must consider the strength of the organization in which the program exists, the opportunities for the program to be integrated into an existing organization, and the leadership of the organization. The strength of the organization in which a program exists is crucial to the program's success. If a program is implemented as part of a larger organization, then the program must align with the mission of the larger organization. A program should complement the organization in which it is being implemented to ensure ongoing support.

If the organization in which the program exists is successful and well implemented, then the program may be able to become institutionalized, which is one path to sustainability. Examples include programs developed and implemented by universities that later become institutionalized and are run as part of the institution with documented success (Cochran et al., 2008).

In cases where a viable community partnership exists, community organizations may be able to combine resources to facilitate a program's ongoing implementation. Together, these organizations may find it easier to seek future grant funds, seek donations, and raise funds. If one partner has significantly more financial resources than the other, it may be possible that program activities become a line item in the larger organization's budget (Paine-Andrews et al., 2000). In this case, the project team needs to work with the agency to ensure proper procedures are followed and the program maintains its integrity.

Organizational leadership is important to sustainability. Specifically, the leader of the organization and whether that person cares and is invested in the program initiatives can be very influential. At times, decisions rest in the hands of a leader and the sustainability of the program will depend on whether the issue is considered important by the leadership of the organization. If a program is part of a larger organization, the project team should educate organizational leaders and produce reports that show results from the program that relate to the organization's mission and objectives.

Broader Community Context

Last, in the broader community context, the project team should consider the importance of the political climate, the socioeconomic status of community members, and the community's participation in the program. Policies are initiatives that affect community priorities, which, in turn, affect community programs (Edberg, 2007). Community needs can be political in nature as well. Grants are political because federal grants are based on the current priorities of the federal government. But in a democratic system, individuals actually can play a role in forming those initiatives through advocacy. The program team needs to be aware of the political factors in the community and advocate as needed.

The socioeconomic status of those being served by the community program is an important aspect for the project team to consider. The socioeconomic status of community members determines whether individuals potentially can pay fees for services or whether there are community members who could donate financial resources. For example, in the case of a poor community, developing a fee-for-service program might not be an appropriate method for promoting sustainability.

As described, the issue of sustainability is complex. Those who engage in sustainability planning for a program or a grant proposal must keep these factors in mind.

Developing a Sustainability Plan: Things to Consider

One of the best ways to explicate sustainability is to develop a sustainability plan. A sustainability plan discusses how the program will continue after grant funding has ended and any long-term impact the program will hope to make beyond the grant funding period (Virginia Board for People with Disabilities, 2007). The sustainability plan includes an overall strategy for program sustainability, specific goals for sustainability, and an action plan to address these goals (U.S. Department of Justice, 2005). It is meant to be an action plan that outlines what needs to be done and who needs to do it to maintain the program. The plan should include goals, objectives, and action steps including the names of persons responsible for specific activities and the date by which these activities must be accomplished.

Many funding agencies require the grant proposal to include the goals for sustainability. Others require a separate sustainability plan focused specifically on goals and action steps to sustain the program. Regardless of whether a sustainability plan is required by the grantor, the grant team should still develop a plan for sustainability (Conrad, 2008).

No one method for developing a sustainability plan exists, but there are certain considerations in common to all. When building a sustainability plan for a program supported by a grant proposal, the project team should first consider the length of the funding period. If the grant is a multiple-year grant, the grant team has a couple of years to plan ahead, but the successful project team always is cognizant of the end of funding. The grant team needs always to be prepared to move forward with a program without funding. In some rare cases, grant funding is promised by a funding agency but is not provided either on time or in subsequent years of the program. If a sustainability plan is in place, it can be initiated and the project team can avoid the negative effects of delayed or missing funding. A project team should never blame a funding agency for lack of program sustainability.

Sometimes grant funding agencies force grant writers to think about sustainability by requiring a discussion of sustainability plans to be included in a grant proposal. In some cases, grantors step down or lessen funding each year to ensure that programs are not becoming dependent on grant funding. In grant planning and budgeting, a program team can propose being granted more money in year 1 and less in the subsequent years to demonstrate their plan for sustainability.

Sustainability planning should include identifying the challenges to sustainability. One question for the project team to pose is: What could cause the program or organization not to be able to sustain itself? Asking this question is difficult but essential and is the core of any sustainability plan. By knowing the challenges, the project team can develop approaches to address them effectively (Akerlund, 2000; Conrad, 2008). The main obstacle to sustainability includes the inability to garner funding to continue the program beyond the grant funding period. Whatever the issues, the project team must address them in an effective and efficient manner.

As a program is implemented, it is helpful for the project team to use strategies to explore what community members and those involved in the program implementation think. This exploration could be a component of the evaluation plan, but it is also important for sustainability. Community members need to remain connected to the program for it to be sustainable (Edberg, 2007). One method of exploring the beliefs and values of the community is simply for the project team to check in and ask. As previously mentioned, a community advisory board could help provide this insight (Akerlund, 2000). However, town hall meetings, community trainings, focus groups, and informal interviews can also help (Dressendorfer et al., 2005). Information gathered in such ways can provide valuable insight into program sustainability and can be carried out as part of program implementation.

BEST PRACTICE HINT

Strategies for garnering community feedback are discussed in Chapter 10 on evaluation planning.
Combine evaluation planning with sustainability planning to maximize time and resources.

Sustainability planning can be difficult because it requires a group of busy people to look to the future. Regardless, addressing sustainability is an essential step in ensuring a program's survival. The best approach is for the project team to start early in program planning and to be prepared for anything. The team can also build a committee or task group that focuses on achieving sustainability (Akerlund, 2000). In some cases, the individuals in this group may be volunteers or members of the project team, and the group should include a community stakeholders and those who have a vision for the future. This group should also include individuals who have used the services and have directly benefited. Including the community ensures that a plan is developed that meets the needs and desires of the community and aids in establishing sustainability.

The sustainability plan needs to be practical and feasible to ensure success. This means that it does not include raising community fees by an exorbitant amount or using strategies that will ultimately lead to problems rather than success. The sustainability committee needs to search for and garner resources continually that will support the program.

Conclusion

Program sustainability is important for multiple reasons and should be the focus of program planning for a program to make a lasting impact. Sustainability requires planning and reflection across many levels. Although there are no right or wrong methods for sustainability planning, the biggest mistake a program team can make is not planning ahead and letting a valuable community service terminate as a result of lack of preparation and thought.

Glossary

Individual sustainability Relies on the buy-in of community members and individuals benefiting from the services to carry on the activities and ongoing participation

Institutional sustainability Relies on how "organizations are brought together to create networks that reinforce program goals and promote coordinated efforts" (Lefebvre, 1990; Shediac-Rizkallah & Bone, 1998, p. 92)

Sustainability The continuation of a community program modified as necessary to meet community needs

Sustainability planning The process by which a program team identifies strategies and roles and responsibilities in a formal plan to maintain the future of the organization

References

Akerlund, K. M. (2000). Prevention program sustainability: The state's perspective. *Journal of Community Psychology, 28*(3), 353–362.

Brennan Ramirez, L. K., Baker, E. A., & Metzler, M. (2008). *Promoting health equity: A resource to help communities address social determinants of health.* Atlanta, GA: U.S. Department of Health and Human Services, Centers for Disease Control and Prevention.

Cochran, T. M., Goulet, C., Black, L. L., Doll, J. D., Ryan-Haddad, A., Furze, J. A., et al. (2008, June). *The impact of community engagement on professional formation in health professions students.* Omaha, NE: Carnegie Academy for the Scholarship of Teaching and Learning (CASTL) Institute.

Community Anti-Drug Coalitions of America. (2008). Coalition resources: Frequently asked questions. Retrieved November 7, 2008, from http://www.cadca.org/Coalition Resources/faq/

Conrad, P. (2008). To boldly go: A partnership enterprise to produce applied health and nursing services researchers in Canada. *Health Care Policy, 3,* 13–30.

Dressendorfer, R. H., Raine, K., Dyck, R. J., Plotnikoff, R. C., Collins-Nakai, R. L., McLaughling, W. K., et al. (2005). A conceptual model of community capacity development for health promotion in the Alberta Heart Health Project. *Health Promotion Practice, 6*(1), 31–36.

Edberg, M. (2007). *Essentials of health behavior: Social and behavior health in public health.* Sudbury, MA: Jones and Bartlett.

Faulk, D., Farley, S., & Coker, R. (2001). After the funding is gone: Evaluating the sustainability of a community-based project. *Nursing and Health Care Perspectives, 22*(4), 184–188.

Fazio, L. (2008). *Developing occupation-centered programs for the community* (2nd ed.). Upper Saddle River, NJ: Prentice Hall.

Gaines, S. K., Wold, J. L., Bean, M. R., Brannon, C. G., & Leary, J. M. (2004). Partnership to build sustainable public health nurse child care health support. *Family and Community Health, 27*(4), 346–354.

Glaser, E. M. (1981). Durability of innovations in human service organizations: A case study analysis. *Knowledge: Creation, Diffusion, Utilization, 3,* 167–185.

Jensen, G. M., & Royeen, C. B. (2001). Analysis of academic-community partnerships using the integration matrix. *Journal of Allied Health, 30,* 168–175.

Lefebvre, R. C. (1990). Strategies to maintain and institutionalize successful programs: A marketing framework. In N. Bracht (Ed.), *Health promotion at the community level.* Newbury Park, CA: Sage.

Paine-Andrews, A., Fisher, J. L., Campuzano, M. K., Fawcett, S. N., & Berkeley-Patton, J. (2000). Promoting sustainability of community health initiatives: An empirical case study. *Health Promotion Practice, 1*(3), 248–258.

Prasad, B., & de L Costello, A. M. (1995). Impact and sustainability of a "baby friendly" health education intervention at a district hospital in Bihar, India. *British Medical Journal, 310,* 621–623.

Resnicow, K., & Botvin, G. (1993). School-based substance use prevention programs: Why do effects decay? *Preventive Medicine, 22,* 484–490.

Scaffa, M. (Ed.). (2001). *Occupational therapy in community-based practice settings.* Philadelphia: F. A. Davis.

Shediac-Rizkallah, M. C. & Bone, L. R. (1998). Planning for the sustainability of community-based health programs: Conceptual frameworks and future directions for research, practice and policy. *Health Education Research, 13,* 87–108.

Shea, S., Basch, C. E., Wechsler, H., & Lantigua, R. (1996). The Washington Heights-Inwood Healthy Heart Program: A 6-year report from a disadvantaged urban setting. *American Journal of Public Health, 86,* 166–171.

Swerissen, H., & Crisp, B. R. (2004). The sustainability of health promotion interventions for different levels of social organization. *Health Promotion International, 19,* 123–130.

Timmreck, T. C. (2003). *Planning, program development and evaluation* (2nd ed.). Sudbury, MA: Jones and Bartlett.

U.S. Department of Justice. (2005). *Developing a sustainability plan for Weed and Seed sites.* Retrieved November 7, 2008, from http://www.ojp.usdoj.gov/ccdo/pub/pdf/ncj210462 .pdf

Virginia Board for People with Disabilities. (2007). *General guidelines for grant proposals.* Retrieved November 7, 2008, from http://www.vaboard.org/downloads/ GeneralGuide-linesGrantProposals.pdf

Wilken, M. (2008). Health Report Card Project: Building community capacity. In C. B. Royeen, G. M. Jensen, & R. A. Harvan (Eds.), *Leadership in interprofessional health education and practice* (pp. 413–426). Sudbury, MA: Jones and Bartlett.

PROCESS WORKSHEET 11-1 **EXPLORING SUSTAINABILITY**

Instructions: Use this worksheet to help to identify aspects of a sustainability plan.

1. What are the challenges to sustainability?

2. What resources are needed for the program to be sustained (funding and so forth)?

3. What resources already exist that support sustainability?

4. What are some viable strategies for sustainability?

PROCESS WORKSHEET 11-2 **SUSTAINABILITY REFLECTION WORKSHEET**

Instructions: Reflect on each component of your program to assist in developing a comprehensive sustainability plan. Focus on sustainability and how each component ties in to the ability to sustain the program.

Program Design and Implementation

Program Component	Reflection
Program effectiveness—How effective is our program?	
Community relationship—How is our relationship with the community?	
Program length—How long do we want this program to be? Do we have long-term goals?	
Funding—Is long-term funding available? If not, how we will garner funding?	
Staff expertise—Are our staff able to be flexible to promote sustainability if programmatic changes occur? Does our staff need training in fund-raising or other areas of sustainability?	

Continues

PROCESS WORKSHEET 11-2 **SUSTAINABILITY REFLECTION WORKSHEET (CONTINUED)**

Organizational Setting

Organizational Component	Reflection
Organization strength—How strong is our organization? Can this organization sustain the program?	
Opportunity for integration—Can we become absorbed in an organization? Can we become institutionalized?	
Organizational leadership—Do we have the right leadership in place to develop a strong sustainability plan?	

Community Context

Community Component	Reflection
Socioeconomic status of community—Can community members afford our services? What can we charge and still sustain?	
Political priorities—What grant opportunities or federal initiatives can support us? What challenges do we face?	
Community participation—Do we have enough participants in the community? Do we have community buy-in that will promote sustainability?	

PROCESS WORKSHEET 11-3 **SUSTAINABILITY PLANNING WORKSHEET**

Instructions: Use this process worksheet to begin to formulate a sustainability plan. Identify goals for sustainability for the program. Then, identify challenges to these goals followed by actions to remedy these challenges to reach the goals.

Sustainability Goal	Challenges to Sustainability	Action Plan

PROCESS WORKSHEET 11-4 **SUSTAINABILITY PLANNING WORKSHEET**

Instructions: Use this worksheet to brainstorm strategies for developing a fee-for-service model.

1. Identify the current program budget amount: _____

2. Identify the amount of funding provided by a grant: _____

3. Subtract the current budget from the grant funding amount: _____
    This number identifies how much money will need to be obtained for ongoing sustainability.

4. Identify the amount of funding from current program revenue: _____

5. What is your service(s) worth? _____

6. How much can people pay for your service(s)? _____

7. Can you charge a fee that will cover your costs? (circle one)   YES   NO

8. Will a sliding scale fee structure work? (circle one)   YES   NO

9. Describe what the fee-for-service would look like.

10. Brainstorm strategies for reducing the program budget.

11. Brainstorm strategies for obtaining funds.

12. Identify any other important elements in developing a fee-for-service model.

PROCESS WORKSHEET 11-5 **COMMUNITY RESOURCES WORKSHEET**

Instructions: Use this worksheet to identify potential contacts for community support.

Corporation	Contact	Procedures	Timeline for Contact	Designated Staff Person

PROCESS WORKSHEET 11-6 **DEVELOPING A SUSTAINABILITY COMMITTEE WORKSHEET**

Instructions: Use this worksheet to identify individuals to include on a sustainability committee or task force.

Name of Task Force: _____

Brainstorm individuals who would be good for a sustainability committee or task force.

Individual	Contact Information	Justification for Committee Membership

PROCESS WORKSHEET 11-7 **SUSTAINABILITY PLAN**

Instructions: Draft a sustainability plan using the following table.

Sustainability Goal	Strategy	Timeline	Person Responsible

Index

Italicized page locators indicate a figure; tables are noted with a *t*.

CPSIA information can be obtained
at www.ICGtesting.com
Printed in the USA
BVHW062120070922
646433BV00002B/11

9 780763 760656